◇ 全国高等中医药院校汉

中医基础理论
第 2 版

主　编　柴可夫

副主编　王玉兴　郭霞珍

主　译　张庆荣

编译委员会（按姓氏笔画排序）
　　　　　　王　彤（北京中医药大学）
　　　　　　王玉兴（天津中医药大学）
　　　　　　刘景峰（辽宁中医药大学）
　　　　　　李　慧（浙江中医药大学）
　　　　　　张立侠（长春中医药大学）
　　　　　　张庆荣（辽宁中医药大学）
　　　　　　柴可夫（浙江中医药大学）
　　　　　　钱俊文（浙江中医药大学）
　　　　　　郭霞珍（北京中医药大学）
　　　　　　戴　红（湖北中医学院）

英语顾问　Sholto（加拿大）

人民卫生出版社

◇Chinese-English Bilingual Textbooks for International Students of Chinese TCM Institutions

Fundamental Theory of Traditional Chinese Medicine

2nd edition

Compiler-in-Chief　　　Chai Kefu
Vice Compiler-in-Chief　Wang Yuxing　Guo Xiazhen
Translator-in-Chief　　Zhang Qingrong

Compiling and Translating Committee (Listed in the order of strokes of their Chinese surname)
　　Wang Tong　(Beijing University of CM)
　　Wang Yuxing　(Tianjin University of TCM)
　　Liu Jingfeng　(Liaoning University of TCM)
　　Li Hui　(Zhejiang University of CM)
　　Zhang Lixia　(Changchun University of TCM)
　　Zhang Qingrong　(Liaoning University of TCM)
　　Chai Kefu　(Zhejiang University of CM)
　　Qian Junwen　(Zhejiang University of CM)
　　Guo Xiazhen　(Beijing University of CM)
　　Dai Hong　(Hubei College of TCM)

Advisor in English　Sholto (Canada)

People's Medical Publishing House

图书在版编目（CIP）数据

中医基础理论/柴可夫主编. 张庆荣主译. —2 版.
—北京：人民卫生出版社，2007.9
全国高等中医药院校卫生部规划汉英双语教材
ISBN 978-7-117-08615-8

Ⅰ.中… Ⅱ.①柴…②张… Ⅲ.中医医学基础-汉英双语教学-中医院校-教材 Ⅳ.R22

中国版本图书馆 CIP 数据核字（2007）第 042373 号

门户网：www.pmph.com	出版物查询、网上书店
卫人网：www.ipmph.com	护士、医师、药师、中医师、卫生资格考试培训

版权所有，侵权必究！

本书本印次封底贴有防伪标。请注意识别。

中医基础理论
第 2 版

主　　编：柴可夫　Chai Kefu
主　　译：张庆荣　Zhang Qingrong
出版发行：人民卫生出版社（中继线 010-59780011）
地　　址：北京市朝阳区潘家园南里 19 号
邮　　编：100021
E – mail：pmph @ pmph.com
购书热线：010-67605754　010-65264830
　　　　　010-59787586　010-59787592
印　　刷：尚艺印装有限公司
经　　销：新华书店
开　　本：787×1092　1/16　印张：21.25
字　　数：472 千字
版　　次：1998 年 10 月第 1 版　2010 年 7 月第 2 版第 4 次印刷
标准书号：ISBN 978-7-117-08615-8/R·8616
定　　价：35.00 元

打击盗版举报电话：010-59787491　E–mail：WQ @ pmph.com
（凡属印装质量问题请与本社销售中心联系退换）

出 版 说 明

1996年,由全国中医药高等教育国际交流与合作学会联合了全国21所中医药高等院校组织编写了全国首套外国进修生教材(汉英双语),并于1998年在我社出版。近十年的教学实践中,本套教材得到了师生的好评,有些院校一直沿用至今。随着当今世界范围内中医药热潮的涌动,中医药在国际上越来越受到人们的关注,逐渐成为中国"输出型"文化而跨出国门,走向世界。因此,来华学习中医药的留学生逐年增多,已形成了一支学习、继承、传播、发展中医药事业不可忽视的力量。为了适应中医药学高水平国际教学的迫切需要,在国家留学基金管理委员会、全国留学生教育管理学会及国家教育部、国家卫生部、国家中医药管理局的关怀指导下,经全国高等医药教材建设研究会、全国中医药高等教育国际交流与合作学会的积极努力,2006年5月开始启动了本套教材的修订工作。

本套教材的修订,在全国高等中医药院校来华留学生卫生部"十一五"规划汉英双语教材编审委员会的指导下,根据留学生教学的实际需要由第一版的6种增补到10种。其编写修订宗旨是:中医基础及临床学科内容的深度和广度适宜、够用,定位在中国中医药学历教育本科段的层次,在"三基"(基础理论、基本知识、基本技能)、"五性"(思想性、科学性、先进性、启发性、实用性)基础上,要求内容更精炼(不涉及学科发展史)、语言更简洁(不引经据典),同时注重突出中医药学科特点;译文准确,名词术语规范,便于汉语水平偏低的留学生学习。

本套教材适用于来华学习中医药的本科生,以及进修生、培训生等。亦适合境内外中医药汉英双语教学使用。

本套教材目录(第一批):

《中医基础理论》(第2版)	主编 柴可夫	主译 张庆荣
《中医诊断学》(第2版)	主编 王天芳	主译 方廷钰
△《中药学》	主编 滕佳林	主译 崔洪江
《方剂学》(第2版)	主编 陈德兴	主译 朱忠宝
△《中医内科学》(第2版)	主编 彭 勃	主译 谢建群
《中医妇科学》	主编 谈 勇	主译 肖 平
《针灸学》(第2版)	主编 沈雪勇 王 华	主译 赵百孝
《推拿学》(第2版)	主编 金宏柱	主译 李照国
《中医养生学》	主编 刘占文 马烈光	主译 刘占文
《医学基础知识导读》	主编 牛 欣	主译 宋一伦

注:△为普通高等教育"十一五"国家级规划教材

Publisher's Note

In 1996, China National Association of International Exchange and Collaboration in TCM Higher Education organized 21 colleges and universities of traditional Chinese medicine in China to compile the first series of textbooks (Chinese-English) for international students. These textbooks were published by the People's Medical Publishing House in 1998 and have been used nearly for ten years to train international students in the colleges and universities of traditional Chinese medicine in China. With the rapid dissemination of traditional Chinese medicine throughout the world, more and more international students come to China every year to study this ancient Chinese system of medicine. To meet the needs of international students of traditional Chinese medicine, the project to revise this series of textbooks began in May 2006 with the support of China Scholarship Council, Chinese Association of Universities and Colleges for Foreign Student Affairs, Ministry of Education of the People's Republic of P.R.C., Ministry of Health of the People's Republic of P.R.C. and State Administration of Traditional Chinese Medicine of P.R.C..

In this revision, four more textbooks were added to the original series so as to equal the level of regular undergraduate education of traditional Chinese medicine in China. The compilation of these textbooks was undertaken on the basis of three essential aspects (essentials of theory, knowledge and techniques), five qualities (theoretical, scientific, advanced, inspiring and practical) and two standards (standard translation and terminology). The contents were concise, excluding much history and quotations from classic texts.

This newly compiled and revised series of textbooks can be used by international students for undergraduate study, advanced study or training purposes in the field of traditional Chinese medicine.

This series of textbook includes the following fascicles (the first set):

Fundamental Theory of Traditional Chinese Medicine (2nd edition)
Compiler-in-Chief: Chai Kefu   Translator-in-Chief: Zhang Qingrong
Diagnostics of Traditional Chinese Medicine (2nd edition)
Compiler-in-Chief: Wang Tianfang   Translator-in-Chief: Fang Tingyu
ΔChinese Materia Medica
Compiler-in-Chief: Teng Jialin   Translator-in-Chief: Cui Hongjiang

Formulas of Traditional Chinese Medicine (2nd edition)
Compiler-in-Chief: Chen Dexing   Translator-in-Chief: Zhu Zhongbao

ΔTraditional Chinese Internal Medicine (2nd edition)
Compiler-in-Chief: Peng Bo   Translator-in-Chief: Xie Jianqun

Gynecology of Traditional Chinese Medicine
Compiler-in-Chief: Tan Yong   Translator-in-Chief: Xiao Ping

Acupuncture and Moxibustion (2nd edition)
Compiler-in-Chief: Shen Xueyong   Translator-in-Chief: Zhao Baixiao
                Wang Hua

Science of Tuina (2nd edition)
Compiler-in-Chief: Jin Hongzhu   Translator-in-Chief: Li Zhaoguo

Health Preservation of Traditional Chinese Medicine
Compiler-in-Chief: Liu Zhanwen   Translator-in-Chief: Liu Zhanwen
                Ma Lieguang

An Introductory Course in Medicine
Compiler-in-Chief: Niu Xin   Translator-in-Chief: Song Yilun

Δ The State Eleventh Five-Year Plan Textbooks for Colleges and Universities

全国高等中医药院校来华留学生卫生部"十一五"规划汉英双语教材编审委员会名单

顾问

  曹国兴（中华人民共和国教育部国际交流与合作司司长）
  张秀琴（国家留学基金管理委员会秘书长　全国高等学校外国留学生教育管理学会会长）
  郑守曾（北京中医药大学校长）
  方廷钰（北京中医药大学教授　全国政协委员）
  胡国臣（人民卫生出版社社长　兼总编辑）
  刘振民（全国中医药高等教育学会秘书长）
  范永升（浙江中医药大学副校长）
  王　华（湖北中医学院院长）
  王之虹（长春中医药大学校长）
  李佃贵（河北医科大学副校长）
  马　骥（辽宁中医药大学校长）
  张俊龙（山西中医学院副院长）
  刘延祯（甘肃中医学院院长）
  左铮云（江西中医学院副院长）
  邓家刚（广西中医学院副院长）
  王彦晖（厦门大学医学院副院长）

主任委员

  吴秀芬（北京中医药大学教授　全国中医药高等教育国际交流与合作学会会长）

副主任委员

  彭　勃（河南中医学院院长　教授　全国中医药高等教育国际交流与合作学会理事）
  谢建群（上海中医药大学常务副校长　党委书记　教授）
  陈盈晖（中华人民共和国教育部科学技术司副司长）
  赵灵山（中华人民共和国教育部国际合作与交流司来华留学工作处处长）
  呼素华（卫生部教材办公室　人民卫生出版社编审）

委员（按姓氏笔画排序）

牛　欣（北京中医药大学国际学院院长　教授　全国中医药高等教育国际交流
　　　　与合作学会副会长）
王洪琦（广州中医药大学国际学院院长　全国中医药高等教育国际交流与合作
　　　　学会副会长）
乐毅敏（江西中医学院国际教育学院院长　教授）
朱忠宝（河南中医学院教授）
孙　勇（卫生部教材办公室　人民卫生出版社编辑）
刘　淼（长春中医药大学国际教育学院院长）
刘占文（北京中医药大学教授）
刘景峰（辽宁中医药大学国际教育学院副院长）
李　军（甘肃中医学院国际处处长）
李　沛（福建中医学院国际合作与交流处处长）
李照国（上海师范大学教授）
应森林（天津中医药大学国际教育学院院长　教授　学会常务理事）
张庆荣（辽宁中医药大学教授）
尚　力（上海中医药大学国际教育学院院长　教授　全国中医药高等教育国际
　　　　交流与合作学会副会长）
罗　萤（福建中医学院党委书记）
周海虹（厦门大学医学院中医系副主任）
房家毅（河北医科大学国际教育学院院长）
赵　熔（南京中医药大学国际教育学院院长　学会常务理事）
赵雪丽（山西中医学院国际教育中心主任）
姚洪武（成都中医药大学外事处副处长　讲师　学会常务理事）
柴可夫（浙江中医药大学国际教育中心主任　教授）
梁　华（黑龙江中医药大学外事处处长　教授　学会常务理事）
崔洪江（山东中医药大学外事处处长　副教授　学会常务理事）
彭清华（湖南中医药大学国际教育学院院长　教授）
傅　萍（湖北中医学院外事处处长）
路　玫（河南中医学院海外教育学院处长　教授　学会常务理事）

Editing Committee of Chinese-English Bilingual Textbooks Included in the Eleventh Five-Year Plan of the Ministry of Health of P.R.C. for International Students of Chinese TCM Institutions

Adivisors

Cao Guoxing (Chief of the International Exchange and Cooperation Department, Ministry of Education, P.R.C.)
Zhang Xiuqin (Secretary-General of China Scholarship Council and Chief of Chinese Association of Universities and Colleges for Foreign Student Affairs)
Zheng Shouzeng (President of Beijing University of CM)
Fang Tingyu (Professor of Beijing University of CM and Member of National Political Consultative Committee)
Hu Guochen (President and Editor-in-General of the People's Medical Publishing House)
Liu Zhenmin (Secretary-General of the National Association of TCM Higher Education)
Fan Yongsheng (Vice President of Zhenjiang University of CM)
Wang Hua (President of Hubei College of TCM)
Wang Zhihong (President of Changchun University of TCM)
Li Diangui (Vice President of Hebei Medical University)
Ma Ji (President of Liaoning University of TCM)
Zhang Junlong (Vice President of Shanxi College of TCM)
Liu Yanzhen (President of Gansu College of TCM)
Zuo Zhengyun (Vice President of Jiangxi College of TCM)
Deng Jiagang (Vice President of Guangxi College of TCM)
Wang Yanhui (Vice President of Medical College of Xiamen University)

Dean

Wu Xiufen (Professor of Beijing University of CM and Chairwoman of China National Association of International Exchange and Collaboration in TCM Higher Education)

Deputy-Dean

Peng Bo (Professor and President of Henan College of TCM and Member of China National Association of International Exchange and Collaboration in TCM Higher Education)

Xie Jianqun (Professor, CPC Branch Secretary and Vice President of Shanghai University of TCM)

Chen Yinghui (Deputy Director-General, Department of Science and Technology, Ministry of Education, P.R.C.)

Zhao Lingshan (Director, Division for International Students, Departement of International Cooperation and Exchanges, Ministry of Education, P.R.C.)

Hu Suhua (Senior Editor of People's Medical Publishing House and the Textbook Office Affiliated to the Ministry of Health of P.R.C.)

Members (Listed in the order of strokes in their Chinese surname)

Niu Xin (Professor and President of International College of Beijing University of CM and Vice Chairman of China National Association of International Exchange and Collaboration in TCM Higher Education)

Wang Hongqi (President of International College of Guangzhou University of CM, Vice Chairman of China National Association of International Exchange and Collabortion in TCM Higher Education)

Le Yimin (Professor and President of International College of Jiangxi College of TCM)

Zhu Zhongbao (Professor of Henan College of TCM)

Sun Yong (Editor of People's Medical Publishing House and the Textbook Office Affiliated to the Ministry of Health of P.R.C.)

Liu Miao (President of International College of Changchun University of TCM)

Liu Zhanwen (Professor of Beijing University of CM)

Liu Jingfeng (Vice President of International College of Liaoning University of TCM)

Li Jun (Director of International Education Center of Gansu College of TCM)

Li Pei (Director of International Cooperation and Exchange Department of Fujian College of TCM)

Li Zhaoguo (Professor of Shanghai Normal University)

Ying Senlin (President of International Education College of Tianjin University of TCM and Standing Member of the China National Association of International Exchange and Collaboration in TCM Higher Education)

Zhang Qingrong (Professor of Liaoning University of TCM)

Shang Li (Professor and President of International College of Shanghai University of TCM, Vice Chairman of China National Association of International Exchange and Collaboration in TCM Higher Education)

Luo Ying (CPC Branch Secretary of Fujian College of TCM)

Zhou Haihong (Deputy Director of TCM Department of Xiamen Medical University)

Fang Jiayi (President of International College of Hebei Medical University)

Zhao Rong (President of International Educational College of Nanjing University of TCM and Standing Member of the China National Association of International Exchange and Collaboration in TCM Higher Education)

Zhao Xueli (Director of International Education Center of Shanxi College of TCM)

Yao Hongwu (Lecturer and Deputy Director of International Affairs Department of Chengdu University of TCM and Standing Member of the China National Association of International Exchange and Collaboration in TCM Higher Education)

Chai Kefu (Professor and Director of International Center of Zhejiang University of CM)

Liang Hua (Professor and Director of Personnel Department of Heilongjiang University of TCM and Standing Member of the China National Association of International Exchange and Collaboration in TCM Higher Education)

Cui Hongjiang (Associate Professor and Director of International Affairs Department of Shandong University of TCM and Standing Member of the China National Association of International Exchange and Collaboration in TCM Higher Education)

Peng Qinghua (Professor and President of International College of Hunan University of TCM)

Fu Ping (Dean of Personnel Department of Hubei College of TCM)

Lu Mei (Director of International Education College of Henan College of TCM and Standing Member of the China National Association of International Exchange and Collaboration in TCM Higher Education)

前 言

中医药学以它独特的理论体系和显著的临床效果,在国际上越来越受到人们的关注。近些年随着世界范围的中医药热潮的涌动,来华学习中医药的留学生逐年增多。为了适应中医药国际交流与合作的需要,加快中医药国际化进程,提高来华学习中医药留学生的教学质量,根据教育部、卫生部、国家中医药管理局等上级领导部门的有关精神,全国中医药高等教育国际交流与合作学会研究决定拟启动"全国高等中医药院校外国进修生教材(1997~1998年出版)"的修订工作。此项工作得到了卫生部教材办公室的高度重视,同时得到了国家教育部国际交流与合作司、国家留学基金管理委员会、全国高等院校外国留学生教育管理学会、全国各高等院校,以及人民卫生出版社的大力支持。随即教材的修订纳入了"卫生部'十一五'规划",并组建了全国高等中医药院校来华留学生卫生部"十一五"规划汉英双语教材编审委员会。本套教材在第一版的基础上,仍然采取汉英两种文字语言的形式出版,即前部分为中文,后部分为中文的英文译文。教材的科目根据留学生教学的需要由原来的6种(《中医基础理论》、《中医诊断学》、《方剂学》、《中医内科学》、《针灸学》、《推拿学》)增补到10种(增加了《中药学》、《中医妇科学》、《中医养生学》、《医学基础知识导读》)。教材的编写针对来华留学生的学习特点及教学需要,以"全国高等中医药院校外国进修生教材(第一版)"为蓝本,参照国内中医药高等院校本科生教学大纲,以及国际中医药从业人员考试大纲和国家中医执业医师考试大纲,同时参考全国高等中医院校五版、七版及二十一世纪课程教材,编写要求坚持"三基"(基础理论、基本知识、基本技能)、"五性"(思想性、科学性、先进性、启发性、适用性)、"三特定"(特定的对象、特定的要求、特定的限制)的基本原则,注重继承与创新、传统与现代、理论与实践、中医与西医的关系,力求做到理论系统、重点突出、简明扼要、临床实用。

本套教材的主编、主译经全国高等中医药院校申报、教材编审委员会根据有关条件严格遴选、确定,最后经卫生部教材办公室审核、确认。教材编写实行主编、主译负责制,编写人员大多为多年从事高等中医药对外教育、具有丰富留学生教学经验的著名专家、教授;英文译者大多为从事中医药专业英语教学研究和汉英双语教学的专家。每种教材的编写均经过编写会、统稿会、定稿会,英文部分均聘请外籍专家审核、修改,最后全套教材的英文稿件又进行了集中统稿、定稿,从而确保了本套教材的编写质量和英文的翻译质量。

中医药走向世界,面临众多层面的跨文化沟通与传播问题,但愿我们这套教材能在弘扬中华民族优秀文化、造福人类健康、促进中国与世界科学文化交流的伟大事业中,做出新的、更大的贡献。

全国中医药高等教育国际交流与合作学会
全国高等中医药院校来华留学生卫生部"十一五"规划
汉英双语教材编审委员会
2007年7月

Foreword

Traditional Chinese medicine (TCM) has a unique theoretical system and is clinically effective. Over the past few decades it has been attracting increasing attention from all over the world. More and more overseas students come to China to learn TCM and there has been a huge upsurge in the learning of TCM worldwide. To meet the needs of these students, accelerate the processes of internationalization of TCM, and improve the quality of education available to overseas students coming to China to learn TCM, these textbooks have been compiled by China National Association of International Exchange and Collaboration in TCM Higher Education in accordance with the wishes of the Ministry of Education of P.R.C., the Ministry of Health of P.R.C., and the State Administration Bureau of TCM of P.R.C.. The Textbook Office Affiliated to the Ministry of Health of P.R.C. has attached great importance to the matter. In addition, the compilation of the textbooks has the support of the following important organizations: International Cooperation and Exchange Department of the Ministry of Education of P.R.C., China Scholarship Council, Chinese Association of Universities and Colleges for Foreign Students Affairs, all the colleges and universities of TCM, and the People's Medical Publishing House. This series of textbooks has been brought into the Eleventh Five-Year Plan of the Ministry of Health of P.R.C. and a new organization, the Editing Committee of Chinese-English Bilingual Textbooks Included in the Eleventh Five-Year Plan of the Ministry of Health of P.R.C. for International Students of Chinese TCM Institutions, was established.

The textbooks have been compiled to conform to the standards of the exam syllabus for international licensed TCM professionals, Chinese licensed TCM physicians, and the 21st century textbooks for TCM universities (referencing the 5th, 6th, and 7th editions). The textbooks are bilingual, with content first in Chinese and then in English. The total is ten textbooks: *Fundamental Theory of Traditional Chinese Medicine, Diagnostics of Traditional Chinese Medicine, Chinese Materia Medica, Formulas of Traditional Chinese Medicine, Traditional Chinese Internal Medicine, Acupuncture and Moxibustion, Science of Tuina, Gynecology of Traditional Chinese Medicine, Health Preservation of Traditional Chinese Medicine, An Introductory Course in Medicine*. The compilers of the textbooks adhered to "three points: basic theories, basic knowledge, and basic techniques"; "five features: the ideological, scientific, advanced, enlightening, and practical"; and "three principles: specific readers, specific requirements, and specific levels". Great attention has been paid to the issues of inheritance and innovation, traditional and modern aspects, theory and practice, and Chinese medicine and biomedicine. It is our aim to make the theories of TCM systematic, presenting key points in concise language that will lead to practical clinical applications.

There was a strict procedure for selecting and translators. Names of compilers and translators had to be approved by the Editing Committee of Chinese-English Bilingual Textbooks Included in the Eleventh Five-Year Plan of the Ministry of Health of P.R.C. for International Students of Chinese TCM Institutions, and The Textbook Office Affiliated to the Ministry of Health of P.R.C.. All candidates selected are experts with years of experience teaching TCM to international students.

Each textbook was repeatedly examined and revised to guarantee quality by numerous committees at multiple stages. The English text was thoroughly reviewed by foreign experts.

Introducing TCM to overseas students in China and abroad meets with many challenges of communication and dissemination of material. We hope this series of textbooks will make great contributions to the development of Chinese culture, the improvement of human health, and the promotion of scientific and cultural exchange between China and the rest of the world.

China National Association of International Exchange and Collaboration in TCM Higher Education
Editing Committee of Chinese-English Bilingual Textbooks Included in the Eleventh Five-Year Plan of the Ministry of Health of P.R.C. for International Students of Chinese TCM Institutions
July, 2007

编写说明

本教材是"全国高等中医药院校来华留学生卫生部'十一五'规划汉英双语教材"系列之一。

中医基础理论是中医学理论体系的重要组成部分，是学习中医各学科知识的基础。本教材主要介绍了中医的基础理论和基本知识，内容包括中医学理论体系的形成和发展、中医学理论体系的基本特点、阴阳五行学说、藏象学说、精气血津液、经络学说、体质学说、病因病机学说、防治原则。

本教材的编写，根据"全国高等中医药院校来华留学生卫生部'十一五'规划汉英双语教材编审委员会"的编写要求，以保持中医药传统特色为宗旨，重视传统中医基础理论的完整性、系统性，指出了这些理论对临床实践的指导意义，使本教材更具有实用价值。同时，又适当吸纳了相关研究的进展内容，结合了编者多年的教学实践经验，以反映中医传统理论的科学性和先进性。为了防止篇幅冗长，在内容详略上进行了适当的处理。

本教材的编写和翻译工作均由教材编译委员会分工完成，其中主编统审中文稿部分，主译统审英文稿部分。教材可供来华留学生、进修生使用，也可作为境内外中医药院校汉英双语教学及中医自修者学习所用。

编写中医汉英双语教材，是一项繁重的工作，尽管我们在编译中作了很多努力，但由于经验不足，水平有限，编写和翻译中可能会存在一些问题，希望大家提出宝贵意见，以便不断修订、改进和提高。

《中医基础理论》编译委员会
2007 年 7 月

Preface

This book is one of the series of bilingual textbooks programmed by the Public Health Ministry for the 11th five plans for Chinese medicine specialized foreign students in college of Chinese medicine and pharmacy in China.

Fundamental theory of Chinese medicine is the important component part of theoretical system of Chinese medicine. It is the basis for studying knowledge of various subjects of Chinese medicine. In this book, the basic theories and knowledge of Chinese medicine are mainly introduced, including the initiating and development of theoretical system of Chinese medicine, the basic characteristics of Chinese medicine theoretical system, yin-yang and the five element theories, visceral picture theory, essence-qi-blood-fluid theory, meridian theory, constitutional theory, etiopathological theory, and principles for prevention and treatment.

According to the demand of Editing Committee for Bilingual Textbooks programmed by The Public Health Ministry for The 11th Five Plans for Chinese Medicine Specialized Foreign Students in College of Chinese Medicine and Pharmacy in China, in the compilation of this book, we take keeping the feature of the traditional Chinese medicine as the aim, emphasize the integrity and systematicness, and point out the guiding role of these theories to the clinical practice, so as to make the book possess more practical value. At the same time, we also draw some contents of advances in relative studies, in combination with the teaching experiences of the authors for many years, so that the scientificness and advancedness of the traditional theory of Chinese medicine can be shown. In order to avoid a large number of the pages, we manage appropriately to give some contents in detail while some others briefly.

The compilation and translation of the book are accomplished through sharing the work by the members of the committee. Of which the Chinese manuscript is examined by the compiler in chief and the English manuscript is done by the translator in chief. The book is mainly for foreign students in China, but it may also serve as a reference book for those engaging in Chinese-English bilingual teaching in college of Chinese medicine and pharmacy, and those who learn Chinese medicine on their own both at home and abroad.

It is a hard work to compile a Chinese-English bilingual textbook. Although we have made a great effort in both compilation and translation, there are definitely some shortcomings or errors because of our insufficient experience and limited learning. Here we earnestly hope to receive any valuable criticism or suggestion from the readers so that we can further revise and improve it.

The Compilation and Translation Committee for
Fundamental Theory of Chinese Medicine
In Hangzhou
July 2007

目 录

1 绪论 ... 3
1.1 中医学理论体系的形成与发展 ... 3
1.1.1 中医学理论体系的形成 ... 4
1.1.2 中医学理论体系的发展 ... 5
1.2 中医学理论体系的基本特点 ... 6
1.2.1 整体观念 ... 6
1.2.2 辨证论治 ... 8

2 阴阳五行学说 ... 10
2.1 阴阳学说 ... 10
2.1.1 阴阳的基本含义 ... 10
2.1.2 阴阳学说的基本内容 ... 10
2.1.3 阴阳学说在中医学中的应用 ... 12
2.2 五行学说 ... 16
2.2.1 五行的基本含义 ... 16
2.2.2 五行特性和五行归类 ... 16
2.2.3 五行学说的基本内容 ... 17
2.2.4 五行学说在中医学中的应用 ... 19

3 藏象学说 ... 23
3.1 五脏 ... 23
3.1.1 心 ... 23
附：脑 ... 25
3.1.2 肺 ... 25
3.1.3 脾 ... 26
3.1.4 肝 ... 28

         3.1.5 肾 …………………………………………………………… 30
         附:女子胞 ………………………………………………………… 32
   3.2 六腑 ……………………………………………………………… 32
         3.2.1 胆 …………………………………………………………… 32
         3.2.2 胃 …………………………………………………………… 33
         3.2.3 小肠 ………………………………………………………… 33
         3.2.4 大肠 ………………………………………………………… 33
         3.2.5 膀胱 ………………………………………………………… 33
         3.2.6 三焦 ………………………………………………………… 34
   3.3 脏腑之间的关系 …………………………………………………… 34
         3.3.1 五脏之间的关系 …………………………………………… 34
         3.3.2 六腑之间的关系 …………………………………………… 37
         3.3.3 脏与腑之间的关系 ………………………………………… 37

4 精气血津液 39

   4.1 精 ………………………………………………………………… 39
         4.1.1 精的含义 …………………………………………………… 39
         4.1.2 精的生成 …………………………………………………… 39
         4.1.3 精的功能 …………………………………………………… 40
   4.2 气 ………………………………………………………………… 41
         4.2.1 气的含义 …………………………………………………… 41
         4.2.2 气的生成 …………………………………………………… 41
         4.2.3 气的运动 …………………………………………………… 41
         4.2.4 气的功能 …………………………………………………… 42
         4.2.5 气的分类 …………………………………………………… 43
   4.3 血 ………………………………………………………………… 45
         4.3.1 血的含义 …………………………………………………… 45
         4.3.2 血的生成 …………………………………………………… 45
         4.3.3 血的运行 …………………………………………………… 46
         4.3.4 血的功能 …………………………………………………… 47
   4.4 津液 ……………………………………………………………… 47
         4.4.1 津液的含义 ………………………………………………… 47
         4.4.2 津液的代谢 ………………………………………………… 47
         4.4.3 津液的功能 ………………………………………………… 48
   4.5 精、气、血、津液之间的关系 …………………………………… 49
         4.5.1 精和气的关系 ……………………………………………… 49
         4.5.2 精和血的关系 ……………………………………………… 50
         4.5.3 气和血的关系 ……………………………………………… 50
         4.5.4 气和津液的关系 …………………………………………… 51

		4.5.5 血和津液的关系	52

5 经络学说 ... 53

5.1 经络的含义和组成 ... 53
- 5.1.1 经络的含义 ... 53
- 5.1.2 经络系统的组成 ... 53

5.2 十二经脉 ... 55
- 5.2.1 十二经脉的名称 ... 55
- 5.2.2 走向、交接、分布、表里关系及流注次序 ... 56
- 5.2.3 十二经脉的循行 ... 58

5.3 奇经八脉 ... 68
- 5.3.1 督脉 ... 69
- 5.3.2 任脉 ... 71
- 5.3.3 冲脉 ... 71
- 5.3.4 带脉 ... 71
- 5.3.5 阴跷脉、阳跷脉 ... 71
- 5.3.6 阴维脉、阳维脉 ... 72

附：经别、别络、经筋、皮部 ... 72

5.4 经络的生理功能 ... 73
- 5.4.1 沟通上下表里，联系全身各部 ... 73
- 5.4.2 运行气血，濡养全身 ... 74
- 5.4.3 感应传导 ... 74
- 5.4.4 调节机体平衡 ... 74

5.5 经络学说在中医学中的应用 ... 74
- 5.5.1 说明病理变化 ... 74
- 5.5.2 指导疾病的诊断和治疗 ... 75

6 体质学说 ... 78

6.1 体质的形成 ... 78
- 6.1.1 体质的生理基础 ... 78
- 6.1.2 体质的构成要素 ... 79
- 6.1.3 影响体质的因素 ... 80

6.2 体质的分类 ... 84
- 6.2.1 传统分类法 ... 84
- 6.2.2 现代分类法 ... 86

7 病因病机学说 ... 88

7.1 病因 ... 88
- 7.1.1 外感病因 ... 89

  7.1.2 内伤病因 ……………………………………………… 91
  7.1.3 病理产物性病因 ………………………………………… 93
  7.1.4 其他病因 ………………………………………………… 94
 7.2 病机 ……………………………………………………… 95
  7.2.1 发病原理 ………………………………………………… 95
  7.2.2 发病类型 ………………………………………………… 97
  7.2.3 基本病机 ………………………………………………… 98

8 防治原则 ……………………………………………… **108**

 8.1 预防 ……………………………………………………… 108
  8.1.1 未病先防 ………………………………………………… 108
  8.1.2 既病防变 ………………………………………………… 109
 8.2 治则 ……………………………………………………… 110
  8.2.1 治病求本 ………………………………………………… 110
  8.2.2 扶正祛邪 ………………………………………………… 113
  8.2.3 重视整体 ………………………………………………… 114
  8.2.4 因异制宜 ………………………………………………… 116

Contents

1 INTRODUCTION **121**

  1.1 Initiation and Development of Theoretical System of Chinese Medicine 121

    1.1.1 Initiation of Theoretical System of Chinese Medicine 123

    1.1.2 Development of Theoretical System of Chinese Medicine 124

  1.2 Cardinal Characteristics of Theoretical System of Chinese Medicine 128

    1.2.1 Conception of Holism 128

    1.2.2 Treatment Determination Based on Syndrome Differentiation 131

2 THEORIES OF YIN-YANG AND THE FIVE ELEMENTS **134**

  2.1 Theory of Yin-Yang 134

    2.1.1 The Basic meaning of Yin-Yang 134

    2.1.2 The Basic Content of Yin-Yang Theory 135

    2.1.3 Application of Yin-Yang Theory in Chinese Medicine 138

  2.2 The Theory of the Five Elements 143

    2.2.1 Fundamental Meaning of the Five Elements 143

    2.2.2 The Characters and the Categorization of the Five Elements 144

    2.2.3 Essential Contents of Theory of the Five Elements 146

  2.2.4 Application of Theory of the Five Elements in Chinese Medicine ·· 149

3 VISCERAL PICTURE THEORY ································ **156**

 3.1 Five *Zang*-Viscera ··· 157
  3.1.1 Heart ··· 157
   Appendix: Brain ··· 159
  3.1.2 Lung ··· 159
  3.1.3 Spleen ··· 163
  3.1.4 Liver ··· 166
  3.1.5 Kidney ·· 170
   Appendix: Womb ·· 174
 3.2 Six *Fu*-Viscera ·· 174
  3.2.1 Gallbladder ·· 174
  3.2.2 Stomach ··· 175
  3.2.3 Small Intestine ··· 175
  3.2.4 Large Intestine ··· 176
  3.2.5 Urinary Bladder ·· 176
  3.2.6 Tri-Jiao ·· 177
 3.3 Relationships among the Viscera ······························· 177
  3.3.1 Relationships among the Five *Zang*-Viscera ··············· 177
  3.3.2 Relationships among the Six *Fu*-viscera ·················· 182
  3.3.3 Relationships between *Zang*-and *Fu*-Viscera ·············· 183

4 ESSENCE, QI, BLOOD AND BODY FLUID ···················· **187**

 4.1 Essence ··· 187
  4.1.1 Concept of Essence ····································· 187
  4.1.2 Production of Essence ·································· 187
  4.1.3 Functions of Essence ··································· 188
 4.2 Qi ·· 190
  4.2.1 Concept of Qi ·· 190
  4.2.2 Production of Qi ······································· 190
  4.2.3 Movement of Qi ······································· 191
  4.2.4 Functions of Qi ·· 192
  4.2.5 Classification of Qi ···································· 194
 4.3 Blood ··· 197
  4.3.1 Concept of Blood ······································ 197
  4.3.2 Production of Blood ··································· 197
  4.3.3 Circulation of Blood ··································· 198

  4.3.4 Functions of Blood ·· 199
 4.4 Body Fluid ·· 200
  4.4.1 Concept of Body Fluid ··· 200
  4.4.2 Metabolism of Body Fluid ·· 200
  4.4.3 Functions of Body Fluid ·· 201
 4.5 Relationships among Essence, Qi, Blood and Body Fluid ············· 203
  4.5.1 Relationship between Essence and Qi ·························· 203
  4.5.2 Relationship between Essence and Blood ······················ 204
  4.5.3 Relationship between Qi and Blood ····························· 204
  4.5.4 Relationship between Qi and Body Fluid ······················· 206
  4.5.5 Relationship between Blood and Body Fluid ··················· 207

5 MERIDIAN THEORY ·· 209

 5.1 Concept of the Meridian and Its Composition ·························· 209
  5.1.1 Concept of the Meridian ·· 209
  5.1.2 Composition of the Meridian System ···························· 210
 5.2 Twelve Meridians ··· 212
  5.2.1 Nomenclature of the Twelve Meridians ························· 213
  5.2.2 Running Course, Interconnection, Distribution, Exterior-Interior
     Relationship and Flow Order ····································· 214
  5.2.3 Running Routes of the Twelve Meridians ······················· 218
 5.3 Eight Extra Meridians ··· 223
  5.3.1 Du Meridian ··· 225
  5.3.2 Ren Meridian ·· 225
  5.3.3 Chong Meridian ··· 226
  5.3.4 Dai Meridian ·· 227
  5.3.5 Yinqiao and Yangqiao Meridians ································ 227
  5.3.6 Yinwei and Yangwei Meridians ································· 228
  Appendix: Meridian Divergences, Divergent Collaterals,
     Meridian Musculatures and Skin Areas ························· 228
 5.4 Physiological Functions of the Meridian System ······················ 230
  5.4.1 Communicating Superiorly, Inferiorly, Exteriorly and Interiorly,
     and Connecting All the Parts of the Body ······················· 230
  5.4.2 Conveying Qi-Blood to Nourish the Whole Body ·············· 232
  5.4.3 Reaction and Conduction ··· 232
  5.4.4 Regulating Functional Balance for the Body ··················· 232
 5.5 Application of the Meridian Theory in Chinese Medicine ············ 233
  5.5.1 Expounding Pathological Changes ······························ 233
  5.5.2 Guiding Diagnosis and Treatment of Disease ··················· 234

6 CONSTITUTIONAL THEORY ... 239

6.1 Formation of Constitution ... 239
6.1.1 Physiological Basis of Constitution ... 239
6.1.2 Essential Component of Constitution ... 241
6.1.3 Factors Affecting Constitution ... 244
6.2 Classification of Constitution ... 250
6.2.1 Traditional Classification ... 250
6.2.2 Modern Classification ... 254

7 ETIOLOGY AND PATHOMECHANISM ... 257

7.1 Etiology ... 257
7.1.1 Exogenous Pathogens ... 258
7.1.2 Endogenous Pathogens ... 264
7.1.3 Pathogens from Pathological Products ... 267
7.1.4 Other pathogens ... 269
7.2 Pathomechanism ... 270
7.2.1 Pathogenesis ... 271
7.2.2 Type of Attack ... 273
7.2.3 Basic Patho-mechanism ... 276

8 PRINCIPLES FOR PREVENTION AND TREATMENT OF DISEASE ... 293

8.1 Principles for Prevention of Disease ... 293
8.1.1 Prevention before a Disease Occurs ... 293
8.1.2 Treatment before a Disease Develops ... 295
8.2 Principles for Treatment ... 296
8.2.1 Treatment Aiming at the Root of a Disease ... 297
8.2.2 Strengthening the Vital and Dispelling the Pathogen ... 301
8.2.3 Attaching Importance to the General Condition ... 303
8.2.4 Treatment Suitable for the Season, Locality and Individual ... 307

中医基础理论

1 绪　　论

中国医药学有着悠久的历史,是中国人民长期同疾病作斗争的经验总结,是中国优秀文化的重要组成部分。在长期的医疗实践中,它逐步形成并发展为独特的、完整的医学理论体系,为中国人民的卫生保健事业和中华民族的繁衍昌盛做出了巨大的贡献。

中国医药学属于生命科学的范畴,是世界医学的重要组成部分,承担着促进生命科学不断前进和创新的使命。中医学独特的医学理论体系和临床诊疗特色,将为世界医学的发展和全人类的健康事业贡献自己的力量。

1.1　中医学理论体系的形成与发展

中医学理论体系的形成可以追溯到战国至秦汉时期,经历了漫长的历史过程。要使零散的、自我意识的、局部的、流传于民间的医学实践知识,上升为具有指导性意义的医学理论知识,成为系统的医学知识体系,需要一定的基础和条件。

(1) 长期医疗经验的积累:社会发展史告诉人们,人类自有生产活动以来就开始了医疗活动。据考证,早在殷代即出现了病名的记载,如癞、疥、蛊、龋、耳鸣、下利、不眠等。再从"疾耳""疾鼻""疾目"等涉及人体器官的病名看,古人对生命活动的认识是与解剖观察分不开的。

至西周及春秋战国时期,对疾病的认识又有了进一步的发展。如先秦文献《山海经》中就记载了 38 种疾病。1973 年底在长沙马王堆三号汉墓出土的医学文献中,除载有五十二病方外,文中提及的病名超过百个。据不完全统计,先秦古籍中所载病名已多达 180 余种。充分说明当时人们对于疾病的认识已经相当深刻,并同时积累了较为丰富的医疗经验,从而为医学理论知识的整理、规律的总结和理论框架的建构提供了直接资料并奠定了实践基础。

(2) 古代哲学思想的影响:哲学是关于世界观和方法论的学说,任何一门自然科学的形成和发展都离不开哲学,必然会受到哲学思想的支配和制约。尤其在自然科学还不很发达的古代,医家们在整理医疗经验、分析规律、归纳特性时,必然要借助于古代哲学的思想和其中蕴涵的方法。

古代哲学观点为医学理论研究提供了思维的框架。尤其是气一元论、阴阳五行等学说,为中医理论体系的形成提供了哲学依据,确立了生命是物质的,是一个阴阳对立统一、运动不息的发展变化过程,疾病可防可治的主导思想;为中医学确立采用整体综合的研究方法、构建独特的中医学理论体系提供了方法;为阐明人与自然的关系、生命的本质、健康与疾病等重大理论问题奠定了基础。从而为散在的、零碎的医疗经验的整理、归纳、总结和研究制定了基本的标准和纲领，使中医学逐步系统化、规范化，理论逐步得到升华，促进了中医学理论体系的形成。毋庸置疑，古代哲学思想是中医学理论体系形成的思想基础。

（3）古代自然科学的渗透：自然科学是关于物质运动规律的理论知识体系，其发展从来就不是孤立的，而是相互渗透、相互影响和相互促进的。具有自然科学属性的中医学，其形成与发展自然也不例外。曾处于领先地位的天文学、历法学、气象学、地理学、物候学、声学、农学、数学、兵法以及生理学、解剖学等自然科学知识，被古代医家用作研究人体生命现象及疾病防治的技术和手段是显而易见的，有些甚至还被吸收、移植乃至融合。可见，古代自然科学的发展为中医学理论体系的形成奠定了科学基础。

1.1.1 中医学理论体系的形成

《黄帝内经》、《难经》、《伤寒杂病论》和《神农本草经》等医学典籍的问世，标志着中医学理论体系的初步形成。

《黄帝内经》一书，著述始于春秋战国，成书于西汉中后期，是众多医家进行搜集、整理、综合而成的现存最早的医学经典。一般认为，现存的《素问》和《灵枢》即是《黄帝内经》的两个部分。该书以医学内容为中心，运用哲学理论和科学知识，以整体观念为指导，阐释了人体内在活动的规律性及人与外在环境的统一性；研究了人的组织结构、生理病理，以及疾病诊断和防治等理论。在《素问》和《灵枢》中有许多内容在当时及其以后较长一段时期内都处于世界领先地位。如在组织结构方面，对人体骨骼和血脉的长度、内脏器官的大小和容积等的记载，基本是符合现代解剖学发现的。在生理方面关于血液的循环运行、人体脏腑多功能的系统认识，以及关于生理、病理方面的整体联系等，对中医学独特的理论体系的构成和思维模式的确立，有着举足轻重的作用。在诊断方面，不仅奠定了望、闻、问、切四诊的方法学基础，而且提出诊断必须结合致病的内外因素加以全面考虑的观点。这些理论至今仍然有效地指导着临床实践。《黄帝内经》的问世标志着中医学由单纯积累经验的阶段，发展到系统的理论总结阶段，它为中医学的发展提供了理论指导和依据。

《难经》原名《八十一难》或《八十一问》。大约著于东汉之前，相传系秦越人所作。全书采用问难答疑的形式，论述了有关脏腑、经络、脉学、病理、针法等内容。该书以基础理论为主，同时分析了一些病症。对经络、命门、三焦的论述，在《黄帝内经》的基础上有所发展，是继《黄帝内经》之后的又一部经典著作。

《伤寒杂病论》为东汉末年张仲景所著。该书总结了东汉以前防治疾病的丰富经验，以六经辨识伤寒，依脏腑论治杂病。该书理、法、方、药齐备，为后世临床医学的发展奠定了基础。这部临床名著被后世誉为"方书之祖"。它的问世标志着中医辨证论治体系的确立。该书后被分为《伤寒论》及《金匮要略》两个部分，前者以外感病为主，后者以内伤杂病为主。

《神农本草经》简称《本经》或《本草经》，约成书于汉代，是中国已知最早的药物学专著。全书收载药物365种，根据药效分为上、中、下三品。上品主养命以应天，中品主养性以应人,下品主治病以应地,成为中国最早的药物分类法。书中还概括地论述了四气(寒、热、温、凉)、五味(酸、苦、甘、辛、咸)、七情和合(单行、相须、相使、相畏、相恶、相反、相杀)等药物学理论。该书的问世是中药理论体系形成的重要标志,为中药学的发展奠定了基础。

1.1.2　中医学理论体系的发展

在《黄帝内经》、《难经》、《伤寒杂病论》和《神农本草经》的基础上,历代医家从不同的角度丰富和发展了中医学的理论体系。

(1) 晋隋唐时期:晋隋唐时期的医药学在以往基础上得到较为全面的发展。特别是在诊断、病源、针灸、方药等方面出现了一批总结性专著。如晋代,太医令王叔和所著《脉经》系统阐述了24种脉象的形态及其所主病症,成为现存最早的脉学专著。著名学者皇甫谧对《素问》、《针经》(即《灵枢》)等书中所论述的经脉、腧穴、针法等加以整理,著成最早的针灸学专著——《针灸甲乙经》。葛洪所著《肘后备急方》对天花、麻疹等传染病已能从发病特点和临床表现上作出诊断。由隋代太医巢元方等人编著的《诸病源候论》(简称《病源》或《巢氏病源》)是一部探讨病源和证候的代表性著作。书中叙述了临床各科疾病的病源和证候,其认识和描述大多是正确的。唐代方药巨著的相继问世令人瞩目。孙思邈所著《备急千金要方》、《千金翼方》和王焘所编《外台秘要》都是以记载名医效方和各种治疗手段为主的传世方书。

(2) 宋金元时期:宋金元时期的医学领域呈现出百家争鸣的活跃气氛,各家学派以独特的学术见解极大地丰富了医学理论和实践。

宋代,陈无择的《三因极一病证方论》提出了著名的"三因学说",将病因具体概括为三个方面,即内因为七情所伤;外因为六淫外感;不内外因为饮食饥饱、叫呼伤气、虫兽所伤、中毒金疮、跌损压溺等。该分类法比较符合临床实际,不但是中医病因学的又一进步,而且深刻影响着后世对病因认识的思维模式。被尊为"儿科之父"的钱乙开创了脏腑证治的先河,以五脏为纲的辨证方法载于《小儿药证直诀》一书之中。钱氏还对某些发疹性疾病如麻疹、痘疹等有了较为明确的认识,并能予以鉴别诊断。

金元时期涌现出各具特色的医学流派,其中最具有代表性的医家是刘完素、张从正、李东垣、朱丹溪,后世尊之为"金元四大家"。

在《素问》病机理论和运气学说的启发下,刘完素提出了疾病多因"火"而发的理论,认为外感"六气皆从火化"、"五志过极皆能化火",治病喜用寒凉方药,被后世称为"寒凉派"。张从正认为,人之所以生病多因邪气内侵所致,邪气散去,疾病即愈,因而倡导治病当以驱邪为要务。治疗多用汗、吐、下诸法,以达到祛邪安正的目的,被后世称为"攻邪派"。李东垣则认为疾病的发生多与脾胃内伤有关。强调脾胃为万物之母,生化之源,脾胃病则百病莫不由之而生,对脾胃升降理论多有阐发,治病以补益脾胃之气为先,故后世称之为"补土派"。另外,由他原创的"阴火"理论和"甘温除热"之法对后世也颇有影响。朱丹溪集刘、张、李三家之说,以杂病证治见长,创见颇多。他对"相火"学说有所发挥,认为疾病的基本病理变化是"阳常有余,阴常不足",主张治宜滋阴降火,故后世称之为"养阴派"。其他人如张元素也对中医理论体系的充实和推进作出了很大的贡献。

(3) 明清时期：由于传染性疾病的肆虐，明清时期出现了研究四时温热病发生、发展规律及其诊治方法的温病学派，这标志着中医学对传染性疾病的探索进入了新阶段。明代医家吴又可著《温疫论》一书，提出了"戾气"学说，认为"温疫"的病原"非风非寒非暑非湿，乃天地间别有一种异气所成"。其传染途径是从口鼻而入。这是对温病（特别是温疫）病因学的重大突破。至清代，著名温病学家叶（天士）、薛（生白）、吴（鞠通）、王（孟英）系统总结了以往有关外感热病的研究成果，突破了"温病不越伤寒"的传统观念，创立了以卫气营血和三焦为核心的温病辨证论治规范，从而使温病学在病因、病机及脉证论治方面，形成了完整的理论体系。应当指出，温病学说和伤寒学说同为治疗外感热病的两大学派，两者是相辅相成的，对临床治疗均有重要的指导作用，迄今为止仍具有较高的研究价值。

此外，明代赵献可、张景岳等提出阴阳肾命学说，清代王清任倡导瘀血致病说、创制活血化瘀系列方剂等，不但为中医基础理论充实了新的内容，而且对中医治疗学的发展也有较大的贡献。

(4) 近现代时期：近代的中国医家一方面着手收集和整理前人经验，一方面在西方医学传入的情况下，试图将中西医论争引导至中西医汇通，进而走向中西医结合的道路。经历了长期论争之后，中西医之间在学术上逐渐沟通。一些有识之士率先提倡中西医汇通。如张锡纯所著《医学衷中参西录》就是一部极具代表性的中西医汇通专著。随着中医药事业的发展，现代中医基础理论的整理和研究都取得了可喜的成绩，已经成为一门独立的基础学科，在理论的系统整理和实验研究等方面都取得了长足的发展。尤其是运用现代科学技术来研究和探讨某些理论的本质，亦显示出一些可喜的苗头。例如关于阴虚、阳虚及寒热本质的研究，肾本质、脾本质的研究，方剂配伍和证候规律的研究等等，都取得了一定的进展，并已引起国内外医学界的极大关注。实践不断证明，中医基础理论的发展势必促进和推动整个中医学的发展和中医理论体系的完善，从而为生命科学研究的深入和发展作出重要的贡献。

1.2 中医学理论体系的基本特点

中医学的理论体系主要包括整体观念和辨证论治两个基本特点。

1.2.1 整体观念

所谓整体，是指事物的统一性和完整性。中医学认为，人体是一个有机的整体，构成人体的各个组成部分之间，在结构上是不可分割的，在功能上是相互协调、相互为用的，在病理上是相互影响的。同时也认识到人与自然环境、社会环境密切相关，人类在能动地适应自然和改造自然的实践中，维持着机体的正常生命活动。这种机体自身整体性和内外环境的统一性的思想，就是中医学的整体观念。

1.2.1.1 人体是一个有机的整体

人体是由若干脏腑组织所构成，各个脏腑组织都有着各自不同的功能，这些功能又都是整体活动的组成部分，从而决定了机体的整体统一性。机体整体统一性的形成是以五脏为中心,配以六腑,通过经络系统的联络作用,把五体、官窍、四肢百骸等全身组织器官联结成一个有机的整体,并通过精、气、血、津液的作用,完成人体统一协调的功能活动来实现的。中医学把所有器官形体组织及其相关功能都包括在五大系统之中。这种五脏一体观指导着中医学对人体生理、病理的研究和认识。

人的正常生理活动一方面依靠脏腑组织发挥各自的功能作用,另一方面又要依靠脏腑组织之间相辅相成的协同作用和相反相成的制约作用,才能维持其生理平衡。每个脏腑都有其各自不同的功能,但又是整体活动下的分工合作与有机配合,这就是局部与整体的统一。

中医学着眼于局部病变所引起的整体病理反应,认为人体某一局部的病理变化,往往与全身脏腑气血的盛衰有关。因而在诊察疾病时可以通过官窍、形体、色脉等外在的变化,来了解和判断脏腑、气血等内在的病变。例如,舌体通过经络可以直接或间接与五脏相通。内在脏腑的虚实、气血的盛衰、津液的盈亏,以及疾病的轻重顺逆,会从舌象变化呈现出来,所以通过观察舌象即可测知内在的功能状态。

对于局部病变,中医学往往从整体出发,确立治则和治法。如心开窍于舌,心与小肠相表里,所以可用清心热、泻小肠火的方法治疗口舌糜烂。其他如眼病从肝治,耳聋从肾治,都是在整体观念指导下确定的治疗原则。

综上可见,中医学在阐述人的生理功能、病理变化,以及疾病的诊断和治疗时,都贯穿着"人体是一个有机的整体"的基本观点。

1.2.1.2 人与环境密切相关

人类生活在自然界,当环境发生变化时,人体必定会随之而发生相应变化。同时,人还与社会环境关系密切,社会环境必然会对人产生影响。当然,人类还会改造社会。

(1) 人与自然的统一性:自然界存在着人类赖以生存的物质条件。当自然界的变化直接或间接地影响到人体时,人体就会产生相应反应。属于生理范围内的,即是生理上的适应性调节;超越了生理范围的,即是病理性反应。

一年之中,春温、夏热、长夏湿、秋燥、冬寒是气候变化的一般规律。生物在气候的影响下,会有春生、夏长、长夏化、秋收、冬藏等适应性变化。人也毫不例外地必须与季节相适应。如春夏季节,阳气发泄,气血趋向于表,表现为皮肤松弛,汗出较多而排尿偏少。机体通过出汗散热调节了自身的阴阳平衡。秋冬季节,阳气收敛,气血趋向于里,表现为皮肤致密,汗出偏少而排尿较多。这样既保证了体内水液代谢的平衡,又不会使人体阳气过多耗散。人的脉象也会随着季节气候而发生适应性变化。如春夏脉象多见浮大,秋冬脉象多见沉小,说明季节气候变化会对人的气血运行产生影响。

即使在一天之内,人的气血阴阳也会随着昼夜晨昏的变化而进行相应调节。如随着清晨太阳升起,人的阳气随之而生,推动着组织器官的功能活动。中午阳气隆盛,生理功能加强。至夜晚则阳气内敛,便于休息,恢复精力。在幅度上昼夜寒温变化虽不如四时季节那样明显,但其对人体生理活动的影响越来越受到医学界的关注。

此外,生存环境的地理差异也是直接影响人体生理功能的一个重要因素。如中国江南多湿热,人的腠理多疏松;北方多燥寒,人的腠理多致密。而一旦易地居处,自然环境突然改变,初期则多有不适,经过一段时间才能有所适应。

自然环境除会直接影响人体生理功能之外,人体发病也常常与自然环境变化密切相关。如四时气候的变化,是生物体进行生、长、化、收、藏的重要条件之一,人类的漫长的进化过程中,已经形成了一整套适应性调节规律。一旦气候剧变,环境过于恶劣,超过了人体正常调节功能的限度,或者机体的调节功能失常,不能对自然环境的变化作出适应性调节时,就会发生疾病。

人与自然存在着统一的整体关系,人的生理病理受到自然界的制约和影响,所以对待疾病要因时、因地、因人制宜,就成为中医治疗学上的重要原则。

(2) 人与社会关系密切:人类除了有确切的自然属性之外,还因存在精神活动而具有社会属性。中医学始终关注着人的社会属性,重视精神活动与脏腑形体的联系,并将其纳入自身的理论体系之中。

社会进步无疑会对人类健康带来很多好处,人均寿命逐年上升,然而,随着物质条件提升,不利于健康的社会问题也在与日俱增。诸如环境污染、食品安全、交通事故、就业困难、紧张焦虑、假冒伪劣、城市老龄化等。

社会的治与乱对人的影响也非常之大。社会安定,人的生活有规律,抵抗力强,发病机会降低,寿命延长。社会动荡,战争频仍,人们流离失所,饥饱无常,劳役过度,瘟疫流行,发病机会明显增加。

个人社会地位的改变,也势必会带来个人物质和精神生活的起伏变化。这对健康所产生的影响也不容小视。因此,不要因贫富、贵贱而影响身心健康。

中医学在长期的医疗实践中,已认识到社会活动对人精神的作用,人的精神对机体健康的反作用,精神活动和生理活动互相联系互为影响。如大怒暴怒则伤肝、大喜暴喜则伤心、思虑过度则伤脾、忧愁不解则伤肺、恐惧太过则伤肾。中医学强调形与神俱、形神相依、形神互动,这是人与社会人文环境整体统一、相互和谐的基础。

1.2.2 辨证论治

所谓辨证,即分析、辨别、认识疾病的证候;所谓论治,即根据辨证结果,研究并制定相应的治则和治法。辨证是决定治疗的前提和依据;论治是治疗疾病的手段和方法,也是对辨证结论是否正确的检验。辨证和论治是诊治疾病过程中相互联系而不可分割的两个阶段,是理论和实践相结合的体现。

在含义上,病、症、证三者是不同的。所谓病,是指有特定病因、发病形式、典型临床表现、发展规律和转归的一种完整的病态过程,如感冒、痢疾、疟疾、中风等。所谓症,包括症状和体征两部分。症状,即患者主观感觉到的不适,如疼痛、眩晕、恶心、乏力等。体征,即病体客观表现出的异常变化,如斑疹、面赤、舌红、脉浮等。另外,广义症状通常也包括体征在内。所谓证,是医生对疾病过程中的某一阶段所作出的病理概括,它包括病因(如风寒、风热、痰饮、瘀血等)、病位(如表里、脏腑、经脉等)、病性(如寒、热等)、病势(如轻、重、缓、急等)以及正邪关系(如虚、实等)等,它标示着当前阶段病理变化的本质。

任何疾病的发生和发展总是要通过一定的症状、体征表现出来,所以症状和体征是疾病表现在外的基本要素,是临床诊断的依据,而不是诊断的结论。能够揭示疾病本质的结论是证。然而,由于证是医生对当前阶段疾病本质所作出的理性判断,所以证的结论与疾病本质之间的符合程度取决于医生的理论水平和实践经验。

在对疾病作出判断的基础上,应把着眼点落实到"证"的辨别,然后才能有针对性地确立治则和治法。以感冒为例,症见恶寒、发热、头身疼痛、脉浮者,属病在表,但由于病因和机体反应性的不同,临床又常呈现出风寒和风热两种不同的情况。只有进一步把感冒的风寒、风热辨别清楚,才能确定是选辛温解表法还是用辛凉解表法。辨证论治的核心是要把握疾病本质与证候表现之间的关系,既要辨病更要辨证,通过治疗"证"而达到治愈疾病的目的。

中医学要求医生能够辨证地看待病和证的关系,既看到同一种病可以概括出若干不同的证,又看到在不同的疾病中可以分析出相同的证,于是形成了"同病异治"和"异病同治"的重要理念。

所谓同病异治,是指同一种疾病,由于发病时间、地区以及患者的反应性不同,或其病情处于不同的发展阶段,所分析出的关于证的结论不同,因而治法亦不一样。仍以感冒为例,因发病季节不同而治法也不尽相同。暑季感冒多由暑湿邪气所致,故治当芳香化浊,祛暑除湿。这与其他季节治以辛凉或辛温解表有所不同。又如麻疹,发病初起,疹邪未透,治宜发表透疹;中期肺热壅盛,则须清解肺热;后期多为余热未尽,肺胃阴伤,则以养阴清热为主。

所谓异病同治,是指不同的疾病,在其发展过程中,由于病机相同,于是可采用相同或相近的治法。例如,胃下垂、久泻脱肛、子宫脱垂是不同的病,倘若均属中气下陷证,即可采用补气升提法予以治疗。

由上可见,中医学治病既重辨病,更重辨证,即着眼于病机的区分。病机相同则采用基本相同的治法;病机不同则必须采用不同的治法。所谓"证同治亦同,证异治亦异",实质上是由于"证"的含义中包含着病机的缘故。这种针对疾病发展过程中不同质的矛盾用不同方法去解决的原则,充分体现了辨证论治的精神实质。

总之,中医学从人体是一个有机整体和人与外界环境密切联系角度出发,来观察人对周围环境的反应状态,并透过临床征象来探究疾病的本质,把握人体反应状态的主要矛盾或矛盾的主要方面,并运用动态平衡理论,采取相应的治疗手段,通过调控而使病者阴阳协调的动态平衡获得重建,达到促使疾病痊愈的目的。辨证论治是中医认识疾病和治疗疾病的基本原则,是中医学对疾病的一种特殊的研究和处理方法,也是中医学的基本特点之一。

思 考 题

- 中医学理论体系是如何形成和发展的?
- 金元四大家各有何学术特点?其在中医学理论体系的发展中起何作用?
- 举例说明人体与自然的统一性。
- 何谓整体观念?其临床意义如何?
- 何谓辨证论治?举例说明"同病异治,异病同治"的精神实质。

2 阴阳五行学说

阴阳五行学说是阴阳学说和五行学说的合称,是中国古代先民用于认识自然和解释自然的世界观和方法论,属于古代哲学范畴。古代医家将阴阳五行学说运用于医学领域,藉以阐明人体生理功能和病理变化,并指导临床诊断与治疗,对中医药学理论体系的形成和发展产生了深刻的影响。时至今日,阴阳五行学说对于中医学理论体系和临床辨证论治的实践应用,仍处于无可替代的地位。

2.1 阴阳学说

2.1.1 阴阳的基本含义

阴阳,是人们对自然界相互关联的事物及现象对立双方相对属性的概括。阴阳的最初涵义是很朴素的,是指日光的向背,向日为阳,背日为阴,后来扩展到气候的冷暖,方位的上下、左右、内外,运动状态的动和静等。通过长期生活实践观察,人们逐渐发现事物都普遍存在着相互对立的阴阳两个方面,进而认识到两者的相互作用促进了事物的发生、发展与转化,因此就以阴阳来解释自然界的各种现象,为阴阳学说的形成奠定了基础。

阴阳学说认为,世间任何事物都可概括为阴和阳两个相互对立的方面,如白昼和黑夜、炎热和寒冷、躁动和静止等等。阴和阳的相互作用是自然界一切事物内部所固有的,自然界一切事物的发生、发展和变化,都是阴和阳运动变化的结果。

阴和阳既可代表相互对立的事物及现象,又可用于分析同一事物内部所存在着的相互对立的两个方面。一般而言,凡是运动着的、外向的、上升的、温热的、明亮的、无形的、功能的皆属于阳;相对静止着的、内守的、下降的、寒冷的、晦暗的、有形的、器质的皆属于阴。以天地而言,天气轻清故属阳,地气重浊故属阴;以水火而言,水寒而润下故属阴,火热而炎上故属阳;以物质的运动变化而言,蒸腾气化者属阳,凝聚成形者属阴。

阴阳学说作为一种方法论被引入医学领域,形成了医用阴阳学说。它把对人体具有推动、温煦、兴奋等作用的归属于阳,对人体具有凝聚、滋润、抑制等作用的归属于阴。

2.1.2 阴阳学说的基本内容

阴阳学说包括阴阳的对立与互根、制约与互用、消长与转化、平衡与失衡等方面的基本内容。

2.1.2.1 阴阳的对立与互根

阴阳对立,是指自然界的一切事物及现象存在着相互对立两个方面的相反属性。如天与地、昼与夜、寒与热、动与静、内与外、升与降、出与入等。阴阳学说认为:天为阳,地为阴;昼为阳,夜为阴;热为阳,寒为阴;动为阳,静为阴;外为阳,内为阴;升为阳,降为阴;出为阳,入为阴。

阴阳互根,是指阴或阳必须以其对方的存在作为自己存在的前提和依据,任何一方都不能脱离对方而单独存在。如上为阳,下为阴,没有上也就无所谓下;同样,没有下也就无所谓上。热为阳,寒为阴,没有热就无所谓寒;同样,没有寒也就无所谓热;外为阳,内为阴,没有外就无所谓内;同样,没有内也就无所谓外。可见阳必须依阴而存,阴必须靠阳而在,任何一方都必须以对方的存在作为自己存在的先决条件。

2.1.2.2 阴阳的制约与互用

阴阳制约,是指相互对立的阴阳双方常可表现出相互抑制和约束的关系。如春、夏、秋、冬四季有温、热、凉、寒的气候变化,春夏之所以温热,是因为阳气上升抑制了寒凉之气;秋冬之所以寒冷,是因为阴气上升抑制了温热之气。这是自然界阴阳之气相互制约的结果。阴阳制约的结果使事物之间或事物内部获得了动态平衡。

阴阳互用,是指相互依存的阴阳双方常可表现出相互资生和促进的关系。以天地云雨为例,地气上升,可将地面的水分挟带至天空而形成云雾;天气下降,可将天空的云雾以雨水的形式下降至地面。云和雨,地气与天气的循环往复过程,即为阴阳互用的过程。所以古有"无阳则阴无以生,无阴则阳无以化"的说法。这种以互根为基础的资生和促进关系,被称为"阴阳互用"。

阴阳的制约与互用虽然是相互矛盾的,但有时却能并存于某些阴阳关系之中。如代谢过程中的合成与分解,功能活动中的兴奋与抑制等,则既相互制约又相互为用。

应当指出,阴阳的制约与互用不具备普适性,也就是说并非所有阴阳双方都具有相互制约或互用的关系。

2.1.2.3 阴阳的消长与转化

事物的阴阳双方不是静止不变的,而是处于不断地运动变化之中。其运动变化包括量变的消长和质变的转化两种形式。

(1) 阴阳消长:消,意为减少、消耗;长,意为增多、增长。阴阳消长具体表现在此消彼长、此长彼消和此消彼亦消、此长彼亦长等方面。①此消彼长,此长彼消:在阴阳制约的条件下,阴或阳任何一方的衰弱,无力制约对方,从而引起对方的增长,甚至亢奋;而任何一方因增长而强盛,势必过度制约对方,从而引起对方的削减,甚至偏衰。以四时气候变化为例,从冬到春及夏,气候由寒冷逐渐转暖变热,此为"阴消阳长";由夏到秋及冬,气候由炎热逐渐转凉变寒,此为"阳消阴长"。一日之内,气温的变化也亦是阴阳消长的结果。平旦之时阳气渐盛,阴气渐衰,气温逐渐增高;日中则阳气隆盛,阴气衰减,气温最高;日西则阳气渐衰,阴气渐盛,则气温逐渐降低;夜半则阴气隆盛,阳气衰减,气温最低。②此消彼亦消,此长彼亦长:在阴阳互用的条件下,阴或阳任何一方的虚弱,无力资生和促进,使对方也随之虚弱;任何一方的旺盛则可助长和促进对方,使对方也随之旺盛。以天地为例,春夏天阳之气由生而旺,地之万物随之生长茂盛;秋冬天阳之气由收而潜,地之万物随之成熟闭藏。

(2) 阴阳转化:在一定的条件下,阴或阳可各自向其相反的方面转化,即阴可以转化为阳,阳也可以转化为阴。阴阳的相互转化,一般表现在事物变化的"物极"阶段。阴阳消长是一个量变过程,而阴阳转化是在量变基础上的质变。

阴阳转化必须具备一定的条件。也就是说,事物如果不发展到一定的程度或阶段,其阴阳属性一般不会发生转化。以四季为例,冬季之阴寒发展到了极致,便具备了转化的条件,阴寒气候就会向阳热方面转化;盛夏之阳热发展到了极致,即具备了转化的条件,阳热气候就会向阴寒方面转化。这里的"极致"就是促使转化的条件。

阴阳的消长(量变)和转化(质变)是运动着的事物发展变化全过程中密不可分的两个阶段,消长是转化的前提,而转化则是消长的结果。

2.1.2.4 阴阳的平衡与失衡

阴阳平衡,是指运动中的阴阳双方,其强弱变化适度,处于和谐匀平的状态。换言之,即阴阳的消长与转化均稳定在一定的范围之内,维持着动态平衡。这是事物自身运动所形成的最佳状态。古人称其为"阴平阳秘"。

事物的运动变化是绝对的、无休止的,但不等于说它是无序或紊乱的。阴阳双方的消长与转化如果能够维持在一定的范围、程度、时间内进行,那么这就属于阴阳的动态平衡状态,一系列重要的过程和变化(如万物的生、长、化、收、藏等)就能得以顺利进行。

阴阳失衡,是指运动中的阴阳双方,其强弱变化太过或不及,超出了动态平衡所限定的范围,导致各种灾变出现的状态。自然界的洪涝干旱、飓风冰雹、地震海啸均属阴阳失衡之列。

阴阳的平衡与失衡是相对而言的。阴阳平衡是阴阳消长与转化处于常态的结果,阴阳失衡是阴阳消长与转化失于常态的结果。阴阳平衡失于维系必然导致失衡,失衡所带来的损失固然巨大,然而失衡毕竟难于长久,而且失衡过后迟早会复归于平衡。自然界本身具有使失衡回归于平衡的自我调控能力。否则,自然界将难以生生不息。

综上所述,阴和阳是对事物及现象相对属性的概括,因而存在着无限可分性;阴和阳之间的相互关系不是孤立的、静止不变的,而是互相联系、互相影响、互为因果的。

2.1.3 阴阳学说在中医学中的应用

2.1.3.1 标识组织结构

阴阳学说认为,人的一切组织结构,既是有机联系的,又是可用阴和阳予以标识的。就大体部位而言,上部为阳,下部为阴;体表属阳,体内属阴。就其背腹四肢而言,则背属阳,腹属阴;四肢外侧为阳,四肢内侧为阴。就脏腑功能而言,则五脏主藏精气、神气而不传化水谷,故为阴;六腑主传化水谷而不藏精气、神气,故为阳。五脏之中又可分阴阳,即心、肺居于上部(胸腔),故属阳;肝、脾、肾位于下部(腹腔),故属阴。具体到各脏内部,则又可分阴阳,如心之心阴、心阳,肾之肾阴、肾阳等。

总之,人体组织结构的上下、内外、表里、前后各部分之间,以及内在脏器之间,均可运用阴阳加以标识。

2.1.3.2 说明生理功能

阴阳学说认为,人的生命活动是由阴阳双方保持协调关系的结果。以脏腑组织与功能活动而言,则脏腑组织属于阴,功能活动属于阳。以营养物质与功能活动而言,则营养物质属于阴,功能活动属于阳。如脾胃功能不佳,便难以完成对营养物质的消化吸收;反之,长期缺乏营养物质供给,脾胃功能将会减退。从气血关系分析,气属阳,血属阴,气能生血、行血和统血,故气的正常有助于血的生化和正常运行;血能生气、载气,血之充沛则又可资助气以充分发挥其生理效应。

生命活动是以物质代谢为基础的,没有物质代谢则无以产生生命活动。生命活动又不断促进着物质代谢。人的功能活动与脏腑组织的关系也就是阴阳相互依存和相互为用的关系。如果阴阳不能相互依存为用而分离,人的生命活动也就终止。

2.1.3.3 阐释病理变化

中医学把阴阳失调作为疾病发生、发展和变化的基本动因,并把它作为所有疾病和各种病理机制的高度概括。

阴阳失调主要表现为某一方的偏盛或偏衰,以及一方对另一方的累及和影响,这些又可统称为"阴阳不和"。如果在此基础上进一步分析,疾病的发生、发展主要涉及到人体的正气和致病的邪气两个方面。所谓"正气",是指人体的正常组织结构、生理功能,以及机体对疾病损害的抵抗、耐受和修复损伤的能力。所谓"邪气",泛指各种致病因素。

正气又可分为阳气和阴液两个方面;邪气也可分为阴阳两类,如六淫中的风、暑、燥、火(热)属于阳邪,而寒、湿属于阴邪。

疾病发生、发展和变化的过程,就是邪正交争、各有胜负的过程。正邪之间相互作用、相互斗争所反映出来的情况,都可以用阴阳的消长失调,即偏胜偏衰进行概括性说明。

(1) 阴阳偏胜:是指阴或阳任何一方过于亢盛及或损及对方所形成的病理变化。一般可有以下情况:

阳胜则热 阳胜,一般是指阳邪致病,或者功能活动中属于阳的一方超过生理限度,达到绝对亢奋的程度,所以都属于阳偏胜。阳偏胜大多为实热性病证。由于阳偏胜常会耗伤体内的阴液,从而引起阴液不足的病理变化,故有"阳胜则阴病"之说。

阴胜则寒 阴胜,一般是指阴邪致病,或者功能活动中偏于阴的一方超过生理限度,达到绝对亢奋的程度,所以都属于阴偏胜。阴偏胜大多为实寒性病证。由于阴偏胜常会损伤体内的阳气,从而引起阳气不足的病理变化,故有"阴胜则阳病"之说。

（2）阴阳偏衰:是指阴或阳任何一方低于正常水平的病理变化。一般可有以下情况:

阳虚则寒 阳虚,一般是指体内阳气虚损,推动和温煦作用明显降低的病理变化。由于阳虚可导致阳不制阴,阴寒之气相对偏盛,表现出虚寒之象。

阴虚则热 阴虚,一般是指体内阴液亏少,滋润和濡养作用明显不足的病理变化。由于阴虚,失去对脏腑组织器官的滋润和濡养,导致阴不制阳,使属于阳的功能活动相对亢奋,表现出虚性亢奋的热象。

（3）阴阳互累:是指当体内阴或阳任何一方虚损到一定程度时,必然就会累及对方,从而引起阴阳俱损的病理变化。主要有以下情况:

阳损及阴 即阳虚达到一定程度时,因阳虚不能化生阴液,可进一步导致阴液亦虚。

阴损及阳 即阴虚达到一定程度时,因阴虚不能滋养阳气,可进一步导致阳气亦虚。

无论是阳损及阴,抑或是阴损及阳,两者最终都表现为阴阳俱损的阴阳两虚证。然而,阳损及阴之阴阳两虚多以阳损为主,阴损及阳之阴阳两虚多以阴虚为主。

（4）阴阳转化:阴证或阳证在一定的条件下可以各自向其相反的方面转化,即阳证可以转化为阴证,阴证可以转化为阳证。如某些外感热病,表现为高热面赤、喘促气粗、烦躁口渴、脉数有力等,属于阳证。由于热毒极盛,严重耗伤元气,在持续高热的情况下,会突然出现体温骤降、面色苍白、四肢厥冷、脉微欲绝等阳气暴脱的危象,此属阳证转化为阴证。再如寒饮中阻患者,本为阴证,由于蕴积日久,寒饮化热,此属阴证转化为阳证。上述情况说明,阴阳转化是有条件的,前者热毒极盛,阳气亡脱,后者寒饮郁久而化热,即是促成阴阳转化的内部条件。

2.1.3.4 指导临床诊断

由于疾病发生和发展的根本原因是阴阳失调,所以,任何病症,尽管其临床表现错综复杂,千变万化,正确的诊断首先要分清阴阳,才能抓住疾病的本质,做到执简驭繁。

在四诊过程中,可分辨色泽、声息、脉象等方面的阴阳属性。

色泽可以分别阴阳,故从色泽可以辨别病情的阴阳属性。色泽鲜明者属阳,色泽晦黯者属阴。

观察呼吸气息的动态,听其发出的声音,也可以区别病情的阴阳属性。语声高亢洪亮,多言躁动者属阳;语声低微,少言沉静者属阴。呼吸气粗者属阳,呼吸微弱者属阴。

脉象也可分阴阳,从部位来分,则寸为阳,尺为阴;以至数分,则数者为阳,迟者为阴;以形态分,则浮、数、洪、大、滑、实者属阳,沉、迟、细、小、涩、虚者属阴。

总之,无论望、闻、问、切四诊,都应以分别阴阳为首务。

在辨证过程中,准确地区分阴阳,从而把握病证的本质属性,方能诊治无误。临床常用的八纲辨证(阴阳、表里、寒热、虚实)是其他各种辨证的纲领,而阴阳又是其中的总纲,以统领其他六纲。即表、热、实属阳,里、寒、虚属阴。辨析阴阳是临床辨证的纲领,大则可以区分整个病症是属阴抑或属阳,小则可分析四诊中某个具体脉症。因此,在临床辨证过程中,分清阴阳是关键。

2.1.3.5 指导疾病治疗

阴阳学说用于指导疾病的治疗最主要的是确定治疗原则和归纳药物的性能。

(1) 确定治疗原则:对阴阳偏胜的治则可概括为"损其有余"。阴阳偏胜,即阴或阳的过盛有余,多为邪气有余的病证。由于阳胜则热,阳胜则阴病,阳热盛易于损耗阴液。阳胜则热属实热证,宜用寒凉药以制其阳,治热以寒,即"热者寒之"。阴胜则寒,阴胜则阳病,阴寒盛易于损伤阳气。阴胜则寒属寒实证,宜用温热药以制其阴,治寒以热,即"寒者热之"。在调整阴阳的偏胜时,应注意有无相应的阴或阳偏衰的情况存在。若其相对一方有所偏衰时,则当兼顾其不足,配合以扶阳或益阴之法。

对阴阳偏衰的治则可概括为"补其不足"。阴阳偏衰,即阴或阳的虚损不足,或为阴虚,或为阳虚。可直接采取滋阴或温阳之法。如果阴虚不能制阳而致阳亢者,属虚热证,一般不能用寒凉药直折其热,须用滋阴壮水法,以抑制阳亢火盛。如果阳虚不能制阴而导致阴盛者,属虚寒证,更不宜辛温发散药以散阴寒,须扶阳益火法,以消退阴霾。

在治疗阴阳偏衰时,根据阴阳互用的原理,还可考虑"阴中求阳,阳中求阴"之法,即在用温阳药时,兼用滋阴药;在用滋阴药时,加用补阳药,以发挥其阴阳互用的生化作用。

总之,治疗的基本原则,是泻其有余,补其不足。阳胜者泻热,阴胜者祛寒;阳虚者扶阳,阴虚者补阴,以使阴阳偏胜偏衰的病理表现,复归于平衡协调的正常状态。

(2) 归纳药物性能:阴阳学说可用于概括药物的性味功能,作为指导临床用药的依据。一般地说,药物性能主要取决于气味功效和升降浮沉。

药性 即指寒、热、温、凉四种药性,又称"四气"。其中寒凉属阴,温热属阳。一般而言,凡能减轻或消除热证的药物大多属于寒凉之性,如黄芩、栀子等。反之,凡能减轻或消除寒证的药物一般属于温热之性,如附子、干姜之类。此外,对药性不甚明显的药物归为平性。

五味 即指酸、苦、甘、辛、咸五味。其中酸味能收能敛,苦味能下能泻,咸味能软能润,故酸苦咸属阴。如乌梅、大黄、芒硝等。辛味能升能散,甘味能补能益,故辛甘属阳。如桂枝、甘草等。另外,有些药物滋味不明显,被称为淡味。如茯苓、薏苡仁。因其味淡,故属阳。还有某些药物有涩味,属阴。尽管药物滋味不止五种,但习惯上仍称为五味。

升降浮沉 凡具有升阳发表、祛风散寒、涌吐、开窍等功效的药物,多上行向外,其性升浮,故属阳;而凡具有泻下、清热、利尿、重镇安神、潜阳息风、消导、降逆、收敛等功效的药物,多下行向内,其性沉降,故属阴。升浮之品如桑叶、菊花等,沉降之药如鳖甲、磁石等。

2.2 五行学说

2.2.1 五行的基本含义

五,在五行中指木、火、土、金、水五种物质。行,是运动的意思。五行,即木、火、土、金、水五种物质的运动。中国古代先民在长期生活实践中,认识到木、火、土、金、水五种物质是人类生活中不可或缺的物质,故称其为"五材"。

五行学说是在"五材"说的基础上,把这五种物质的属性加以抽象推演,用来说明自然界中的一切事物及现象之间相互资生、相互制约的运动变化的一门学说。

中医学运用五行特性、归类以及生克规律,来概括脏腑组织的功能属性,阐释五脏系统的内在联系,藉以说明人的生理、病理及其与外在环境的相互关系等,从而指导辨证论治,达到预防和治疗疾病的目的。

2.2.2 五行特性和五行归类

2.2.2.1 五行特性

五行特性是古人在对木、火、土、金、水五种物质的朴素认识基础上,进行抽象升华而逐渐形成的理论含义。主要用于分析各种事物的五行属性和研究事物之间的相互联系。对五行特性的认识已超越了五种具体物质的本身,而具有更为广泛的哲学涵义。

木的特性:古人称"木曰曲直"。曲直,是指树木的枝干能曲能直,向上向外舒展。因而引申为具有生长、升发、条达舒畅等作用或性质的事物,均归属于木。

火的特性:古人称"火曰炎上"。炎上,是指火具有温热、上升的特性。因而引申为具有温热、升腾等作用或性质的事物,均归属于火。

土的特性:古人称"土爰稼穑"。爰,通"曰"。稼穑,是指土地可播种和收获农作物。因而引申为具有生化、承载、受纳等作用或性质的事物,均归属于土。

金的特性:古人称"金曰从革"。从革,是指金可顺从人意,改变其状。因而引申为具有清洁、肃降、收敛等作用或性质的事物,均归属于金。

水的特性:古人称"水曰润下"。润下,是指水具有滋润和向下的特性。因而引申为具有寒凉、滋润、向下运行等作用或性质的事物,均归属于水。

2.2.2.2 五行归类

对事物及现象进行五行归类的依据是五行特性,方法包括直接归类和间接推衍两种。

(1) 直接归类:是将某事物及现象的部分特性直接与五行特性相类比,从而得出该事物及现象的五行属性。如与木的特性相类似的事物,则归属于木;与火的特性相类似的事物,则归属于火;等等。如东方为日出之地,富有生机,与木的升发、生长特性相类,故归属于木;南方气候炎热,植物繁茂,与火的炎上特性相类,故归属于火;西方为日落之处,其气肃杀,与金的肃杀、潜降特性相类,故归属于金;北方气候寒冷,虫类蛰伏,与水的寒冷、闭藏特性相类,故归属于水;中央气候适中,四季分明,长养万物,统御四方,与土的生化、承载特性相类,故归属于土。

(2) 间接推衍:当某事物及现象已被纳入某一行之后,与该事物及现象存在密切联系者均可随之一并纳入。如长夏多湿,由于湿与长夏关系密切,所以湿也随长夏的归类而被纳入土行。秋季多燥,由于燥与秋关系密切,所以燥也随秋的归类而被纳入金行。

无论是直接归类还是间接推衍,被归纳于同一行中的各种事物及现象之间,必然存在着这样或那样的内在联系。这种内在联系的基础是同一行的所有事物及现象都具有近似该行的某些特性。

现将自然界和人体的五行属性归类为表 2-1。

表 2-1　五行归类表

自 然 界							五行	人 体								
五音	五时	五味	五色	五化	五气	五季	五方 || 五脏	五腑	五体	五华	五志	五官	五液	五声	五脉
角	平旦	酸	青	生	风	春	东	木	肝	胆	筋	爪	怒	目	泪	呼	弦
徵	日中	苦	赤	长	暑	夏	南	火	心	小肠	脉	面	喜	舌	汗	笑	洪
宫	日西	甘	黄	化	湿	长夏	中	土	脾	胃	肉	唇	思	口	涎	歌	缓
商	日入	辛	白	收	燥	秋	西	金	肺	大肠	皮	毛	悲	鼻	涕	哭	浮
羽	夜半	咸	黑	藏	寒	冬	北	水	肾	膀胱	骨	发	恐	耳	唾	呻	沉

可以看出,以五行特性来分析、归类和推演络绎,就把自然界千变万化的事物,归结为木、火、土、金、水的五行系统。对人体来说,也即是将人体的各种组织和功能,归结为以五脏为中心的五个生理系统。

2.2.3　五行学说的基本内容

(1) 五行的生克制化:①五行相生:指五行中的某一行对另一行的资生和助长。相生次序是:木生火、火生土、土生金、金生水、水生木。在五行的相生关系中,任何一行都有"生我"和"我生"两个方面的关系,生我者为"母",我生者为"子",所以五行相生关系也称为"母子关系"。以木为例,由于木生火,故木为火之母,而木由水所生,故木为水之子。②五行相克:指五行中的某一行对另一行的克制和约束。相克次序是:木克土、土克水、水克火、火克金、金克木。在五行的相克关系中,任何一行都有"克我"和"我克"两个方面的关系(见图 2-1),我克者为我"所胜",克我者为我"所不胜"。以木为例,克木者为金,金为木之所不胜;木克者为土,土为木之所胜。

五行的相生与相克是不可分割的两个方面。具体体现在"生中有克"和"克中有生"。如木能生火,也能克土;土能生金,又能克水。这种生中寓制,制中寓生,相反相成,并保持生克相对平衡,是事物正常发生和发展的保证。

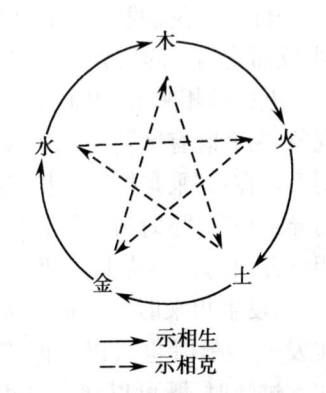

图 2-1　五行生克规律示意图
→ 示相生
--→ 示相克

五行的相生相克反映着自然界的正常现象。五行系统结构的各部分都不是孤立的,而是密切相关的,每一部分的变化,都必然影响着其他部分的状态,同时又受着五行系统结构整体的影响与制约。

(2) 五行的生克异常

1) 相生异常:由于五行相生关系异常是发生在母子之间的,故又称"母子相及"。母子相及包括母病及子和子病及母两种情况。

母病及子:是指五行中作为母的一行异常,影响到作为子的一行,导致母子两行都异常的情况。母病及子一般是在母行虚弱的情况下,导致子行亦不足,结果母子两行皆不足。如水为母,木为子,水不足则不能生木,导致母子俱虚,水竭木枯。

子病及母:是指五行中作为子的一行异常,影响到作为母的一行,导致子母两行都异常的情况。子病及母会出现虚实两种类型。一种是子行太过,引起母行亦亢盛,结果子母两行皆亢盛。如火为子,木为母,火旺引起木亢,导致木火俱亢这种情况称之为"子病犯母";另一种是子行不足,累及母行,引起母行亦不足,导致子母两行俱不足,如木为子,水为母,木不足引起水亏,导致木水俱不足,这种情况称之为"子盗母气"。

2) 相克异常:五行相克关系异常主要表现为相乘和相侮两种情况。

相乘:乘,有以强凌弱之意。五行相乘是指五行中某"一行"对被克的"一行"克制太过,从而引起一系列的异常相克反应。引起相乘的原因不外乎两个方面:一是某"一行"过于强盛,于是造成对被克制的"一行"克伐太过,导致被克的"一行"虚弱。如木过于强盛,则克土太过,造成土的不足,即称为"木乘土"。二是某"一行"过于虚弱,因而导致"克我"一行显得相对太过,使自身难以承受原先克它的"一行"相对较强的克制,从而使其更加衰弱。如木本无太过,其克土之力也仍在正常范围。但由于土本身的不足,于是形成了木克土的力量相对增强,使土更加不足,即称为"土虚木乘"。

相侮:侮,有欺负、欺侮之意。五行相侮是指五行中某"一行"对克我的"一行"实行反向克制,从而引起一系列的异常相克反应。引起相侮的原因也不外乎两个方面:一是某"一行"过于强盛,非但不受"克我"之行的克制,反而对原来"克我"的"一行"实施反向欺侮,所以反侮也称反克。如木本受金克,但在木过于强盛时,非但不受金的克制,反而对金进行反克,称为"木侮金"。二是某"一行"过于虚弱,因而导致"我克"一行相对太过,"我克"一行非但不受我的克制,反而对我施以反克。如金本身十分虚弱,不仅失于对木的克制,反而受到木的反克,称为"金虚木侮"。

五行的相乘和相侮都是异常相克现象,两者既有区别又有联系。两者区别表现在:相乘是按五行相克次序发生的异常克制;相侮则是与五行相克次序相反方向的异常克制。两者联系表现在:当发生相乘时也会同时发生相侮;在发生相侮时也可以同时发生相乘。如木过强时,既可以乘土又可以侮金;金虚时,既可以受到木侮,又可以受到火乘。以木为例图示如图 2-2:

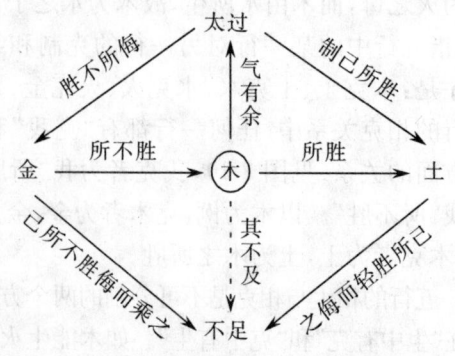

图 2-2 五行相乘相侮关系示意图

2.2.4 五行学说在中医学中的应用

中医学应用五行学说，就是用事物属性的五行归类方法及其相生相克的变化规律，解释五脏的生理功能、病理现象，并指导临床诊断与治疗。

2.2.4.1 说明生理功能及其相互关系

五行学说将人体的内脏分别归属于五行，以五行特性来说明五脏的生理功能特点。如肝喜条达，有疏泄之能，木有生发的特性，故以肝属"木"；心阳有温煦的作用，火有阳热的特性，故以心属"火"；脾为生化之源，土有生化万物的特性，故以脾属"土"；肺气主肃降，金有清肃、收敛的特性，故以肺属"金"；肾有主水、藏精的功能，水有润下的特性，故以肾属"水"。通过间接推衍，与五脏有生理联系的五腑、五体、五华、五志、五窍、五液等也都一并随五脏而归属于相应的五行之中了。

五行学说还可用以说明人的脏腑组织之间生理功能的内在联系。如五行"相生"可用于说明五脏之间的资生关系。如肾（水）之精以养肝（木），为水生木；肝（木）藏血以济心（火），为木生火；心（火）之热以温脾（土），为火生土；脾（土）化生水谷精微以充肺（金），为土生金；肺（金）通调水道以助肾（水），为金生水。五行"相克"可用于说明五脏之间的制约关系。如肺（金）清肃下降可抑制肝（木）的上亢，为金克木；肝（木）的条达可防止脾（土）气的壅滞，为木克土；脾（土）的运化可以防止肾（水）的泛滥，为土克水；肾（水）上承，可防止心（火）过于亢烈，为水克火。

此外，人与外界环境四时、五气，以及饮食五味等的关系，也都是运用五行学说来加以说明的。所以，五行学说应用于生理在于说明人的脏腑组织之间以及人与外在环境之间相互联系的统一性。

2.2.4.2 阐释病理变化及其相互影响

五行学说可用于说明在病理情况下脏腑之间的相互影响，其所采用的是五行生克异常规律。如肝病如果传脾，为"木乘土"；脾病如果影响到肝，为"土侮木"；肝脾同病，互相影响，即木郁土虚或土壅木郁；肝病还会影响心，为"母病及子"；影响到肺，则为"木侮金"；影响到肾，为"子病及母"。肝病是这样，其他脏器的病变也是如此，都可以用五行生克异常的关系来加以说明。

2.2.4.3 指导临床诊断

人的内脏功能活动及其相互关系的异常变化，通常可从外部征象反映出来。五脏与五色、五味以及脉象变化，在五行分类归属上有着一定联系，所以在诊断疾病时可综合四诊所得的资料，根据五行所属及其生克规律来推断病情。如面见青色，喜食酸味，脉见弦象，可初步诊断为肝病；面色赤色，口苦，脉象洪数，可以初步诊断为心火亢盛。脾虚病人，面见青色，为木虚土乘；心气虚弱者，面见黑色，为火虚水乘等。

2.2.4.4 指导疾病治疗

（1）指导确定治则和治法

1）根据相生规律确定治则和治法：根据相生规律确定治则是补母和泻子，主要用于相生关系失常的病证。

补母：该原则主要适用于母子关系失调的虚证。如肾阴不足，不能滋养肝木，而导致肝阴不足，肝阳亢逆者，称为水不生木或水不涵木，其治则不但要治肝，而且同时滋补肾阴。肾为肝母，肾水可以生肝木，故单治肾即可以涵敛肝阳。又如肺气亏虚发展到一定程度，可以影响脾的健运，从而导致脾虚。脾土为母，肺金为子，土能生金，故可以用母子同治的方法进行治疗。此即"虚则补其母"的含义。

泻子：该原则主要适用于母子关系失调的实证。如肝火炽盛，有升无降，而见肝病实证时，其治疗则可兼用泻心之法，肝木是母，心火是子，故泻心火则有助于泻肝火。此即"实则泻其子"之含义。

根据相生规律制定的常用治法主要有滋水涵木、金水相生、培土生金、益火补土等。

滋水涵木法：又称滋肾养肝法、滋补肝肾法。该法是通过滋补肾阴以养肝阴，从而达到涵敛肝阳的治疗方法，主要适用于肾阴亏损而致肝阴不足，甚则肝阳偏亢之证。临床可见头目眩晕，两眼干涩，耳鸣颧红，口干，五心烦热，腰膝酸软，男子遗精，女子月经不调，舌红少苔，脉弦细数等症。

金水相生法：又称补肺滋肾法、滋养肺肾法。该法是滋补肺肾阴虚的一种治疗方法，主要适用于肺虚不能输布津液以滋肾，或肾阴不足，精气不能上荣于肺，以致肺肾阴虚之证。临床可见咳嗽气逆，干咳或咳血，音哑，骨蒸潮热，盗汗，遗精，腰酸腿软，身体消瘦，口干舌红少苔，脉细数等症。

培土生金法：又称补脾益肺法。该法是指补脾益气而达到补益肺气的一种治疗方法，主要适用于脾虚胃弱不能滋养肺气而致肺脾虚弱之证。临床可见久咳不已，痰多清稀或痰少而黏，食欲减退，大便溏薄，肢倦乏力，舌淡，脉弱等症。

益火补土法：又称温肾健脾法或温补脾肾法，是指用温壮肾阳以补助脾阳的方法。适用于肾阳衰微而致脾阳不振的脾肾阳虚（即"火不生土"）之证，以及部分脾阳不振之证。临床可见下腹冷痛，五更泄泻，畏寒肢冷，舌淡胖，苔白滑，脉沉微等症。

应当指出，如按五行相生规律，则心属火，脾属土，火生土即是心生脾。"火不生土"本应理解为心火不生脾土。但自从命门学说兴起之后，这个概念有所改变。临床上多将此"火"专指肾阳（或命门之火），很少再指心火了。治疗上用温壮肾阳以助脾阳之法也的确有较好的疗效。但是，补心益脾之法，亦有其当用之证，故亦不应废弃。

2）根据相克规律确定的治则和治法：根据相克规律确定的治则包括抑强和扶弱。

抑强：即抑其太过，是指抑制过亢之脏，使被乘或被侮之脏功能易于恢复的治则。如肝气横逆犯胃或乘脾所出现的肝胃不和或肝脾不和，成为木亢乘土之证，治应疏肝、平肝为法；若是脾胃壅滞，影响及肝，导致肝失条达疏泄者，则成土壅木郁之证，是为相侮（反克）之证，其治法则当以运脾和胃为主。抑制其强，则被克者功能自然易于恢复。

扶弱：即扶其不及，是指扶助被乘或被侮之脏的功能，使双方力量对比恢复均衡的治则。主要适用于相克力量不及，或因虚被乘，或因虚被侮所致之证。如肝虚气郁,累及脾胃,受纳运化失调,则称为木不疏土,治宜补肝、和肝为法,兼顾健脾和胃。总之,扶助其弱,则有助于恢复其制约关系的协调。

根据相克规律临床常用的治法主要有抑木扶土、培土制水、佐金平木、泻南补北等。

抑木扶土法:又称疏肝健脾法。该法是通过疏肝健脾以治疗肝气亢逆、脾虚失运病证的一种方法,主要适用肝郁脾虚之证,临床可见胸闷胁胀、不思饮食、腹胀肠鸣、大便或溏,或见脘痞胀痛、嗳气、矢气等症。

培土制水法:又称健脾温肾利水法。该法是通过温运脾阳或健脾温肾方法,用以治疗水湿停聚的一种方法,主要适用于脾虚不运或脾肾阳虚,水湿泛滥之证,临床可见下肢水肿、腹部胀满、舌淡胖、脉弦滑等症。

佐金平木法:又称泻肝清肺法。该法是通过清肃肺气,以抑制肝火亢盛的一种治疗方法,主要适用于肝火亢逆,灼伤肺金,影响肺气清肃之"木火刑金"证候。临床可见胁痛口苦,咳嗽咯血,或痰中带血,急躁烦闷,脉弦数等症。

泻南补北法:又称泻火补水法、滋阴降火法或壮水制火法。该法即泻心火、补肾水的一种治疗方法,主要适用于肾阴不足,心阳偏亢,水火失济,心肾不交病证。临床可见腰膝酸软,心烦失眠,遗精,心悸健忘,或潮热盗汗等症。

应当指出,肾为水火之脏,肾阴虚亦能使相火偏亢或妄动,从而出现性功能亢奋,可见梦遗、耳鸣、喉痛、咽干等症。此属肾脏本身之阴阳偏盛、偏衰,不能与五脏相互关系之水不制火混为一谈。

(2) 指导精神疗法:五行的生克关系对于精神疗法具有一定的指导意义。精神疗法主要适用情志失调病证。情志生于五脏,五脏之间有着生克关系,所以情志之间也存在着这种关系。正是由于在生理上人的情志变化有着相互抑制的作用,而在病理上和内脏亦有着密切关系,故在临床上即可以运用情志之间的制约关系来达到调整情志、治疗疾病的目的,称之为五志相胜法。如:

悲为肺志,属金;怒为肝志,属木。金能克木,故悲能胜怒。

恐为肾志,属水;喜为心志,属火。水能克火,故恐能胜喜。

怒为肝志,属木;思为脾志,属土。木能克土,故怒能胜思。

喜为心志,属火;忧为肺志,属金。火能克金,故喜能胜忧。

思为脾志,属土;恐为肾志,属水。土能克水,故思能胜恐。

(3) 指导针灸取穴:五行学说还可用于指导针灸取穴。在针灸疗法中,手足阴经的"五输穴"与五行相配,则为井穴属木,荥穴属火,输穴属土,经穴属金,合穴属水,手足阳经的"五输穴"与五行相配,则为井穴属金,荥穴属水,输穴属木,经穴属火,合穴属土。针灸治疗时,根据病证,按五行生克规律选穴施治。如肝虚之证,据"虚则补其母"的治则,取肾经合穴(水穴)阴谷,或取本经的合穴(水穴)曲泉进行治疗。肝实之证,据"实则泻其子"的治则,取心经荥穴(火穴)少府,或取本经荥穴(火穴)行间予以治疗。

五行生克规律对指导临床具有一定意义,然而并非适合所有病证,要根据具体情况灵活运用。

综上所述,阴阳学说和五行学说虽然各有侧重,各有特点,但两者相互关联,在医学领域中综合运用才能较完整地说明人的生理病理等关系。在实际运用过程中,论阴阳则往往联系到五行,言五行又常常离不开阴阳。阴阳学说和五行学说相结合不仅可以说明事物矛盾双方的一般关系,而且可以说明事物间相互联系、相互制约的较为具体和复杂的关系,从而有利于解释复杂的生命现象和病理过程。

思考题

- 阴阳学说的基本内容包括哪些方面?试简述之。
- 何谓阴阳的消长与转化?阴阳的消长、转化有何联系?
- 试以阴阳学说来说明人体的组织结构和生理活动。如何运用阴阳学说指导疾病的诊断和治疗?
- 何谓五行与五行学说?五行学说对事物是如何进行五行归类的?
- 五行的生克规律有哪些内容?
- 如何运用五行学说说明脏腑的生理功能和相互关系?

3 藏象学说

"藏象"一词出自《素问·六节藏象论》。藏,是指藏于体内的内脏;象,是指表现于外的生理、病理征象。

藏象学说,是通过考察人体外在的生理和病理征象,以测知人体内脏的生理功能、病理变化及其相互关系的学说。中医学认为,人体是一个有机的整体,内脏各有外候,与形体诸窍具有特定的联系。因此,内脏虽然隐藏在体内,但其生理功能、病理变化在外有一定的征象,通过考察相关的外在征象,即可推测内脏的功能状况。如通过观察面色、舌色、脉象、胸部感觉等外在征象便可了解内脏心之主血功能是否正常。

藏象学说以内脏为其主要的研究内容。根据内脏的生理功能特点,可分为脏、腑和奇恒之腑。脏,即心、肺、脾、肝、肾,合称为五脏,其共同的生理功能是化生和贮存精气,特点是"满而不实";腑,即胆、胃、小肠、大肠、膀胱、三焦,合称为六腑,其共同的生理功能是受盛和传化水谷,特点是"实而不满"。此外,还有奇恒之腑,即脑、髓、骨、脉、胆和女子胞。奇者异也,恒者常也。奇恒之腑的形态大多为中空而似腑,但生理特点却为贮存精气而似脏;似脏非脏,似腑非腑,故称之为"奇恒之腑"。

藏象学说虽然以一定的解剖学知识为基础,但主要是在中国古代哲学思想的指导下,通过整体观察、"以象测藏"、"司外揣内"而探知内脏的活动。因此,藏象学说中的脏腑,不单纯是指解剖学脏器,更重要的是指生理功能。中医脏腑与西医脏器的名称虽然大致相同,但其内涵却大不一样。中医藏象学说中的一个脏腑的生理功能,可能包含着西医学中几个脏器的生理功能;而西医学中的一个脏器的生理功能,亦可能分散在中医藏象学说的几个脏腑的生理功能之中。

3.1 五脏

3.1.1 心

心位于胸中,主要生理功能为主血和藏神。心与小肠通过经脉相互络属,构成表里关系。心在体合脉,其华在面,在志为喜,在窍为舌,在液为汗。心对整个人体生命活动起着主宰的作用,故称为"君主之官"、"五脏六腑之大主"。

3.1.1.1 心的主要生理功能

(1) 主血:心主血功能包括心主行血和生血两个方面。①心主行血:是指心气具有推动和调控血液在脉道中运行的作用。血液在脉道中周流不息有赖于心气的作用。心气通过推动血液的运行和调控脉道的舒缩,维持血流顺畅、脉道通利。因此,心气充沛,心主血功能正常,则面部红润,胸部舒畅,脉搏和缓有力;反之,心气不足,心主血功能失常,则血流不畅,脉搏无力,甚则发生气血瘀滞,血脉受阻,而见面色晦黯,唇舌青紫,心前区憋闷和刺痛,以及脉象结、代、促、涩等病症。②心主生血:血液主要由营气和津液所化生,而营气和津液在化生为血液的过程中需要心阳的作用,方能变化而赤成为血液,即所谓"奉心化赤"。

心既主行血,又能生血,从而保证全身组织得到血液的充分濡养。

(2) 藏神:心藏神是指心具有主司人的精神情志等心理活动和主宰全身生命活动的作用。人的精神情志活动虽与五脏密切相关,由五脏协同完成,但总由心主宰。心藏神,神能驭气,心神驾驭协调各脏腑之气的运行以达到推动和调控五脏六腑的生理功能。心藏神的功能正常,则精神振奋,神志清晰,思维敏捷,反应灵敏,脏腑组织功能协调,全身安康;反之,心藏神的功能异常,则可出现失眠,多梦,神志不宁,谵狂,或可出现反应迟钝、健忘、精神委顿、昏迷等临床表现,还可影响其他脏腑组织的功能活动,即所谓"心动则五脏六腑皆摇",甚至危及到人体的生命。

心藏神的生理功能与心主血的生理功能密切相关。心藏神,能调节心气推动血液在脉道中运行的作用,有助于心主血;而心主血,为神志活动提供了物质基础,有助于心藏神,因为血液是神志活动的主要物质基础。因此,心主血的功能异常,必然会出现心神的病变;反之,心藏神的功能异常,也可以出现血行的变化。

3.1.1.2 心与体、志、窍、液的关系

(1) 在体合脉,其华在面:脉即脉道,为气血运行的通道。心在体合脉是指全身的血脉由心所主。心与脉直接相连,脉道的舒缩依赖于心气的调控。心气充沛,则脉搏和缓有力、节律调匀;心气不足,则脉搏细弱无力。其华在面,是指心的生理功能状况,可以显露于面部的色泽变化。心合脉,而面部的血脉极为丰富,所以心气旺盛,血脉充盈,则面部红润有泽;心气不足,则可见面色㿠白、晦滞;心血亏虚则可见面色无华;心血瘀阻则可见面色青紫等。

(2) 在志为喜:心的生理功能和情志"喜"密切相关。适度的喜属于良性刺激,有助于心主血等生理功能。但喜乐过度,则可使心神涣散,出现喜笑不休,精神失常等临床表现。此外,心藏神,故不仅过喜伤心,而且五志过极均能扰及心神。

(3) 在窍为舌:心与舌通过经络相互联系,"手少阴之别……循经入于心,系舌本",心的功能状况影响并反映于舌,故心在窍为舌。心主血、藏神的功能正常,则舌质红润柔活,味觉灵敏,语言流利。心主血功能异常,心血亏虚,则舌质淡白;心阳不足,则舌质淡胖;心血瘀阻,则舌质黯紫或有瘀斑;心藏神的功能异常,则可见舌蜷、舌强、语謇或失语等病症。

(4) 在液为汗:心在液为汗,是指汗液与心血、心神关系密切。汗为津液所化生,津液与血又同源互化,津液渗入脉内可生成血液,血液渗出脉外可化为津液,而血又为心所主,心血充盛,津液充足,汗化有源;又心藏神,汗的生成、排泄受心神的调节,如精神紧张可出汗,故称汗为心液。

附：脑

脑，又名髓海，位居颅内。

脑主要生理功能是主持生命活动、精神意识和感觉运动。脑主持生命活动、精神意识和感觉运动功能正常，则人体生命力旺盛，精神饱满，意识清楚，感觉、运动灵敏；反之，脑主持生命活动、精神意识和感觉运动功能失常，则人体生命活动障碍，精神委靡，意识模糊，感觉迟钝，运动迟缓。

3.1.2 肺

肺位于胸腔，左右各一，主要生理功能为主呼吸之气、主全身之气、通调水道和朝百脉。肺与大肠通过经脉相互络属，构成表里关系。肺在体合皮，其华在毛，在志为悲(忧)，在窍为鼻，在液为涕。肺在脏腑中位置最高，覆盖诸脏，故有"华盖"之称。肺叶娇嫩，与外界息息相通，易受邪侵，故又有"娇脏"之称。

肺气的运动主要表现为宣、降两种形式。宣，即宣发。肺气宣发是指肺气能向上升宣和向外发散。肺气宣发的生理作用，主要体现在三个方面：一是排出体内的浊气；二是将脾转输来的水谷精微和津液上输于头面，外达于肌表；三是宣发卫气于肌肤，以温分肉，充皮肤，调节腠理之开阖，控制汗液的排泄。因此，肺气失宣，便可出现咳嗽，恶寒，无汗等异常表现。降，即肃降。肺气肃降是指肺气能向下通降，并保持呼吸道清肃洁净。肺气肃降的生理作用，也主要体现在三个方面：一是吸入自然界的清气；二是将脾转输至肺的水谷精微和津液向下、向内布散至其他脏腑等组织；三是肃清肺和呼吸道内的异物，以保持呼吸道的洁净。因此，肺气不降，便可出现呼多吸少、喘息气逆等异常现象。

肺气宣发和肃降，是相反相成的两个方面。在生理情况下，相互依存和相互制约；在病理情况下，则又常常相互影响。肺气宣发和肃降正常，则呼吸均匀调畅，水液输布正常。二者的功能一旦失去协调，就会发生"肺气失宣"和"肺失肃降"的病变，出现胸闷、咳嗽、气喘、咳痰等异常表现。

3.1.2.1 肺的主要生理功能

（1）主呼吸之气：肺主呼吸之气是指肺具有吸入自然界的清气，呼出体内的浊气，实现人体与外界环境之间气体交换的作用。肺主呼吸之气，实际上是肺气宣发、肃降运动在体内外气体交换过程中的具体表现。肺气宣发，呼出浊气；肺气肃降，吸入清气，从而保证肺主呼吸功能的正常进行。肺气失宣或不降，则必将影响到肺的呼吸运动，从而出现胸闷、咳喘等异常表现。

（2）主全身之气：肺主全身之气是指肺具有主持全身之气的生成和运行的作用。肺主全身之气，首先体现于主全身之气的生成。全身之气主要由宗气和元气构成，而宗气主要由肺吸入的清气与脾胃运化的水谷精气相结合而成。宗气在肺中生成，积于胸中。肺主呼吸之气，影响宗气的生成，进而影响全身之气的生成。其次，肺主全身之气，还体现于对全身的气机具有调节作用。肺的呼吸运动过程，即是气的升降出入运动过程，肺有节律的一呼一吸，对全身之气的升降出入运动起着重要的调节作用。

肺主全身之气的功能与肺主呼吸之气的功能是密不可分的,并取决于肺主呼吸之气的功能。肺主呼吸之气,一呼一吸,呼浊吸清,促进气的生成,调节气的升降出入运动,从而保证了人体新陈代谢的正常进行。肺主全身之气的功能正常,则全身之气的生成和运行方能正常;反之,肺主全身之气的功能异常,则会出现声低气怯、肢倦乏力等气虚之症和全身之气升降出入运动失调的异常表现。

(3) 通调水道:通,即疏通;调,即调节;水道,即水液运行和排泄的通道。肺主通调水道是指肺具有疏通和调节体内水液输布、运行和排泄的作用。肺主通调水道的功能,实际上是肺气宣发、肃降运动在水液代谢方面的具体体现。肺气宣发,不但将津液升宣、布散至头面和肌表,而且能宣发卫气,司腠理之开合,调节汗液的排泄;肺气肃降,不但将津液向下输送至其他脏腑等组织,而且能将脏腑代谢所产生的浊液下输至肾,成为尿液生成之源。肺主通调水道功能正常,水液代谢方能正常;反之,肺主通调水道功能减退,就可发生水液停聚而出现水湿痰饮等病变。

肺在脏腑中位置最高,参与调节体内的水液代谢,故称"肺为水之上源"。

(4) 朝百脉:朝即朝向、聚会的意思。肺朝百脉是指全身的血液,通过百脉而会聚于肺,通过肺的呼浊吸清,进行气体的交换,然后通过肺气宣降运动,将富含清气的血液再通过百脉输送到全身。

血液运行,虽由心气推动,然肺有助心行血的作用。血液的运行,有赖于气的推动。肺主全身之气的生成与运行,肺气充沛,气的生成与运行正常,有助于血运顺畅。反之,肺气虚衰,不能辅助心脏运行血液,血行不畅,则可出现胸闷心悸,唇青舌紫等气虚血瘀之象。

3.1.2.2 肺与体、志、窍、液的关系

(1) 在体合皮,其华在毛:皮毛为全身之表。肺具有宣发卫气,输精于皮毛等生理功能,保证了皮毛得到卫气和水谷精微的温养和润泽,故肺与皮毛关系密切。肺气充盛,宣发卫气、输精于皮毛功能正常,则皮肤致密,毫毛光泽;反之,肺气虚衰,无力宣发卫气、水谷精微于皮毛,则可出现多汗,易于感冒,或皮毛憔悴、枯槁等现象。

(2) 在志为悲(忧):悲与忧同属于肺志。悲忧属于不良刺激的情志变化,对于人体的影响,主要是使气不断地消耗。即所谓"悲则气消"。由于肺主气,所以悲忧易伤肺。过度悲忧,可出现呼吸气短等肺气不足之象。反之,肺气虚衰,人体对不良刺激的耐受能力下降,则易于产生悲忧的情志变化。肺与悲忧之志相互影响,故肺在志为悲(忧)。

(3) 在窍为鼻:鼻为呼吸之气出入的通道,与肺相通,故肺在窍为鼻。鼻的通气与嗅觉功能正常,有赖于肺气的作用。肺气宣畅,则鼻窍通利,嗅觉灵敏;反之,肺气失宣,可见鼻塞,嗅觉不灵敏等表现。由于肺开窍于鼻,所以外邪袭肺,多由鼻而入。

(4) 在液为涕:涕即鼻涕,鼻为肺窍,故肺在液为涕。肺中精气充足,则鼻涕润泽鼻窍而不外流。若肺寒,则鼻流清涕;肺热,则鼻涕黄浊;肺燥,则鼻干。

3.1.3 脾

脾位于膈下,主要生理功能为主运化、升清和统血。脾与胃通过经脉相互络属,

构成表里关系。脾在体合肉,主四肢,其华在唇,在志为思,在窍为口,在液为涎。脾将水谷化为精微,为后天生命活动和气血生成提供了物质保障,故称为"后天之本"、"气血生化之源"。

3.1.3.1 脾的主要生理功能

(1) 主运化:运,即转运;化,即消化。脾主运化是指脾具有把水谷转化为水谷精微,并将水谷精微吸收、转输至全身的作用。脾主运化,可分为运化水谷和运化水液两个方面。

运化水谷 脾主运化水谷是指脾气具有促进对食物的消化和食物精微的吸收,并对吸收的食物精微进行输布的作用。食物的消化虽在胃肠道中进行,但必须依赖于脾的运化作用,方能将食物化生为精微;食物精微又必须依赖于脾的运化,方能被吸收,并上输于肺,布散至全身。脾主运化食物功能旺盛,则机体的消化、吸收、输布功能健全,才能为化生精、气、血、津液提供足够的养料,才能使脏腑、经络、四肢百骸,以及筋肉皮毛等组织得到充分的营养,从而进行正常的生理活动;反之,若脾主运化食物的功能减退,则机体的消化、吸收、输布功能即因之而失常,可出现腹胀、便溏、食欲不振等脾失健运,以及倦怠、消瘦等气血生化不足之象。

运化水液 脾主运化水液是指脾气具有吸收、转输津液,调节水液代谢的作用。脾气有助于将人体所摄入的水液吸收,并把吸收的水液输布至全身,以发挥滋润、濡养作用;并可将体内多余的水分,及时地转输至肺和肾,通过肺、肾等气化功能,化为汗和尿排出体外。因此,脾主运化水液功能健旺,既保证全身组织得到津液的滋润,又可防止水液在体内异常停滞。如果脾主运化水液功能减退,必然导致水液在体内的停滞,从而产生水湿痰饮等病理产物。

脾主运化食物和运化水液两个方面可分而不可离,二者相互联系,相互影响。脾主运化功能,为气血生成提供了物质保障,对维持人体生命活动至关重要,故要善于保护脾、使脾气健运,气血充足,不易受邪。

(2) 主升清:升,上升;清,即水谷精微等营养物质。脾主升清是指脾气上升,将其运化所得的水谷精微等营养物质上输于心、肺、头目,并通过心、肺的作用,化生气血,以营养全身。脾主升清,是和胃主降浊相对而言。"脾宜升则健,胃宜降则和"。脾气升,胃气降,升降相因,人体的消化、吸收功能才能正常。此外,正由于脾气上升,才能维持人体内脏处于相对恒定的位置,防止其下垂。若脾气不能升清,则水谷精微等营养物质不能上输于心、肺,气血生化无源,头目失于气血营养,可出现神疲乏力,头目眩晕等病症;若脾气无力升举,反而下陷,则可见久泄脱肛、内脏下垂等病症。

(3) 主统血:统,即统摄。脾主统血是指脾气具有统摄血液在脉中运行,防止其逸出脉外的作用。脾之所以能主统血,与脾主运化而为气血生化之源密切相关。脾气健运,气血生化有源,则气血充盛,气充盛则气的固摄血液作用就健全,血液就不会逸出脉外而致出血;反之,脾虚失运,气血生化乏源,则气血亏虚,气亏虚则气的固摄血液功能就减退,从而导致血逸脉外,产生出血现象。由于脾气主升、在体合肉,所以脾不统血多表现为便血、尿血、崩漏等下部出血及肌衄等病症。

3.1.3.2 脾与体、志、窍、液的关系

(1) 在体合肉,主四肢,其华在唇:全身的肌肉和四肢,都需要依靠脾所运化的水谷精微来营养,故脾在体合肉,主四肢。脾主运化功能正常,肌肉、四肢得到水谷精微的营养,则肌肉丰满发达,四肢活动轻劲有力。脾主运化功能障碍,肌肉、四肢失去水谷精微的营养,必致肌肉瘦削,四肢软弱无力,甚至萎弱不用。口唇的色泽,与全身气血是否充盈有关;而脾为气血生化之源,口唇的色泽可以反映脾气功能的盛衰,所以脾其华在唇。脾主运化功能正常,气血就充盈,口唇则红润光泽;反之,脾主运化功能失常,则气血虚少,可出现口唇淡白无华等异常表现。

(2) 在志为思:思,即思虑。思虑过度,会影响气的正常运动,导致气滞和气结,尤易导致气结于中,影响脾主运化和升清的功能,可出现不思饮食,脘腹胀闷,头目眩晕等病症,故称脾在志为思。

(3) 在窍为口:脾主运化,脾气健运,则口味、食欲正常,即所谓"脾气通于口,脾和则口能知五谷矣"。若脾失健运,则可出现食欲减退,并可见口淡,口甜,口腻,口苦等异常的感觉。食欲、口味等与脾主运化功能密切相关,故脾在窍为口。

(4) 在液为涎:涎为口津,口为脾窍,故脾在液为涎。脾主运化、升清功能正常,则津液上行于口而为涎,以助饮食物的吞咽和消化。若脾胃不和,则导致涎液化生异常。

3.1.4 肝

肝位于上腹部,右胁之内,主要生理功能为主疏泄和主藏血。肝与胆通过经脉相互络属,构成表里关系。肝在体合筋,其华在爪,在志为怒,在窍为目,在液为泪。肝性主升、主动,喜条达而恶抑郁,故有"刚脏"之称。

3.1.4.1 肝的主要生理功能

(1) 主疏泄:疏,即疏通;泄,即发散。肝主疏泄是指肝具有疏通、畅达全身气机的作用。气机,即气的运动。肝主疏泄功能,对各脏腑组织之气升降出入运动起着重要的调节作用,以保持全身气机的通畅,进而促进精血津液的运行输布、脾胃的运化、胆汁的分泌排泄、情志的调畅、男子排精和女子行经等,对人体产生广泛的影响。肝主疏泄作用主要表现在以下方面:

调畅气机 肝的生理特点是主升、主动。肝主疏泄,其疏,可使气机疏通、畅达;其泄,可使气布散而不郁。因此,肝主疏泄功能正常,则气机调畅,气血和调,经络通利,脏腑活动正常。若肝主疏泄功能异常,既可表现为肝的疏泄不及,则气的升发不足,气机的疏通和畅达就会受到阻碍,从而形成气机不畅,气机郁结的病理变化,出现胸胁、两乳或少腹等局部的胀痛不适等病理现象;又可表现为肝的疏泄太过,则气的升发过亢,气的下降不及,从而形成肝气上逆的病理变化,出现头目胀痛,面红目赤,易怒等病理表现,甚则血随气逆,而导致吐血,咯血等血从上溢的病理变化。

促进血液与津液的运行 血液和津液属阴主静,其运行输布有赖于气的推动。肝主疏泄功能正常,气的升降出入运动就能调畅,血液的运行和津液的输布也随之顺

畅。反之,肝气郁结就会导致血行障碍,形成瘀血;肝气上逆,迫血上涌,则可出现吐血、咯血等出血现象。肝主疏泄功能失常,也可导致津液代谢障碍,形成水湿痰饮等病理变化。

促进脾胃的运化功能 脾气主升,胃气主降,升清降浊,升降相因,脾胃运化功能方能正常,而肝主疏泄功能正常,是脾胃之气正常升降的一个重要条件。肝主疏泄功能正常,气的运动才能条达、疏畅,脾气才能升,胃气才能降,脾胃运化功能才能正常。肝主疏泄功能异常,则不仅会影响脾的升清,在上则为眩晕,在下则为腹泻;而且还会影响胃的降浊,在上则为呕逆、嗳气,在中则为脘腹胀满、疼痛,在下则为便秘。

有助于胆汁的分泌排泄 胆汁是肝之余气所化生,胆汁的分泌与排泄受肝主疏泄功能的影响。肝主疏泄功能正常,气机调畅,则胆汁能够正常地分泌与排泄,从而有助于脾的运化和胃的腐熟功能。肝气郁结,则可影响胆汁的分泌与排泄,从而出现胁下胀满、疼痛,口苦,纳食不化,甚则黄疸等病理表现。

调畅情志 正常的情志活动,主要依赖于气血的正常运行。肝主疏泄,有助于气机通畅,气能行血,气畅则血畅,气血运行正常,情志活动的物质基础得到保障,则心情开朗舒畅。反之,肝的疏泄不及,则肝气郁结,心情易于抑郁,稍受刺激,则抑郁难解;肝的疏泄太过,气的升发过亢,则心情易于急躁,稍有刺激,则易于发怒。

有助于男子排精和女子行经 男子排精和女子行经与肝主疏泄功能有密切的关系。肝主疏泄功能正常,气机调畅,则男子精液排泄通畅有度,女子月经周期正常,经行通畅;反之,肝主疏泄功能失常,气机失调,则男子排精失畅,女子经期紊乱,经行不畅。

(2) 主藏血:肝主藏血是指肝具有贮存血液、调节血量和防止出血的作用。肝主藏血功能,首先体现在肝能贮存一定的血量,以制约肝之阳气,防止其升发太过,以维护肝主疏泄功能的正常进行。其次,肝储藏了一定的血液,在肝主疏泄功能的配合下,便可以根据人体生理变化情况,有效地调节各部分组织的血液需要量,人动则血运行于诸经,人静则血归于肝。此外,肝主藏血还有助于血液收摄于血脉之中,以防止血液无故流失。故有"肝者,凝血之本"之说。因此,肝不藏血,不仅可出现肝血不足、阳气升泄太过等病变,而且还可以导致各种出血病症。

肝主藏血,其体属阴;肝主疏泄,其用属阳,故有"肝体阴而用阳"之说。肝主疏泄功能与肝主藏血功能相互为用,肝主疏泄,气机调畅,则血能正常地归藏和调节;肝主藏血,血藏于肝,涵养肝气,勿使肝之阳气过亢,则肝能正常地疏泄。

3.1.4.2 肝与体、志、窍、液的关系

(1) 在体合筋,其华在爪:筋,即筋膜。肝在体合筋,主要是由于人体筋膜有赖于肝血的滋养。肝血充盛,筋膜得以滋养,则运动有力而灵活。若肝血衰少,筋膜失养,则表现为筋力不健,运动不利,还可出现手足振颤,肢体麻木,屈伸不利,甚则瘛疭等症。爪,即爪甲,乃筋之延续。爪甲同样需要肝血的滋养。肝血的盛衰,可影响爪甲的荣枯,故肝之华在爪。肝血充足,则爪甲坚韧明亮,红润光泽。若肝血不足,则爪甲软薄,枯而色夭,甚则变形脆裂。

(2) 在志为怒:怒是人在情绪激动时的一种情志变化。过怒可使气血上逆,阳气

升泄。由于肝主疏泄,阳气升发,为肝之用,故肝在志为怒。怒易伤肝,过怒可致肝之升发太过,血随气逆,出现呕血,甚则猝然昏不知人。反之,肝阴不足,肝阳无制,则心情稍有不顺,即易发怒。

(3) 在窍为目:足厥阴肝经上连目,肝之气血循肝之经脉上注于目,以维持目的视觉功能。肝血充足,肝气调和,则目能视物辨色。反之,肝血不足,则两目干涩,视物不清或色盲;肝经风热,则目赤痒痛;肝火上炎,则目赤生翳;肝阳上亢,则头目眩晕;肝风内动,则目斜上视等。

(4) 在液为泪:泪从目出,肝开窍于目,故肝在液为泪。肝之气血调和,则泪液濡润目而不外溢。若肝血不足,可见两目干涩;而在风火赤眼、肝经湿热等情况下,可见目眵增多、迎风流泪等病症。

3.1.5 肾

肾位于腰部,左右各一,主要生理功能为藏精、主水和主纳气。肾与膀胱通过经脉相互络属,构成表里关系。肾在体合骨,其华在发,在志为恐,在窍为耳及二阴,在液为唾。肾藏先天之精,为生命之源,故称为"先天之本"。

3.1.5.1 肾的主要生理功能

(1) 主藏精:肾主藏精是指肾具有贮存精气的作用。肾为封藏之本,主藏精。肾所藏之精包括"先天之精"和"后天之精"。"先天之精"来源于父母的生殖之精,与生俱来,藏于肾中。"后天之精"来源于脾胃运化生成的水谷之精。人出生以后,脾胃运化而生成的水谷之精经脾气的转输作用,输送至各脏,则成为脏之精。各脏腑之精支持其生理功能后的剩余部分,则输送至肾,以充养"先天之精"。"先天之精"和"后天之精"相互融合,组成了肾精。肾精是化生肾气的物质基础。

肾主藏精,主要是不使肾中精气无故流失,从而为精气在体内能充分发挥其应有的生理效应创造良好的条件。

肾中精气的生理效应首先是促进机体的生长、发育和生殖。人体存在生、长、壮、老、已的生命规律,生命的整个过程都受肾中精气盛衰的影响。人从幼年开始,肾中精气逐渐充盛,则出现齿更发长;到了青壮年,肾中精气进一步充实,乃至盛极,则出现真牙生,筋骨坚,身体盛壮;而至老年,肾中精气逐渐衰减,则出现面色憔悴,发堕齿槁,筋骨失健,形体衰老。由此可见,肾中精气决定着人体生长发育过程。人体生殖器官发育及其生殖能力同样受肾中精气盛衰的影响。人体生长至青春时期,随着肾中精气充盛到一定程度,便可产生一种具有促进生殖器官发育成熟和维持生殖功能作用的精微物质,称作天癸。于是,男子出现排精,女子出现行经,人体具备了生殖能力。其后,肾中精气不断充盈,人体不断产生天癸物质,从而维持了生殖功能。而从中年进入老年,肾中精气由盛转衰,天癸随之减少,以至竭绝,则生殖能力也随之衰退,以至丧失。由此可见,决定生殖功能的根本因素在于肾中精气的盛衰,故有"肾主生殖"之说。肾中精气充盛,则生长发育正常,生殖功能健全;反之,肾中精气不足,小儿则生长发育不良,成人则早衰,并可出现生殖功能低下等病症。因此,优生优育、养身保健和防止衰老等应注重对肾中精气的调养。

其次,肾中精气对人体各脏腑的生理活动起着推动和调节作用。肾精化为肾气,肾气又表现为肾阴和肾阳两个方面的生理效应:肾阴起着凉润、宁静、抑制等作用,肾阳起着温煦、推动、兴奋等作用。肾藏先天之精,为生命之源,肾阴和肾阳则为各脏腑阴阳之本。五脏六腑之阴,依赖肾阴得以滋生;五脏六腑之阳,依赖肾阳得以壮大。肾阴和肾阳相互制约,相互为用,维护着各脏腑阴阳的平衡,保证了机体代谢和生理活动的正常进行。如果由于某些原因,造成肾阴虚,则可出现内热、眩晕、耳鸣、腰膝酸软、遗精、舌红少津等;造成肾阳虚,则可出现疲惫乏力,形寒肢冷,腰膝冷痛和萎弱,小便清长或不利或遗尿失禁,舌质淡,以及性功能减退和水肿等病症。肾阴和肾阳对人体生命至关重要,故肾阴又称为"真阴"、"元阴",肾阳又称为"真阳"、"元阳"。

(2) 主水:肾主水是指肾具有主持和调节体内水液的输布和排泄,维持水液代谢平衡的作用。水液代谢是通过胃的摄入,脾的运化和转输,肺的宣发和肃降,肾的蒸腾气化,以三焦为通道,输送到全身;经过代谢后的水液,则化为汗液、尿液等排出体外。在整个水液代谢过程中,涉及到多个脏腑的一系列生理活动,而肾中精气起着主持和调节的作用。肾中精气分化的肾阴和肾阳是机体各脏腑阴阳的根本,维护着各脏腑阴阳的平衡,从而保证各脏腑正常地参与水液代谢。此外,水液代谢过程中,脏腑形窍产生的浊液通过三焦下输于肾。到达肾的浊液,在肾的气化作用下,分为清浊二部分,清者回吸收,再由脾气的转输,上达于肺,再度参与水液代谢;浊者通过肾的气化作用形成尿液,下输膀胱,并在肾与膀胱的气化作用下排出体外。可见,尿液的生成和排泄,与肾的蒸腾气化直接相关;而尿液的生成和排泄,在维持体内津液代谢平衡方面至关重要。若肾中精气的蒸腾气化失常,则可引起尿液的生成和排泄异常,出现尿少、水肿等病理现象。

(3) 主纳气:纳,即摄纳。肾主纳气是指肾具有摄纳肺所吸入的清气,保持吸气深度的作用。人体的呼吸功能,虽为肺所主,但肺吸入的清气,必须经肾气的摄纳潜藏,才能保持一定的深度。正常的呼吸运动依靠肺肾协同完成,故有"肺为气之主,肾为气之根。肺主出气,肾主纳气"之说。肾中精气充盛,摄纳有权,则呼吸均匀和调;反之,肾中精气不足,摄纳无权,则呼吸表浅,可出现动辄气喘,呼多吸少等病理现象。肾主纳气功能,实际上是肾主封藏在呼吸运动中的具体体现。

3.1.5.2 肾与体、志、窍、液的关系

(1) 在体合骨,生髓,其华在发:骨即骨骼,具有支撑人体,保护内脏和进行运动的功能。肾藏精,精生髓,髓居于骨中以养骨,故肾在体合骨。肾精充盛,髓化有源,骨得髓养,则骨骼健壮。若肾精不足,骨髓空虚,骨失髓养,小儿则囟门迟闭,骨软无力;老人则骨质脆弱,易于骨折。

"齿为骨之余",牙齿同样依赖肾精的充养。肾精充盛则牙齿坚固;反之,肾精不足则小儿齿迟,成人齿松、脱落。

发有赖于精血的滋养。肾藏精,精化血,精血旺盛,则发长而润泽;反之,肾虚,精血不足,则发失滋养,枯槁脱落,故其华在发。

骨、齿、发与肾中精气关系密切,骨、齿、发的生长状态反映了肾中精气的盛衰,故

是判断人体生长发育状况和衰老程度的客观标志。

(2) 在志为恐：恐是一种恐惧、害怕的情志活动。肾与恐关系密切,是古人长期观察所得。肾居下焦,肾精化生肾气,肾气必须上行,通过中焦、上焦方能布散至周身。"恐则气下",人在恐惧的状态中,肾气不得上行,反而下走,影响了肾气的正常布散,故肾在志为恐。

(3) 在窍为耳及二阴：肾在窍为耳是指耳的听觉灵敏程度与肾中精气的盈亏密切相关。即所谓"肾气通于耳,肾和则耳能闻五音矣"。肾精生髓,"脑为髓之海",肾中精气充盈,髓海得养,听觉才能灵敏;反之,肾中精气不足,髓海失养,则听力减退,耳鸣,甚则耳聋。

二阴,即前阴和后阴。前阴是排尿和生殖的器官,后阴是排泄粪便的通道。人的生殖功能,有赖于肾中精气的充盈。而尿液和粪便的排泄,与肾的气化、调节功能也密切相关。故有"肾开窍于二阴"之说。

(4) 在液为唾：唾为肾精所化,有滋润口舌的作用。肾精通过足少阴肾经上达舌下之金津、玉液二穴,分泌而出即为唾,故肾在液为唾。由于唾出于肾,若咽而不吐,则能回滋肾中精气。若多唾或久唾,则易耗损肾精。

附：女子胞

女子胞,又名胞宫、子宫,位居小腹部,下口与阴道相连。

女子胞主要生理功能是主持月经,孕育胎儿。产生月经和孕育胎儿是脏腑、天癸、经脉、气血作用于女子胞的结果,故女子胞功能正常与否直接影响月经的产生和胎儿的孕育。女子胞功能正常,则月经、胎孕正常;反之,女子胞功能失常,则月经紊乱,胎孕异常。

女子胞的生理功能与脏腑、经脉等均有关,其中与心、肝、脾、肾,以及冲脉、任脉的关系尤为密切。

3.2 六腑

3.2.1 胆

胆位于右胁下,附于肝之短叶间。胆的主要生理功能为贮存和排泄胆汁。

胆与肝相连,肝之余气化生胆汁,汇集于胆,由胆贮存。胆汁精纯、清净,称为"精汁",故胆又有"中精之府"之称。贮存于胆的胆汁,在肝主疏泄功能的控制和调节下排泄入肠中,以助水谷之消化和吸收。肝主疏泄功能正常,胆汁排泄畅达,水谷之消化和吸收则正常;反之,肝主疏泄功能失常,胆汁排泄不畅,则影响水谷之消化和吸收,可出现胁下胀痛、食欲减退、腹胀等病症;若胆汁上逆,则可见口苦、呕吐黄绿苦水等病症;若胆汁外溢,则可出现黄疸。

此外,胆尚有主决断的作用,能判断事物,作出决定。

在形态上,胆中空有腔,与其他五腑相类,故属六腑;在功能上,胆贮存精汁,又与五脏"藏精气"相似,故又为奇恒之腑。

3.2.2 胃

胃位于上腹部,上连食道,下通小肠。胃的主要生理功能为受纳和腐熟水谷。

受纳水谷是指胃具有接受和容纳饮食水谷的作用。水谷入口,在胃气的作用下容纳于胃中,故胃有"太仓"、"水谷之海"之称。

腐熟水谷是指胃具有将饮食水谷初步消化,形成食糜的作用。容纳于胃中的水谷经胃气的腐熟作用,得以初步消化,形成食糜。胃主受纳、腐熟水谷功能正常,则纳食正常。若胃主受纳、腐熟水谷功能失常,则可出现纳食不佳、嗳腐食臭等病症。

受纳水谷是腐熟水谷的基础。水谷入胃,经过胃的腐熟,形成食糜后,必须流畅地下行入小肠,以进一步消化、吸收,同时也为胃继续受纳创造条件,故胃主通降,以降为和。胃失通降,胃气郁滞,则可出现食欲不振、脘腹胀闷疼痛、大便秘结等症状。若胃气不仅失于通降,进而形成胃气上逆,则可出现嗳气、恶心、呕吐、呃逆等病症。

3.2.3 小肠

小肠位于腹中,其上口与胃相接,下口与大肠相连。小肠的主要生理功能为受盛化物和泌别清浊。

受盛,即是接受,以器盛物。化物,即消化、化生。受盛化物是指小肠接受经胃下传之食糜以盛纳之,保持食糜在其内停留较长的时间,以利进一步消化,将水谷化生为精微。若小肠受盛化物功能异常,则可出现腹胀、腹泻、便溏表现。

泌,即分泌;别,即分别。小肠泌别清浊是指小肠能将其消化后的饮食水谷,分别为水谷精微和食物残渣两个部分,并将水谷精微吸收,把食物残渣输送至大肠。在吸收水谷精微的同时,小肠还吸收了大量的水液,故有"小肠主液"之说。若小肠泌别清浊功能异常,则可导致水谷混杂而出现便溏、泄泻等表现。

小肠受盛化物和泌别清浊的功能在水谷化为精微的过程中至关重要。小肠受盛化物和泌别清浊功能必须和脾气运化功能协同配合,方能顺利完成。

3.2.4 大肠

大肠位于腹中,其上接小肠,下连肛门。大肠的主要生理功能是传化糟粕。大肠接受经过小肠泌别清浊后所剩下的食物残渣,再吸收其中多余的水液,形成粪便,并将粪便向下传送,经肛门而排出体外。大肠的传化糟粕作用,是对小肠泌别清浊功能的承接,并与胃气的通降、肺气的肃降和肾气的气化功能有关。若大肠传化糟粕功能失常,则可出现粪便质、量和排便次数等的异常变化。由于大肠可以对食物残渣中多余的水液进行再吸收,故有"大肠主津"之说。

3.2.5 膀胱

膀胱位于下腹部,其上通过输尿管与肾相通,其下接尿道。膀胱的主要生理功能是贮尿和排尿。尿液为水液在肾的气化作用下所化生,下输于膀胱,由膀胱贮存。尿液在膀胱内潴留至一定程度时,即可排出体外。膀胱的贮尿和排尿功能,受肾气的调控。肾气充盛,则膀胱开合有度,贮尿和排尿功能正常。若肾气不固,则可出现遗尿、甚则小便失禁；若肾之气化失司，则可出现排尿不畅，甚则癃闭。

3.2.6 三焦

三焦是上焦、中焦、下焦的合称。三焦的含义有二：一是指六腑之一的三焦，即脏腑之间和脏腑内部的间隙互相沟通所形成的通道。二是单纯的部位含义，即膈以上为上焦，膈至脐为中焦，脐以下为下焦。

作为六腑之一的三焦，其主要生理功能，一是通行元气，二是运行水液。元气根源于肾，通过三焦而输布到五脏六腑，充沛于全身，以发挥其生理效应。全身的水液代谢，是由肺、脾胃、肾和膀胱等诸脏腑的协同作用而完成的，但必须以三焦为通道，才能正常地升降出入。如果三焦水道不通利，则肺、脾、肾等输布调节水液的功能就难以实现其应有的生理效应。

如果将三焦作为单纯的部位含义，则上焦（包括心、肺两脏和头面部）的生理功能为主气的升发和宣散。《灵枢经·营卫生会》将此概括为"上焦如雾"。中焦（包括脾、胃、肝、胆等脏腑）的生理功能为消化饮食物，吸收和输布水谷精微以化生气血。《灵枢经·营卫生会》将此概括为"中焦如沤"。下焦（包括小肠、大肠、肾和膀胱）的生理功能为主排泄糟粕和尿液。《灵枢经·营卫生会》将此概括为"下焦如渎"。

3.3 脏腑之间的关系

人体是一个有机的整体，脏腑之间存在着相互资生、相互制约、相互为用、相互协调的密切关系。

3.3.1 五脏之间的关系

3.3.1.1 心与肺

心与肺的关系，主要表现在血液运行和呼吸运动两个方面。

血液运行，有赖于心气的推动，也有赖于肺气的辅助；肺朝百脉，助心行血，保证血液的正常运行。若肺气不足或壅塞，不能正常辅心行血，可致心血瘀阻，血行不畅。

肺司呼吸，吸清呼浊，维持正常的呼吸运动；而心主行血，血行正常，肺得血养，肺司呼吸功能方能正常。若心气虚弱，无力行血，血行不畅，则可影响肺司呼吸功能，出现胸闷、咳喘等症。

宗气主要依靠肺吸入的清气与脾胃运化的水谷精气相结合而成。宗气既能走息道而司呼吸，又能贯心脉而行血气，从而加强了血液运行和呼吸运动之间的相互联系。

3.3.1.2 心与脾

心与脾的关系，主要表现在血液生成和血液运行两个方面。

心主行血，供血以养脾，维持脾正常的运化功能；脾主运化，为气血生化之源，脾气健运，血液化生有源，保证血液充盈。若心血不足，可影响脾主运化功能；反之，脾气虚弱,血之化源不足,则血虚而心失所主。

心主行血,心气推动血液在脉道中运行;脾主统血,脾气统摄血液,使之行于脉中而不逸出。二者相反相成,保证血液的正常运行。若心气虚弱,无力行血,则可致气虚血瘀等病证;若脾气不足,无力摄血,则可致气虚出血等病症。

3.3.1.3 心与肝

心与肝的关系,主要体现在血液运行的相互协调和精神活动的相互为用。

心主行血,血运正常,则肝有所藏;肝主藏血,贮存血液、调节血量和防止出血,贮调相宜,则心有所主。两者相互配合,共同维持血液的正常运行。病理上,心血与肝血常相互影响,从而出现心肝血虚证或心肝血瘀证等病变。

心主神志,主宰着人的精神情志活动;肝主疏泄,调畅气机,使气血调和,情志舒畅。两者相互为用,共同维持正常的精神情志活动。若心主神志与肝主疏泄功能失常,则人体精神情志活动异常,可出现精神恍惚,情绪抑郁,或心烦失眠、急躁易怒等病症。

3.3.1.4 心与肾

心与肾的关系,主要表现为"水火既济"和"精神互根"。

心位于胸中,五行属火,故为阳;肾位于腰部,五行属水,故为阴。就阴阳水火的升降理论而言,居上者宜降,居下者宜升。故心火宜下降以暖肾水,肾阴宜上升以济于心阴,而制心阳。若心火不能下降于肾,肾水不能上济于心,则可出现"心肾不交"的病理变化。

心藏神,神能驭精;肾藏精,精能化神。精与神互根互用,精为神的物质基础,神为精的外在表现。若肾精不足,化神乏源,可出现精神不振,思维迟钝等病症;反之,神不安守,易致精不得藏,可出现遗精、梦交等病症。

3.3.1.5 肺与脾

肺与脾的关系,主要体现在气的生成和水液代谢两个方面。

肺吸入的清气和脾运化的水谷精气,是生成气的主要物质基础,两者结合,化为宗气。宗气是全身之气的重要组成部分,因此,肺司呼吸功能和脾主运化功能对气的生成具有重要作用。病理上,肺气虚与脾气虚常相互影响,从而出现肺脾两虚之证。

肺通调水道,疏通和调节水液的输布、运行和排泄;脾运化水液,保证水液的生成和输布。脾输布水液,是肺通调水道的前提。脾肺协调配合,维持水液的正常代谢。若脾主运化水液功能失常,水湿内生,常可影响及肺,肺失宣降,从而出现痰饮咳喘等病变。

3.3.1.6 肺与肝

肺与肝的关系,主要体现在气机升降的相互协调。

肝主升,肺主降;肝气升发,肺气肃降。升降协调对全身气机的顺畅具有重要的调节作用。病理上,肝肺病变常相互影响。肝气上逆,肝火上炎,耗伤肺阴,可致肺气失于肃降；反之，肺失清肃，燥热内盛，伤及肝阴，阴不制阳，可致肝阳上亢。

3.3.1.7　肺与肾

肺与肾的关系，主要表现在呼吸运动和水液代谢方面的相互为用。

肺司呼吸，吸入清气，呼出浊气，实现体内外气体的交换；肾主纳气，肺司呼吸功能需要肾主纳气功能的协助，才能保持吸气的深度，防止呼吸表浅，保证呼吸运动的均匀和调。病理上，肺气久虚，肃降失司，与肾气不足，摄纳无权常相互影响。

肺主通调水道，肺疏通、调节水液输布、排泄的功能有赖于肾的气化作用；肾主水，气化升降水液的功能，离不开肺气肃降，使水液下归于肾的作用。肺肾相互为用，维持着水液代谢的正常进行。若肺肾功能失调，则水液代谢障碍，可出现水肿等病变。

此外，肺肾阴气相互资生，肺阴充足，下输于肾，使肾阴充盈；肾阴充盈，上滋于肺，使肺阴充足。病理上，肺阴不足与肾阴虚损常互为因果，相兼为病。

3.3.1.8　肝与脾

肝与脾的关系，主要表现在水谷运化和血液运行两个方面。

脾主运化，具有把水谷化为精微，并将精微吸收、转输至全身的功能；肝主疏泄，调畅气机，协调脾升胃降，并疏利胆汁，有助于脾的运化功能。若肝失疏泄，气机不畅，可致脾失健运，出现肝脾不和之证。

脾主统血，脾气统摄血液而使之不逸出脉外；肝主藏血，肝血充足，肝体得养，则疏泄正常，气机条达，而使气机调畅，血行无阻。肝脾相互协作，保证血液既顺畅运行，又不逸出脉外。若肝脾受损，统藏失司，可致血行异常，出现出血等病症。

3.3.1.9　肝与肾

肝与肾的关系，主要表现为精血互化和藏泄互用。

肝藏血，肾藏精。肾精是化生血液所需要的基本物质之一，血液的化生有赖于肾中精气的充盛；肾中精气的充盛，也有赖于肝血的滋养。肝血与肾精生理上相互为用，病理上相互影响。肝血不足可导致肾精亏虚，肾精亏虚也可导致肝血不足，从而出现头昏目眩，耳鸣耳聋，腰膝酸软等肾精肝血两亏病症。

肝主疏泄，肾主封藏，相反相成。肝气疏泄，有助于肾气开合有度；肾气闭藏，可防止肝气疏泄太过。二者相互为用，协调女子的月经来潮和男子的排精功能。若肝肾泄藏失调，女子则月经紊乱；男子则阳痿、遗精、滑泄，或阳强不泄等。

此外，肝肾阴阳之间关系密切，肾阴滋养肝阴，进而制约肝阳，维持阴阳平衡。若肾阴亏虚，不能滋养肝阴，可致肝肾阴虚，肝阳上亢，出现眩晕，中风等病证。

3.3.1.10　脾与肾

脾与肾的关系，主要体现在先后天相互资生和水液代谢相互协同。

肾为先天之本，脾为后天之本。脾气健运，化生水谷精微，有赖于肾气的资助和推动；肾中精气的充盈，也有赖于水谷精微的培育和补养。病理上，脾虚与肾亏常相互影响,导致脾肾两脏皆不足。若脾肾气虚,则可出现腹胀便溏,或大小便失禁,或虚喘乏力等病症;脾肾阳虚,则可出现畏寒腹痛、腰膝酸冷、五更泄泻、完谷不化等病症。

脾主运化,输布水液,防止水湿泛滥;肾主水,主持和调节水液的输布和排泄。脾肾相互协同,共同维持水液代谢的平衡。若脾肾两虚,水湿内停,则可出现尿少浮肿,腹胀便溏,腰膝酸软等病症。

3.3.2 六腑之间的关系

六腑之间的关系,主要表现在对水谷的消化、吸收、传导以及糟粕的排泄过程中的相互联系和配合。

水谷入胃,经胃的腐熟,下传到小肠,经小肠的受盛化物和泌别清浊,清者在脾的作用下转输至全身;浊者下传到大肠,经燥化和传导作用,形成粪便,排出体外。渗入膀胱的水液,经气化作用排泄于外而为尿;在上述水谷消化、吸收和糟粕的排泄过程中,还有赖于胆排泄胆汁以助消化、三焦疏通水道以行水液的作用。六腑不断地受纳、消化、传导水谷并排泄糟粕,宜通不宜滞,故有"六腑以通为用"之说。

六腑功能上相互协调,病理上相互影响。如胆火炽盛,常可犯胃,致使胃失和降,出现呕吐苦水等病症;胃热伤津,导致大便燥结,大肠传导不利。

3.3.3 脏与腑之间的关系

3.3.3.1 心与小肠

手少阴心经属心络小肠,手太阳小肠经属小肠络心,心与小肠通过经脉相互络属,构成表里关系。

心阳下降于小肠,阳气温煦,有助于小肠受盛化物和泌别清浊;小肠吸收水谷精微,上奉于心,化赤为血,以养心脉。心与小肠在功能上相互为用,病理上相互影响。若心火亢盛,可移热于小肠,出现心烦、舌赤生疮,尿少、尿热、尿赤、尿痛等病症。

3.3.3.2 肺与大肠

手太阴肺经属肺络大肠,手阳明大肠经属大肠络肺,肺与大肠通过经脉相互络属,构成表里关系。

肺气清肃下降,有助于大肠传导糟粕;大肠传导通畅,有利于肺气清肃下降。若肺气失于肃降,津不下达,则大肠津亏,肠燥便秘;若大肠传导失畅,腑气不通,也可影响肺气宣降,出现胸满、咳喘等病症。

3.3.3.3 脾与胃

足太阴脾经属脾络胃,足阳明胃经属胃络脾,脾与胃通过经脉相互络属,构成表里关系。

胃主受纳,脾主运化,纳运相依。胃的受纳和腐熟水谷,是脾主运化的前提;脾主运化,转输精微,为胃继续纳食提供了条件。

脾气升,胃气降,脾升与胃降互为前提,升降相因,协同完成布散精微和传导糟粕的作用。

脾为脏属阴,喜燥恶湿;胃为腑属阳,喜润恶燥;燥湿相济,阴阳调和,纳运、升降方能协调正常。

脾与胃在功能上相互为用,病理上相互影响。若脾为湿困,脾气不升,脾失健运,可影响胃之受纳与和降,可出现纳呆、腹胀、恶心、呕吐等病症;反之,饮食伤胃,胃失和降,可影响脾之升清与运化,可出现腹胀、泄泻等病症。

3.3.3.4 肝与胆

足厥阴肝经属肝络胆,足少阳胆经属胆络肝,肝与胆通过经脉相互络属,构成表里关系。

胆汁源于肝之余气,胆汁分泌和排泄受肝之疏泄功能的调控,肝的疏泄功能正常,则胆汁分泌与排泄正常;反之,胆汁排泄通畅,也有利于肝气疏泄。若肝气郁滞,则胆汁分泌、排泄失常;胆腑湿热,胆汁排泄失畅,则影响肝气疏泄,从而出现肝胆郁滞、肝胆湿热以及肝胆火旺等病证。此外,肝主谋虑,但要做出决断,又取决于胆,两者密切配合。

3.3.3.5 肾与膀胱

足少阴肾经属肾络膀胱,足太阳膀胱经属膀胱络肾,肾与膀胱通过经脉相互络属,构成表里关系。

膀胱为水腑,主要功能是贮尿和排尿,但膀胱的贮尿功能有赖于肾的固摄作用,膀胱的排尿功能有赖于肾的气化作用。若肾化无力或固摄无权,则膀胱排尿、贮尿障碍,可出现尿少、尿闭或尿失禁等病症。肾为水脏,肾的主水功能也受膀胱贮尿与排尿功能的影响。若膀胱贮尿与排尿功能异常,可影响肾的气化或固摄功能,可出现尿色质、数量等改变。

脏与腑之间的关系,除脏与相表里的腑之间存在密切联系,脏与非表里的其他腑之间也存在着联系。如肝主疏泄影响着胃气通降,肝气得疏则胃气得降;肝失疏泄,则胃失和降,可出现胸胁、胃脘胀痛,呃逆嗳气,吞酸嘈杂等肝胃不和的病变。

思考题

- 何谓藏象和藏象学说?
- 五脏、六腑、奇恒之腑有何区别?
- 试述五脏的主要生理功能。
- 试述六腑的主要生理功能。
- 试述脏与脏、脏与腑之间的关系。

4 精气血津液

精、气、血、津液是构成人体和维持人体生命活动的基本物质,由人体脏腑经络及组织器官功能活动所化生。因此,精、气、血、津液与脏腑经络及组织器官之间在生理、病理上关系非常密切。

4.1 精

4.1.1 精的含义

精是体内的一类精微物质。其含义有广义和狭义之分。广义之精泛指由气而化生的构成人体和维持人体生命活动的精微物质,包括气、血、津液、髓以及水谷精微等;狭义之精是指藏于肾中具有繁衍后代作用的生殖之精,是促进人体生长发育和生殖功能的基本物质。

4.1.2 精的生成

人体之精根源于先天而充养于后天,故从精的生成来源而言,有先天与后天之分。

4.1.2.1 先天之精

先天之精禀受于父母,是构成胚胎的原始物质。父母遗传的生命物质是与生俱来的精,谓之先天之精。古人通过对人类生殖繁衍过程的观察和体验,认识到男女生殖之精的结合能产生一个新的生命个体。然而在胚胎形成之后,直至胎儿发育成熟,全赖女子胞中气血的养育。因此,先天之精为原始生命物质,主要秘藏于肾。

4.1.2.2 后天之精

后天之精来源于水谷,又称"水谷之精"。人出生之后,要依赖脾胃对饮食物的消化吸收,将饮食精华生为水谷精微,以营养各个脏腑组织,才能维持正常的生命活动。由于这部分精微来源于后天,故称为后天之精。

人体之精虽有先天和后天之分,但两者相互依存,相互促进。先天之精必须不断得到后天之精的充养才能维持正常的生理作用,而后天之精的生成要依靠先天之精的活力资助。因此,无论是先天之精还是后天之精的匮乏,均能产生精虚不足的病理变化。

4.1.3 精的功能

人体之精具有繁衍生命、生长发育、生髓化血、濡养脏腑、生气化神等作用。

4.1.3.1 繁衍生命

生殖之精是生命起源的原始物质,通过男女两性的交合,便可产生一个新的生命个体,因而生殖之精具有繁衍后代的作用。由先天之精与后天之精合化而成的生殖之精藏于肾中,组成肾中精气,随着肾中精气的不断充盛,形体逐渐发育成熟,到一定年龄便产生了"天癸",于是便具备了繁衍生命的功能。因此,肾中精气不仅包含生殖之精,而且还能化生肾气以促进生殖。这一给予后代的生命遗传物质,即是新生命的"先天之精"。肾精充足则生殖能力强;肾精不足就会影响生殖能力。故补肾填精是临床上治疗男子不育和妇女不孕等生殖问题的重要方法。

4.1.3.2 生长发育

肾中精气具有促进人体生长发育的作用。人出生后,随着肾中精气的不断充盛,人体不断生长、发育直到成熟,然后随着肾中精气的不断衰退,人体逐渐衰老。因而,随着精气由盛到衰的变化,人体呈现出生、长、壮、老、已的生命规律。若肾精充盛,则人体生长发育正常;若肾精不足,则出现生长发育迟缓、五软、五迟等病变。

4.1.3.3 生髓化血

肾藏精,精生髓,髓分为脑髓和骨髓。脑髓能够养脑,故脑髓充盈,则意识清楚,思维灵敏,言语清晰等。骨赖髓养,故肾精充足,骨髓充满,则骨骼坚固有力,运动轻捷。齿为骨之余,牙齿亦赖肾精所生之髓来充养。肾精充足则牙齿坚固而有光泽。若肾精亏虚,不能生髓,则骨骼失养,牙齿松动脱落;髓海不足,则头昏眩晕,神疲健忘,智力减退。

精生髓,髓可化血,是血液生成的来源之一。肾精充盈则肝有所养,血有所充,精足则血旺,精亏则血虚,故有"精血同源"之说。临床上用血肉有情之品如鹿角胶、龟甲等补益精髓可以治疗血虚之证。

4.1.3.4 濡养脏腑

精能滋润濡养人的各脏腑组织官窍。先天之精与后天之精充盛,则全身脏腑组织官窍得到充养,各种生理功能得以正常发挥。如果先天禀赋不足,或后天之精化生障碍,则肾精亏虚,五脏之精也会随之而衰,脏腑组织官窍得不到精的濡养和资助,其功能则不能正常发挥,甚至衰败。如肾精有损,则见生长发育迟缓或未老先衰;肺精不足,则见呼吸障碍,皮肤失润无泽;肝精不足,肝血不充,筋脉失养,则见拘挛、震颤或抽搐等症。

4.1.3.5 生气化神

先天之精可以化生先天之气(元气),水谷之精可以化生谷气,再加上由肺吸入的自然清气,综合而成一身之气。气不断地推动和调控人的新陈代谢,维系生命活动。精不但生气还能化神,精是神的物质基础。只有积精,才能全神,这是生命存在的根本保证。反之,精亏则神疲,精亡则神散。神健则身全,神疲则身病,神散则生命休矣。

4.2 气

中医学关于"气"的理论源于古代哲学的"气一元论",其原本是对自然界及其物质本原的一种抽象认识。"气一元论"认为气是构成世界的最基本物质,自然界的一切事物都是由气的运动变化而产生的。当这一观点渗透到医学领域后,促使医学家将其与医学知识相结合,从而构筑起中医气学理论。

4.2.1 气的含义

人体之气是构成人体和维持人体生命活动的、具有很强活力并运行不息的精微物质。

气是构成人体的基本物质。既然万物皆由气所构成,那么人也不例外。人的躯体是以气为基本物质,由气之抟聚而成,所以有"气聚则形存,气散则形亡"之说。

气是维持人体生命活动的基本物质。人的全部生命活动都是在气的作用下得以进行的。所以,气对人的生命活动来说至关重要,被视为人体生命的根本。

气是具有很强活力并运行不息的精微物质。气所具有的活力主要表现在激发和推动脏腑功能以及精血津液的运行等方面。因此,中医学常以气的运动变化来阐释人的生命活动。

4.2.2 气的生成

人体之气的生成来源可分为先天与后天两个方面:人在出生之前,从父母身体所禀受的精微之气,称为"先天之气";人在出生之后,从自然界所获得的精微之气(如自然界的清气和饮食中的营养物质等),称为"后天之气"。

人体之气的生成主要依靠肺、脾胃和肾等脏腑生理功能的综合作用,将先天之精与后天之精结合起来而生成为人体之气。其中,先天精气藏之于肾,自然清气受制于肺,水谷精气有赖脾胃。肺、脾胃、肾三个环节的生理功能正常与否,相互间协调和谐与否,往往直接影响着气的生成。其中,脾胃最为关键。

4.2.3 气的运动

气作为具有很强活力并运行不息的精微物质,它流行于周身,内至五脏六腑,外达组织官窍,无处不到,时刻推动和维持着人的各种生理活动。因此,气的运动决定着生命活动的状态。

气的运动又可称作"气机"。气的运动形式,通常可概括为升、降、出、入四种基本形式。升,是指气由下向上的运动;降,是指气由上向下的运动;出,是指气由内向外的运动;入,是指气由外向内的运动。就人体而言,气的升降出入运动是普遍存在、不容间断的。如肺的呼吸过程,呼浊是由肺向上,经咽喉、鼻孔、皮毛等,将浊气排除体外,故呼气既是出又是升;吸清是由体外向内,经鼻孔、咽喉等,将清气吸入于肺,故吸气既是入又是降。

应当指出,脏腑之气的升降出入运动,具体到某个脏腑往往有所侧重。五脏之中肝、脾以升为主,心、肺以降为主;六腑之中除胆气主升外,皆以和降为顺。从整体来看,升降出入之间是协调平衡的。如肝主升发与肺主肃降,脾主升清与胃主降浊,肺主出气与肾主纳气,心火下降与肾水上济,等等。

气的升降出入运动在人的生命活动中至关重要。通过气的运动能够调节人的生理功能,使其达到相对协调平衡的状态。具体表现在:一方面通过气的升降出入运动而使人的脏腑经络及形体官窍在生理功能方面和谐有序。如肾中精气、水谷精气以及自然清气都必须经过升降出入,以三焦为通道,敷布全身,发挥其各种生理效应。精血津液等必须依赖气的运动,而运行不息,营养滋润脏腑组织及形体官窍。另一方面通过身体内外之气的交换,即吸收天地之精气,排出体内浊气及代谢终末产物,而使人体之气不断更新与补充,以维持生命活动,并调节人的生理平衡。如果气的升降出入运动遭到破坏,脏腑组织及形体官窍之间失去协调平衡,就会出现各种病理变化。

气的升降出入运动畅通无阻、协调平衡,称为"气机调畅"。反之,若气的升降出入运动受阻,或失去和谐,则称为"气机失调"。

气机失调的表现常见有五种形式,即:①气滞,指气的运动不畅,或阻滞不通,又可称为"气机不畅"或"气机郁阻";②气逆,指气的上升太过或下降不及或横行逆乱;③气陷,指气的下降太过或上升不及;④气闭,指气不能外达而结聚于内;⑤气脱,指气不能内守而大量外逸。

4.2.4 气的功能

人体之气既是维持生命活动的源泉,又是脏腑经络和组织器官功能活动的动力。气在人的生命活动中所发挥的作用一般可概括为六个方面。

4.2.4.1 推动作用

气是具有很强活力的精微物质。气以其自身活力和运动,能够激发和推动人的生长发育以及脏腑经络和组织器官的生理功能,能够促进和推动血、津液等液态物质的生成及运行。若体内之气充沛,则功能健旺正常、生机盎然;若体内之气虚馁,则脏腑功能减退、精血津液代谢失常,甚至生长发育迟缓,表现出以功能低下为特征的各种病理状态。

4.2.4.2 温煦作用

气的温煦作用,是指气可以产生热能,而使身体温暖,消除寒冷。具体表现在三个方面:①保证人体维持相对恒定的体温;②有助于脏腑经络、形体官窍的生理功能;③有助于精血津液等的正常输布而不致凝滞,促进机体的新陈代谢。如果因气虚而失于温煦,则四肢不温、畏寒怕冷,功能低下,精血津液等运行迟缓。

4.2.4.3 防御作用

气的防御作用,是指气具有护卫肌表,防御外邪侵袭,或与入侵之贼邪抗争,驱邪外出的能力。当致病邪气侵犯人体时,气具有与病邪作斗争,驱邪外出的功能。当邪气侵入于某一部位时,机体便会将气调动聚集于患病部位,发挥与外邪抗争的作用。气的防御作用正常,则邪气不易入侵;或虽有邪气侵入也不易发病;即使发病也容易治愈。若气的防御作用减退,则机体抗病能力就会随之下降,外邪易乘虚而入,使机体罹患疾病。

4.2.4.4 固摄作用

固摄有固护、统摄、约束之义。气的固摄作用是指气对血液、津液、精液等液态物质具有固护、统摄、约束,防止其无故流失的作用。具体表现在三个方面:①固摄血液,使血液运行于脉内而不外逸;②固摄汗液、唾液、尿液,控制其分泌排泄量,使其有序地排出,以防止体液丢失过多;③固摄精液,使之闭藏而不妄泄。若气虚而固摄作用减弱,可导致体内液态物质大量流失。如气不摄血则出血;气不摄津则多汗、多尿或小便失禁、口流涎唾;气不摄精则遗精滑泄。此外,对大便泄利、脱肛、妇女白带过多及孕妇滑胎失固等病证多与气失固摄有关。

4.2.4.5 营养作用

气的营养作用,主要体现在三个方面:①通过行于肌腠的卫气,对体表组织起到充养作用;②通过经络之气,起到输送营养,濡润组织器官的作用;③通过营气化生血液,以营养全身。

4.2.4.6 气化作用

气的气化作用,是指气具有通过运动而产生和促进各种物质和能量变化的功能。体内精微物质的相互化生、精微物质转化为各种功能,以及体内废物的排泄等,都依赖于气的气化。气化是生命活动最基本的特征。如果气化失常,则影响饮食物的消化吸收,影响精气血津液之间的正常转化,影响汗、尿及粪便的排泄,形成各种代谢失常的病变。

4.2.5 气的分类

由于人体之气的生成、分布及功能不同,因而又有元气、宗气、营气、卫气等不同名称。现分述如下:

4.2.5.1 元气

元气是指人体最根本、最重要的气,是人体生命活动的原动力。所以,元气又名原气、真气。

(1) 元气的生成与分布:元气主要由肾中所藏的先天之精所化生,并不断得到脾胃所化生的水谷精气的充养和培育。因此,元气的盛衰除与先天禀赋有直接关系外,后天的饮食状况、身体锻炼、精神调摄等也会对元气产生影响。对于先天不足而元气虚弱者,往往可以通过后天培育而使元气得到充盛。元气下藏于肾,通过三焦而布达于全身,内则五脏六腑,外则形体官窍,无处不到。

(2) 元气的功能:元气的生理功能主要体现在两个方面:①推动和调节人的生长发育与生殖功能。②激发、推动和调控脏腑经络及组织器官的生理活动。其中,元阳能助长一身之阳气,元阴能滋养一身之阴气。元气充沛则人的生长发育及生殖能力正常,脏腑功能旺盛,抗病能力强健。若因先天禀赋不足,或因后天调摄失当,久病不愈,肾中精气渐衰,元气化生乏源,或因元气耗损太过,均可导致元气虚衰而产生各种病变。

4.2.5.2 宗气

宗气是指积于胸中之气,是人体后天的根本之气。因胸中为宗气汇聚之处,故称其为"气海"。

(1) 宗气的生成与分布:宗气是由肺所吸入的自然清气与脾胃所化生的水谷精气相互结合而成的。宗气聚集于胸中,通过上出呼吸道,贯注心脉及沿三焦下行的方式布散周身。宗气一方面上出于肺,循喉咙而走息道,推动呼吸;另一方面贯注心脉,推动血行。三焦是诸气运行的通道,宗气还可沿三焦向下,蓄于丹田,以资先天元气,并由气街注入足阳明经。

(2) 宗气的功能:宗气的生理功能主要体现在三个方面:①走息道以行呼吸。凡语言、声音、呼吸的强弱,均与宗气的盛衰有关。②贯心脉以行气血。凡心搏的节律与强弱,气血的运行,肢体的寒温与活动能力,以及视听感觉等都与宗气盛衰有关。③蓄丹田以资先天。宗气对先天元气有重要的资助作用。借三焦通道,宗气自上而下,蓄积丹田,可资先天元气。若宗气不足则表现为呼吸短促微弱、语音低微、含糊不清、脉律不齐、血行缓慢、肢体不温、行动乏力等。

4.2.5.3 营气

营气是指运营于脉中,具有营养作用的气。营气在脉中是血的重要组成部分,与血可分而不可离,故常以"营血"相称。营气与卫气相对而言,属于阴,故又有"营阴"之称。

(1) 营气的生成与分布:营气是由水谷精微中最精纯、最富含营养的部分所化生。营气运行于脉内,循脉运行全身,内入脏腑,外达肢节,终而复始,营周不休。

(2) 营气的功能:营气的生理功能主要体现在两个方面:①化生血液。营气富含营养,注于脉中,则成为血液的重要组成部分,因此,营气是血液生成的主要物质基础。②营养全身。营气由水谷精微中含有丰富营养的精纯部分所化生,营气循脉流行于全身,可为脏腑经络及组织器官的生理活动提供必需的营养物质。

营气化生血液和营养全身的生理作用是相互关联的,若营气亏少则会引起血液亏虚以及全身脏腑经络及组织器官得不到充足的营养,生理功能就会逐渐衰退。

4.2.5.4 卫气

卫气是指运行于脉外,具有护卫机体作用的气。卫气与营气相对而言,属于阳,故又有"卫阳"之称。

(1) 卫气的生成与分布:卫气是由水谷精微中慓疾滑利的部分所化生。由于卫气慓疾滑利,运行迅速,活力较强,所以不受脉的约束,外而行于皮肤肌腠,内而胸腹脏腑,布散全身。

(2) 卫气的功能:卫气的生理功能可概括为三个方面:①护卫肌表。卫气布达于肌表,起着抵御外邪侵袭的功能,集中体现了气的防御作用。②温煦机体。卫气布散周身,内至脏腑,外达肌肤,对脏腑经络、肌肉皮毛发挥着温煦作用。既有助于脏腑的生理活动,又可使肌肉充实、皮肤润泽。③调节腠理开阖。卫气布散于肌表,根据生理活动的需要调节腠理开阖,控制汗液的排泄,以维持体温的相对恒定。

营气与卫气虽同源于水谷精微,但在性质、分布及生理功能方面有所区别。营气性质精纯,行于脉内,具有化生血液和营养全身的功能,故属阴;卫气性质慓疾滑利,行于脉外,具有护卫肌表和温煦机体的功能,故属阳。营气与卫气之间必须协调互济,才能正常发挥各自的生理功能。

人体之气除上述之外,还有"脏腑之气"、"经络之气"等,它们都是由元气所派生的,是元气分布于某脏某腑或某经某络,并与水谷精气或自然界清气相合,则成为某脏某腑或某经某络之气。临床上可根据这些脏腑经络的功能状况,来判断相应脏腑经络之气的盛衰。

4.3 血

4.3.1 血的含义

血是指循行于脉中并具有较强营养与滋润作用的红色液态物质。

正常情况下,血液是沿着相对密闭的脉道循行而不逸出脉外的。周身之血均运行于脉道之内,故又称脉为"血府"。若因某些原因,使血液逸出脉外,称为"出血",逸出脉外之血,称为"离经之血"。

4.3.2 血的生成

一般而言,血液是由营气和津液化合而成,此外,精也可转化为血。

4.3.2.1 水谷精微化生血液

饮食物经过胃的腐熟和脾的运化,转化为水谷精微,其精纯部分化生成为营气;营气注入于脉中,并与津液相合而成为血液。由于营气是水谷中最为精纯的部分所化生,从而确保了血液中含有极为丰富的营养成分。由于津液也是血的重要组成部分,并起到维持和调节血液总量、稀释血液和滑润脉道的作用,从而确保了血量的充足和血液的恒久运行。营气与津液是生成血液的主要物质基础。饮食物营养丰富和脾胃功能健旺是血液生成的重要保证,故有"脾胃为气血生化之源"之说。

4.3.2.2 精生血

精能化血缘于精系生命之源,而且精血同类,互生互化。人之始生,必从精始,而血即精之属。精藏之于肾,肾精充盈必输泄滋养于肝,肝主藏血,精归于肝则化为血。精血之间相互资生和转化,突出反映了肝肾在生理功能上的密切关系,故有"肝肾同源"和"精血同源"之说。若肝肾功能衰弱,尤其是当肾精亏耗或肾阴不足时,血液的化生就会受到影响,形成血虚之证。

总之,血液的生成主要依赖于脾胃的运纳功能,并在心、肝、肾等脏的生理功能配合作用下得以充盈不衰。

4.3.3 血的运行

血在脉中,运行不休,如环无端,营养全身,以供人体生命活动的需要。

4.3.3.1 维持血液正常循行的条件

(1) 气的推动和固摄作用:血在脉道中循行必须依赖气的推动作用。只有气的充沛,血运才能获得足够的动力。同时,血的运行还必须依赖气的固摄作用。只有气的充沛,血才不会逸出脉外。因此,气的推动和固摄作用协调平衡是维持血液正常循行的重要保障。

(2) 脉道的完整与通畅:脉为血之府,脉道完整无损与滑润通畅是血液运行的重要条件。若遇跌打损伤,常会导致脉道破损而出血;饮食失宜,痰浊内阻,则常导致脉道壅阻,轻则血运不畅,重则闭塞不通。

(3) 血的质量与寒温:血的质与量往往会直接影响血的循行。如血质的稠与稀、血量的多与少,都会引起血运变化。津少血稠则血行迟滞,血量不足则血行失畅。血为流动的液态物质,遇寒则凝,得温则行,逢热则妄行,所以,寒温也是影响血液循行的常见因素之一。

4.3.3.2 心肺脾肝与血液循行的关系

心、肺、脾、肝四脏对维持血的正常循行起着重要的作用。

(1) 心主行血:心气是血液循行的主要动力。血能正常地在脉道中按照一定方向循行主要依靠心气的推动作用。

(2) 肺朝百脉:肺主一身之气,尤其决定着宗气的盛衰。宗气贯心脉以行气血。循行于周身的血脉均汇聚于肺,血液在肺中经过吐故纳新之后,再经心运向周身血脉。肺直接参与了血的循行,成为辅助心脏,推动血液循行的又一基本动力。

(3) 脾主统血:血液循行于脉内而不逸出脉外,主要是脾气对血的固摄作用。脾气充盛,不仅血之生化有源,而且能统摄血液,不致逸出脉外。

(4) 肝主藏血:肝通过贮藏血液和调节血量,可使脉中有效循环血量维持恒定,以防止血液妄行而逸出脉外。另外,肝主疏泄,调畅气机,也是确保血液和调畅行的重要因素之一。

总之,血液正常运行主要是在心、肺、脾、肝等脏功能的相互配合下完成的。具体而言,推动血行的是心;促进血行、保持脉道通畅的是肺与肝;贮藏、统摄血液,防止血逸脉外的是肝与脾。此外,保持血脉温暖舒展的是心阳与肾阳。

4.3.4 血的功能

血是富含营养和阴津的生命物质,其功能主要体现在两个方面:

4.3.4.1 营养和滋润作用

血液运行脉中,内至五脏六腑,外达肌肤官窍,无所不至,运行不息,从而不断地对全身发挥营养和滋润作用,以保证生命活动的需要。血液充盛,脏腑得养,则面色红润,肌肉壮实,毛发和皮肤润泽,感觉灵敏,运行自如。若血液亏虚,营养和滋润作用减弱,则多见面色苍白无华,头晕目眩,毛发干枯脱落,皮肤粗糙,肢体麻木或屈伸不利,妇女月经减少、迟至,甚至闭经等。

4.3.4.2 精神活动的物质基础

血液是精神活动的主要物质基础,人的精神活动必须得到血液的营养。血液充盈则人的精神振奋,思维敏捷,神志清晰,感觉灵敏,活动自如。若血液亏虚,血脉失于调和流畅,可出现不同程度的神志病变。表现为失眠多梦,烦躁健忘,神志恍惚,精神委靡,甚至谵妄、狂乱或不省人事等。

此外,血液还是化生精液、月经、乳汁的物质基础。

4.4 津液

4.4.1 津液的含义

津液是体内一切正常水液的总称。主要存在于脏腑形体、组织器官之内。此外,某些正常分泌物,如胃液、肠液、涕液、涎唾等在未排出体外之前也都属于津液的范畴。津液遍布全身,在脉内则是血液的组成部分;在脉外则是渗灌于脏腑器官以及组织间隙的体液。

津液可细分为津和液两部分。二者虽同源于饮食,生成于脾胃,流布于脉之内外,但在性状、分布和功能方面有所区别。一般地说,津是指性状较为清稀,流动性较大,主要布散于体表皮肤、肌肉和孔窍,并可渗入血脉,而成为血的组成部分,能起到滋润作用的部分;液是指性状较为稠厚,流动性较小,主要灌注于骨骼、关节、脏腑、脑髓以及皮肤等组织,能起到濡养和滑润作用的部分。

津和液并无本质的区别,而且在代谢过程中能够相互补充、相互转化,所以往往统称为"津液"。只是在"伤津"和"脱液"的病证中必须辨别清楚。

4.4.2 津液的代谢

津液的代谢包括生成、输布和排泄。

4.4.2.1 津液的生成

津液主要来源于饮食物,包括日常饮水以及食物中所含的水分。津液的生成涉及多个脏腑的生理活动。具体而言,主要是靠胃、脾、肝以及大、小肠消化、吸收饮食水谷中的水分和营养而生成。其过程是:经过胃的受纳,脾的运化,肝的疏泄,小肠的泌别清浊以及大肠主津等生理活动,而完成津液的生成过程。其中,脾胃功能尤为突出。

综上可见,津液的生成取决于两个方面:一是要有充足的来源作为生成津液的物质基础;二是消化、吸收功能的正常发挥,促使摄入的水分和营养化生为津液。若水饮摄入不足,或脾胃等脏腑功能虚弱,均会导致津液生成不足,引起津液缺乏。

4.4.2.2 津液的输布

津液生成后,在脾的运化作用下,一方面将部分津液直接布散四周,另一方面将大量津液向上转输于肺。上达于肺的津液,在肺的宣发作用下,进一步向上向外布散;在肺之肃降作用下,进一步向下向内输布。经代谢后的水液下达于肾。肾主水,肾阳的蒸腾气化作用可对其蒸清泌浊,蒸其清者而复归于脾肺,再度敷布;泌其浊者而化为尿液,注入膀胱。此外,三焦水道的通畅以及肝气的条达都有助于津液的输布。

4.4.2.3 津液的排泄

津液被人体利用后,其剩余水分及代谢废物需要适时地排出体外。其排泄途径主要有四:①通过皮肤排出汗液:肺主宣发,可将津液输布至体表皮毛,经阳气蒸腾而化为汗液,经汗孔排出体外;②通过膀胱排出尿液:尿液是津液代谢的终末产物,贮于膀胱,经过肾和膀胱的气化而排出体外,这是体内废液最为重要的排泄途径;③通过粪便挟带部分水液:在大肠排出的粪便中,也带有部分废液;④通过呼气带走水分:肺司呼吸,肺在呼气的过程中,也会不断散发出水分。

总之,津液的代谢需要多个脏腑的综合调节,其中尤以肺、脾、肾三脏最为关键。若此三脏功能失调,就会影响津液的代谢过程,从而产生痰饮、癃闭、水肿等诸多病证。

4.4.3 津液的功能

4.4.3.1 滋润与濡养作用

津液广泛分布于脏腑官窍及形体肢节。津液不仅拥有大量水分,而且含有多种营养物质,对全身起着滋润与濡养作用。如布散于体表,则肌肤丰润,毛发光泽;输注于孔窍,则孔窍通利灵敏;灌注于关节,则屈伸自如;注留于骨髓,则骨骼坚强;渗入于脉中,则扩充血量、滑利脉道;进入于脏器,则滋养脏腑。

4.4.3.2 化生与调节作用

津液是血液的重要组成部分之一。在心阳作用下,津液与营气结合,化生血液,环周全身,发挥着津液的滋润和濡养作用。另外,津液还有调节血液浓度的作用。在血液浓度偏高时,津液就渗入脉中,起着稀释血液,补充血量的作用。在机体津液偏低时,血中津液则可从脉中渗出脉外,起着补充津液,纠正脱水的作用。借助脉内外津液的渗透移行,机体可根据生理或病理的变化来调节血液浓度,维持正常的有效血量,并使血脉滑利顺畅,有利于血液的循行。

4.4.3.3 调节与中和作用

津液性质属阴,故又可称"阴液",对机体有调节阴阳、协调寒热、平衡体温的作用。阴可制阳,故津液充沛则虚火难升,津液不足则热盛燥干。在寒冷时,皮肤汗孔闭合,津液不能借汗外泄,而下注膀胱,使小便增多;在炎热时,皮肤汗孔大开,津液外泄以助散热解暑,津液减少下行,使小便减少。在机体丢失水分时,可通过补充饮料或服用生津止渴之品予以纠正。

津液属液态物质,故有中和作用。津液可中和稀释体内的毒素或偏颇的性味,以减少刺激和损伤,加速排泄。津液的中和作用对于维持人的生理功能是不容小视的。

4.4.3.4 排泄废物的作用

津液通过代谢过程,能将机体各部的代谢产物借排泄尿、汗、粪等途径适时地排出体外,从而保证机体生理活动的正常进行。若这种功能发生障碍,致使代谢产物潴留体内,则可产生多种病理变化。

4.5 精、气、血、津液之间的关系

虽然精、气、血、津液在性状、生成、分布及功能上各具不同特点,但均为构成人体和维持人体生命活动的基本物质。因此,它们之间在生理上相互依存、相互促进、协调平衡;在病理上又相互影响、相互累及。

4.5.1 精和气的关系

精与气相比,气主动,属阳;精主静,属阴。两者之间有着密切的关系,具体表现在精能化气、气能生精和气能摄精三个方面。

4.5.1.1 精能化气

人体之精在气的激发推动下可化生为气。五脏之精化生五脏之气,而藏于肾中的先天之精化为元气,水谷之精化为谷气。精为气化生的本源,精足则人身之气充盛,分布到脏腑经络,则脏腑经络之气亦充足;五脏之精充足则五脏之气化生充沛,能推动和调控各脏腑形体官窍的生理活动。故精足则气旺,精亏则气衰。临床中,精虚及失精患者常常同时见到气虚之象。

4.5.1.2 气能生精

气的气化功能旺盛则能促进精的化生。肾中所藏之精以先天之精为基础,且赖

后天水谷之精的不断充养才得以充盛。只有全身脏腑之气充足，功能正常，才可以运化吸收饮食水谷之精微，使五脏六腑之精充盈，流注于肾而藏之。因而，精的化生依赖于气的充盛。

4.5.1.3 气能摄精

气不但能促进精的化生，且又能固摄精，使精聚而充盈，不致无故耗损外泄，这是气之固摄作用的体现。若气虚失化则精亏不足，若气虚失摄则妄泄失精，临床上对此常采用补气生精、补气固精等法治之。

4.5.2 精和血的关系

精与血均属液态生命物质。由于精血之间具有相互资生和相互转化的关系，所以有"精血同源"之说。

4.5.2.1 精能生血

精是化生血液的基本物质之一。五脏之精融入血液，则化而为血。肾中之精在肾的气化作用下，入肝则化而为血。水谷之精在脾的气化作用下，精纯部分化为营气，清稀部分化为津液，营气与津液在心阳的作用下，变化而赤，入脉则化为血液。在治疗肝血不足时，兼用补肾益精之法，常能获得理想的效果。

由于肾主藏精，所以肾精化血的意义尤显重要。肾精化血，荣养毛发，故称肾"其华在发"，又称"发为血之余"。因此，肾精亏耗则会兼见血虚之象，出现头发枯槁脱落之候。

4.5.2.2 血能化精

血液以后天水谷精微为主要生成来源，肾中之精也有赖于后天水谷精微的不断充养。因此，血液也可化生为精，以不断充实和滋养肾之所藏，使肾中之精保持旺盛不衰。故血充则精足，血少则精亏。

4.5.3 气和血的关系

气属阳，无形而善动，主推动温煦；血属阴，有形而宁静，司营养濡润。二者相反相成，相互为用，相互资生，不可相离须臾。气与血的这种关系，通常概括为"气为血之帅，血为气之母。"气为血之帅是气对血的作用，包括气能生血、行血、摄血三个方面；血为气之母是血对气的作用，包括血能养气和载气两个方面。

4.5.3.1 气能生血

气能生血是指气参与并促进着血的生成。具体体现在两个方面：①营气是血的主要组成部分：营气营运于脉中，既是促进血液生成的基本物质，又是与渗注于脉的津液相结合的动力；②脏腑之气化生血液：即通过脾胃、小肠、心肺等脏腑之气的作用，从饮食物中转化为水谷精微，进一步转化为营气和津液，化赤为血，以及肾精所化生的血等等，每个环节都离不开气的运动变化。由于气旺则血充，气虚则血少，所以气虚常会进一步导致血虚，出现头晕目眩、少气懒言、乏力自汗、面色无华、心悸怔忡、失眠健忘、舌淡而嫩、脉细弱等气血两虚之象。

4.5.3.2 气能行血

气能行血是指气的推动作用是血液运行的原动力。血属阴而主静,其运行有赖于气的推动。具体而言,心主行血,心气是推动血液循行的基本动力;肺主气而朝百脉,肺气是心主行血的主要辅助力量;肝主疏泄而调畅气机,肝气是保持血行通畅的重要环节。此三脏功能协调,则血流畅通无阻。

若气虚推动乏力或气机郁滞等,都可引起血行迟缓,甚则凝涩不行而形成瘀血。此外,气机逆乱,也可导致血行异常,如气逆则血溢,气陷则血泄。

4.5.3.3 气能摄血

气能摄血是指气具有统摄血液在脉道中循行,防止其逸出脉外的功能。这是气之固摄作用的具体体现之一,主要与脾气对血的统摄作用有关。若脾气虚弱,统摄失职,则常常会导致各种出血症,如便血、皮下出血、妇女崩漏等。临床上称这类现象为"气不摄血"或"脾不统血"。

4.5.3.4 血能养气

血液含有丰富的营养,可为气的化生和功能活动提供物质基础,使气得到及时而适当的补充。故血液盈满充足,则气得以滋养。若血虚日久,无以养气,则必然导致气虚。

4.5.3.5 血能载气

气无形而善动,故必须附着于有形主静之血,才能发挥其应有的生理效应。故血液盈满充足,则气得以运载。若血液大量丧失,则会导致气随血脱。

4.5.4 气和津液的关系

气无形而动,属阳;津液有质而静,属阴。两者关系可概括为气为津主和津能载气。其中,气为津主是指气对津液的作用,包括气能生津、行津、摄津三个方面。

4.5.4.1 气能生津

气能生津是指气具有促进津液生成的效应。津液是由摄入的饮食物,经脾胃之气的消化吸收而生成的,所以脾胃之气充足,消化吸收功能健旺,则津液化生充盛;相反,若脾胃之气虚弱,消化吸收功能减退,则津液化生不足,故有"气旺津充"和"气弱津少"等说法。

4.5.4.2 气能行津

气能行津是指气具有推动津液输布和排泄的效应。通过气的推动,津液可输布于全身;通过气的气化,津液代谢的终末产物可适时地排出体外。津液的输布与排泄离不开肺、脾、肾、三焦等脏腑的气化功能和协同作用。若上述脏腑之气不足或气的升降出入异常,致使津液的输布和排泄障碍,内生水湿痰饮等病理产物,称为"气不行水"。

4.5.4.3 气能摄津

气能摄津是指气具有固摄津液,防止其无故流失的效应。这是气之固摄作用的具体体现之一,主要关系到肺卫之气对汗液和肾气对尿液的调节与控制作用。若肺肾气虚而固摄失职,就势必导致体内津液异常流失,发生多汗、多尿等病象。

4.5.4.4 津能载气

津能载气是指津液对气具有运载的功能。气必须依附于津液,才能存在于体内并流布至全身,故有"津能载气"之说。具体体现在两个方面:一是脉内津液,作为血的组成部分,能运载营气;二是脉外津液,流行贯注,能运载卫气。由于津能载气,故在多汗、多尿、大吐、大泻等津液大量流失时,气亦随之外脱,从而形成"气随津脱",出现气短息微、身倦乏力、脉微细等症。由于津液是气的载体,因而在病理上还可表现为津停气阻,即因水液停滞而妨碍到气的运行。

4.5.5 血和津液的关系

血与津液均为液态物质,同属于阴,都来源于水谷精微,具有滋润和濡养作用。由于血之与津有分有合,有入有出,相互资生,相互转化,所以血与津液的关系可概括为"津血同源"。

4.5.5.1 血能化津

血液通常是运行于脉内的。而当血液中的津液成分渗出脉外,与营气分离,便可融入脉外的津液之中。如若血液亏耗,尤其是在失血过多时,脉中血少,脉外津液会大量渗入脉内,以补偿有效血量的减少,从而造成脉外津液的相对不足,出现口渴、咽燥、尿少、肤干等症。因此,对失血者不宜采用汗法,以防津液与血液进一步耗竭的恶性后果。

4.5.5.2 津能生血

运行于脉外的津液渗入脉内,在心阳的作用下,与营气结合,便成为血液的组成部分。当水饮摄入不足,脾胃功能虚弱,或大汗、大吐、大下,或严重烧烫伤等造成脉外津液不足时,脉内的津液成分就会大量渗出,从而造成有效血量骤减,血液相对变稠,进而形成"津枯血燥"或"津亏血瘀"等病理变化。因此,对津亏者不可妄行破血、放血等疗法。

思考题

- 何谓精?精的生成来源有哪些?
- 气的生成与哪些脏腑关系较为密切?
- 何谓气机?其基本形式如何?
- 气的生理功能有哪些?
- 血的运行主要与哪些脏腑密切相关?
- 津液的输布主要与哪些脏腑关系密切?

5 经络学说

经络学说,是研究人体经络系统的含义、构成、循行分布、生理功能、病理变化及其与脏腑形体官窍、气血精神之间相互联系的基础理论,是中医学理论体系的重要组成部分。经络学说与脏腑理论共同构成中医理论体系的核心。

经络学说贯穿于人体生理、病理及疾病的诊断和防治各个方面,与阴阳五行、藏象、精气血津液等理论相互辅翼,它深刻地阐释人体的生理活动和病理变化,对临床各科,尤其是针灸、推拿、气功等都起到极其有效的指导作用。

5.1 经络的含义和组成

5.1.1 经络的含义

经络是由经脉和络脉及连属部分所组成,是运行全身气血,联络脏腑肢节,将五脏六腑、四肢百骸、五官九窍、皮肉筋脉等组织器官联结成一个有机的整体,是人体组织结构的重要组成部分。经络不但是有机体内部相互联系的通路,也是机体和自然界相应、维持体内外环境协调统一的桥梁,机体脏腑组织通过经络时时刻刻都在与自然界进行着物质、能量、信息的交流,以确保人体生命活动的正常进行。

经,有路径的意思;络,有网络的意思。经脉是主干,络脉是分支。后世医家多认为:经脉大多循行于深部,行于分肉之间;络脉循行于较浅的部位,有的络脉还显现于体表。经脉较粗大,络脉较细小。经脉以纵行为主,有一定的循行径路,而络脉则纵横交错,网络全身。但实际上,经脉虽然多"伏行于分肉之间",也常显露于体表;络脉虽有"浮而常见"者,而更多的则是分布于脏腑组织之中。而且,经脉也有横行者,如带脉;络脉呈网络状,纵横交错,必然也有纵行者。

经脉和络脉是构成经络系统的主体部分,担负着运行气血、联络沟通等作用,把人体所有的脏腑、器官、孔窍以及皮肉筋骨等组织联结成一个统一的有机整体。

5.1.2 经络系统的组成

经络系统在内连属于脏腑,在外连属于筋肉、皮肤。

经络可分为正经、奇经和经别三大类。正经有十二条,包括手三阴经、手三阳经、足三阳经、足三阴经,合称"十二经脉"或"十二正经",是气血运行的主要通道。十二经脉有一定的起止、一定的循行部位和交接顺序,在肢体的分布和走向有一定的规律，与体内脏腑有直接的络属关系，相互之间也有表里关系。十二正经是气血在经脉中运行的必经之路。

奇经有八条，即任、督、冲、带、阴维、阳维、阴跷、阳跷，合称"奇经八脉"，有统率、联络和调节十二经脉中气血的作用。奇经八脉与十二经脉不同，它与脏腑没有直接

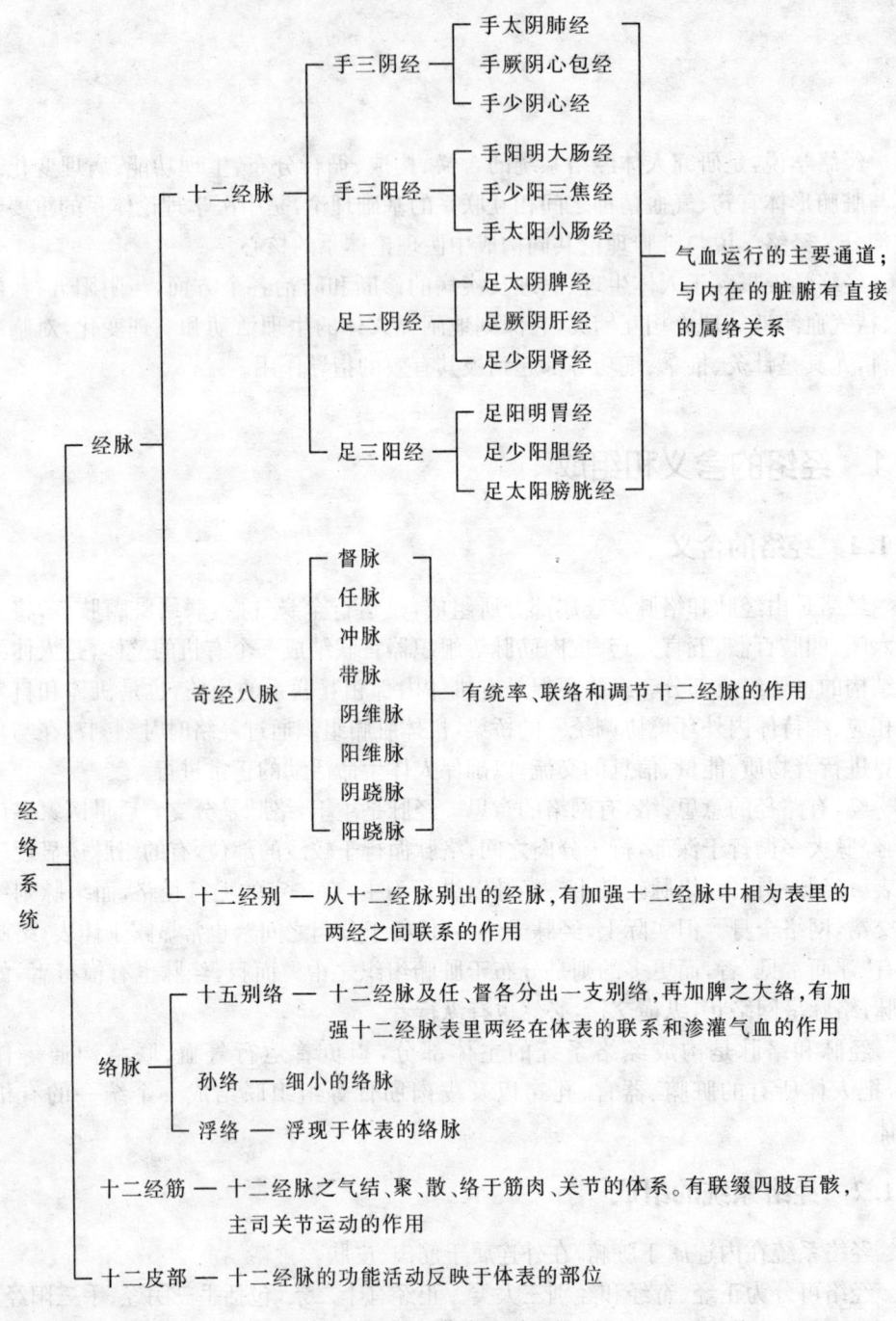

```
                        ┌ 手太阴肺经
                ┌ 手三阴经 ┼ 手厥阴心包经
                │        └ 手少阴心经
                │        ┌ 手阳明大肠经
                ├ 手三阳经 ┼ 手少阳三焦经
                │        └ 手太阳小肠经         气血运行的主要通道；
        ┌ 十二经脉┤        ┌ 足太阴脾经         与内在的脏腑有直接
        │       ├ 足三阴经 ┼ 足厥阴肝经         的属络关系
        │       │        └ 足少阴肾经
        │       │        ┌ 足阳明胃经
        │       └ 足三阳经 ┼ 足少阳胆经
        │                └ 足太阳膀胱经
        │                ┌ 督脉
  ┌ 经脉┤                │ 任脉
  │     │                │ 冲脉
  │     │                │ 带脉
  │     ├ 奇经八脉───────┤              ─ 有统率、联络和调节十二经脉的作用
  │     │                │ 阴维脉
经│     │                │ 阳维脉
络│     │                │ 阴跷脉
系│     │                └ 阳跷脉
统│     │
  │     └ 十二经别 ─ 从十二经脉别出的经脉，有加强十二经脉中相为表里的
  │                 两经之间联系的作用
  │
  │     ┌ 十五别络 ─ 十二经脉及任、督各分出一支别络，再加脾之大络，有加
  │     │          强十二经脉表里两经在体表的联系和渗灌气血的作用
  ├ 络脉┤
  │     │ 孙络 ─ 细小的络脉
  │     └ 浮络 ─ 浮现于体表的络脉
  │
  ├ 十二经筋 ─ 十二经脉之气结、聚、散、络于筋肉、关节的体系。有联缀四肢百骸，
  │           主司关节运动的作用
  │
  └ 十二皮部 ─ 十二经脉的功能活动反映于体表的部位
```

图 5-1　经络系统图

的属络关系,相互之间也无表里关系,故称为"奇经"。

十二经别是从十二经脉别出的经脉,它们分别起自四肢,循行于体腔脏腑深部,上出于颈项浅部。阳经的经别从本经别出而循行体内后,仍回到本经;阴经的经别从本经别出而循行体内后,却与相为表里的阳经相合。十二经别的作用,主要是加强十二经脉中相为表里的两经之间的联系,还由于它通达某些正经未循行到的器官与形体部位,因而能补正经之不足。

除此之外,并有无数络脉布满全身,络脉是经脉的分支,有别络、浮络和孙络之分。别络是较大的和主要的络脉,有本经别走邻经之意。十二经脉与督脉、任脉各有一支别络,再加上脾之大络,合为"十五别络"。别络的主要功能是加强相为表里的两条经脉之间在体表的联系,通达某些正经所没有到达的部位,可补正经之不足,还具有统领一身阴阳诸络的作用。浮络是循行于人体浅表部位而常浮现的络脉。其分布广泛,没有定位,起着沟通经脉,输达肌表的作用。孙络是最细小的络脉,属络脉的再分支,分布全身,难以计数。

经筋和皮部,是十二经脉与筋肉和体表的连属部分。人体的经筋是十二经脉之气"结、聚、散、络"于筋肉、关节的体系,是十二经脉的附属部分,有联缀四肢百骸、主司关节运动的作用。全身的皮肤,是十二经脉的功能活动反映于体表的部位,也是经络之气的散布所在,所以,把全身皮肤分为十二个部分,分属于十二经,称"十二皮部"。

以上十二经脉、奇经八脉、十二经别、别络、孙络、浮络及经络所连属的经筋、皮部等,共同组成经络系统(见图5-1),成为不可分割的整体。

5.2 十二经脉

十二经脉是经络系统的核心部分。经络系统的十二经别以及络脉等都是从十二经脉中分出,彼此联系,相互配合而协同发挥作用的。

5.2.1 十二经脉的名称

十二经脉即手三阴经(肺、心包、心)、手三阳经(大肠、三焦、小肠)、足三阳经(胃、胆、膀胱)、足三阴经(脾、肝、肾)的总称。它们是经络系统的主体,故又称为"正经"。十二经脉对称地分布于人体的两侧,分别循行于上肢或下肢的内侧或外侧,每一经脉又分别隶属于一脏或一腑,因此十二经脉的名称各不相同。十二经脉中每一经脉的命名是根据脏腑、手足、阴阳而定的,它们分别隶属于十二脏腑,各经都用其所属脏腑的名称,结合循行于手足、内外、前后的不同部位,根据阴阳学说而给予不同名称,并根据阴阳衍化的道理分为三阴三阳,定出了手太阴肺经、手阳明大肠经等十二经脉名称。

具体来说,行于上肢,起于或止于手的经脉,称"手经";行于下肢,起于或止于足的经脉,称"足经"。分布于四肢内侧面的经脉,属"阴经";分布于四肢外侧面的经脉,属"阳经"。阴经隶属于脏,阳经隶属于腑。按照阴阳的三分法,阴分为三阴:太阴、厥阴、少阴;阳分为三阳:阳明、少阳、太阳。胸中三脏,肺为太阴,心包为厥阴,心为少阴,其经脉皆行于上肢,故肺经称为手太阴经,心包经称为手厥阴经,心经称为手少阴经,并依次分布于上肢内侧的前、中、后线;与此三脏相表里的大肠、三焦和小肠,则分属阳明、少阳和太阳,其经脉分别称为手阳明经、手少阳经和手太阳经,并依次分布于上肢外侧的前、中、后线。腹中三脏,脾为太阴,肝为厥阴,肾为少阴,其经脉皆行于下肢,故分别称为足太阴经、足厥阴经和足少阴经,并依次分布于下肢内侧的前、中、后线(在下肢内踝尖上8寸以下,足厥阴经在前缘,足太阴经在中线);与此三脏相表里的胃、胆和膀胱,则分属阳明、少阳和太阳,其经脉分别称为足阳明经、足少阳经和足太阳经,依次分布于下肢外侧的前、中、后线(表5-1)。

表5-1 十二经脉名称分类表

	阴经(属脏)	阳经(属腑)	循行部位(阴经行内侧,阳经行外侧)	
手	太阴肺经	阳明大肠经	上肢	前缘
	厥阴心包经	少阳三焦经		中线
	少阴心经	太阳小肠经		后缘
足	太阴脾经*	阳明胃经	下肢	前缘
	厥阴肝经*	少阳胆经		中线
	少阴肾经	太阳膀胱经		后缘

* 在小腿下半部和足背部,肝经在前缘,脾经在中线。在内踝尖上8寸处交叉后,脾经在前缘,肝经在中线。

5.2.2 走向、交接、分布、表里关系及流注次序

5.2.2.1 走向与交接规律

十二经脉的手三阴经,从胸腔内脏走向手指端,与手三阳经交会;手三阳经,从手指走向头面部,与足三阳经交会;足三阳经,从头面部走向足趾端,与足三阴经交会;足三阴经,从足趾走向腹部和胸部,在胸部内脏与手三阴经交会。如此,手经交于手,足经交于足,阳经交于头,阴经交于胸腹内脏,十二经脉就构成了"阴阳相贯,如环无端"的循环路径(图5-2)。

十二经脉的交接有三种方式:

其一,相为表里的阴经与阳经在四肢末端交接。相为表里的阴经与阳经共6对,都在四肢末端交接。其中相为表里的手三阴经与手三阳经交接在上肢末端(手指),相为表里的足三阳经和足三阴经交接在下肢末端(足趾)。如手太阴肺经和手阳明大肠经在示指端交接,手少阴心经和手太阳小肠经在小指端交接,手厥阴心包经和手少阳三焦经在无名指端交接;足阳明胃经和足太阴脾经在足大趾交接,足太阳膀胱经和足少阴肾经在足小趾交接,足少阳胆经和足厥阴肝经在足大趾爪甲后交接。

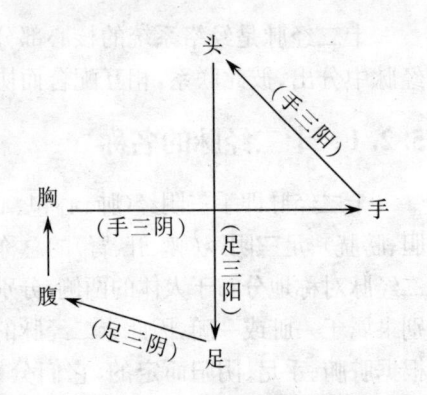

图5-2 十二经脉走向交接规律示意图

其二,同名手足阳经在头面部交接。同名的手足阳经有3对,都在头面部交接。如手阳明大肠经与足阳明胃经交接于鼻翼旁,手太阳小肠经与足太阳膀胱经交接于

目内眦,手少阳三焦经与足少阳胆经交接于目外眦。

其三,足手阴经在胸部交接。足手阴经,又称"异名经",也有3对,交接部位皆在胸部内脏。如足太阴脾经与手少阴心经交接于心中;足少阴肾经与手厥阴心包经交接于胸中;足厥阴肝经与手太阴肺经交接于肺中。

5.2.2.2 分布与表里关系

十二经脉在体内的分布虽有迂回曲折、交错出入的状况,但基本上是纵行的。除足阳明胃经外,阴经均行于四肢内侧及躯干的胸腹面,阳经均行于四肢外侧及躯干的背面。手经行于上肢;足经行于下肢。十二经脉在身体不同部位的分布特点如下:

在四肢部,阴经分布在内侧面,阳经分布在外侧面,内侧分三阴,外侧分三阳。上肢内侧为太阴在前,厥阴在中,少阴在后;上肢外侧为阳明在前,少阳在中,太阳在后;下肢内侧,内踝尖上8寸以下为厥阴在前,太阴在中,少阴在后;内踝尖上8寸以上则太阴在前,厥阴在中,少阴在后;下肢外侧为阳明在前,少阳在中,太阳在后。在头面部,阳明经行于面部、其中足阳明经行于额部;太阳经行于面颊部、头顶及头后部;少阳经行于头侧部。诸阴经并不都是皆到颈部、胸中而还,其中手少阴心经、足厥阴肝经均上达目系,足厥阴肝经与督脉会于头顶部,足少阴肾经上抵舌根,足太阴脾经连舌本、散舌下,均行达头面之深部或巅顶。在躯干部,手三阳经行于肩胛部;足三阳经则阳明经行于前(胸、腹面);太阳经行于后(背面);少阳经行于侧面。手三阴经均从腋下走出,足三阴经均行于腹面。循行于腹面的经脉,自内向外的顺序为足少阴、足阳明、足太阴、足厥阴。另外,十二经脉循行于躯干胸腹面、背面及头面、四肢,均是左右对称地分布于人体两侧,每侧十二条。左右两侧经脉除特殊情况外(如手阳明大肠经在头面部走向对侧),一般不走向对侧,相为表里的阴阳两经在体内与脏腑相互属络。

十二经脉通过经别和别络互相沟通,组合成6对表里相合关系。即手太阳小肠经与手少阴心经相表里,手少阳三焦经与手厥阴心包经相表里,手阳明大肠经与手太阴肺经相表里,足太阳膀胱经与足少阴肾经相表里,足少阳胆经与足厥阴肝经相表里,足阳明胃经与足太阴脾经相表里。相为表里的两条经脉,都在四肢末端交接,都分别循行于四肢内外两个侧面的相对位置(足厥阴肝经与足太阴脾经在下肢内踝上8寸处交叉后,变换前后位置;足太阴在前缘,足厥阴在中线),分别络属于相为表里的脏腑。

十二经脉的表里关系,不仅加强了表里两经的联系,而且使相为表里的脏腑在生理上得以相互配合,在病理上亦相互影响,如肺经受邪影响大肠腑气不通而便秘,心火亢盛循经下移小肠而见尿痛、尿赤等;在治疗上,根据表里经的经气互相沟通的原理,相为表里的两条经脉的腧穴可交叉使用,如肺经的穴位可用以治疗大肠或大肠经的疾病。

5.2.2.3 流注次序

十二经脉是气血运行的主要通道,它们首尾相贯、依次衔接,因而脉中气血的运行也是循经脉依次传注的。由于全身气血皆由脾胃运化的水谷之精化生,故十二经脉气血的流注从起于中焦的手太阴肺经开始,依次传至足厥阴肝经,然后再传手太阴肺经,首尾相贯,如环无端。其流注次序如下(图5-3):

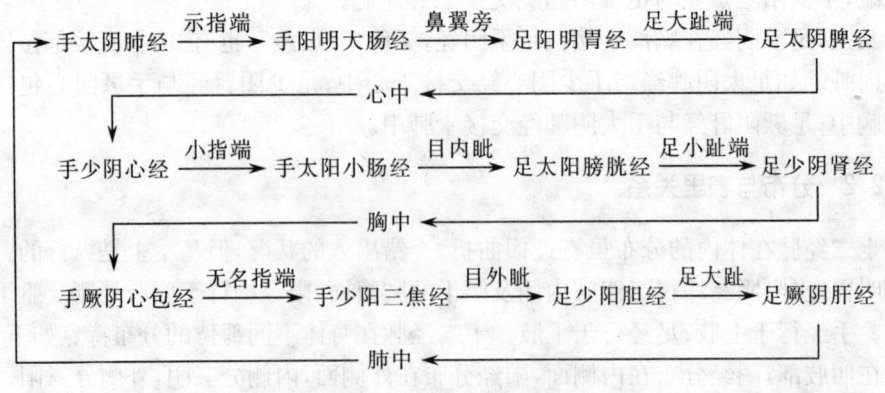

图 5-3 十二经脉流注次序图

5.2.3 十二经脉的循行

5.2.3.1 手太阴肺经

起于中焦,下络大肠,还循胃口(下口幽门,上口贲门),通过横膈,属肺,至喉部,横行至胸部外上方(中府穴),出腋下,沿上肢内侧前缘下行,过肘窝,入寸口,上鱼际,直出拇指之端(少商穴)。

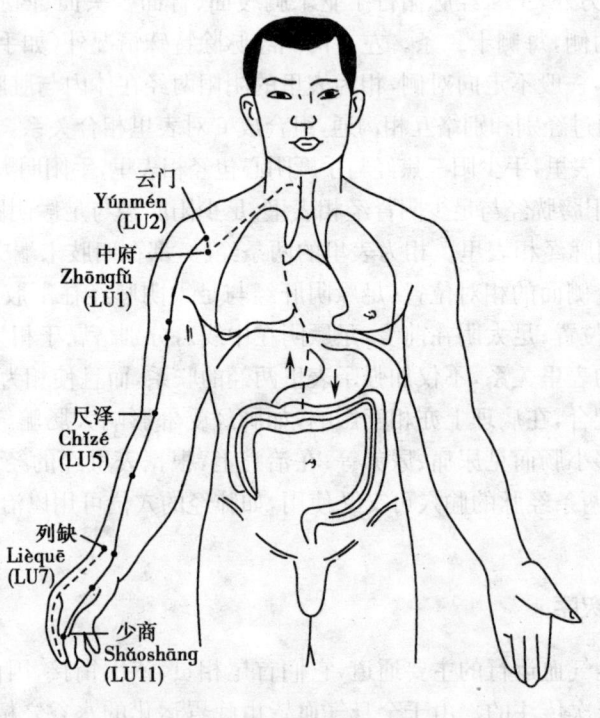

图 5-4 手太阴肺经示意图

Fig. 5-4 The Lung Meridian of Hand Taiyin

分支：从手腕的后方(列缺穴)分出，沿掌背侧走向食指桡侧端(商阳穴)，交于手阳明大肠经(图 5-4)。

5.2.3.2 手阳明大肠经

起于食指桡侧端(商阳穴)，经过手背行于上肢伸侧前缘，上肩，至肩关节前缘，向后到第七颈椎棘突下(大椎穴)，再向前下行入锁骨上窝(缺盆)，进入胸腔络肺，向下通过横膈下行，属大肠。

分支：从锁骨上窝上行，经颈部至面颊，入下齿中，回出挟口两旁，左右交叉于人中，到对侧鼻翼旁(迎香穴)，交于足阳明胃经(图 5-5)。

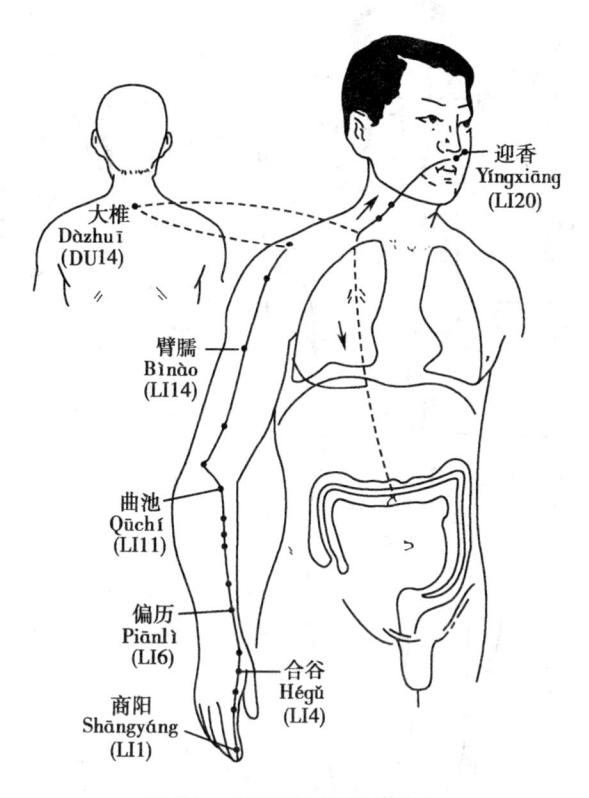

图 5-5　手阳明大肠经示意图
Fig. 5-5　The Large Intestine Meridian of Hand Yangming

5.2.3.3 足阳明胃经

起于鼻翼旁(迎香穴)，夹鼻上行，左右侧交会于鼻根部，旁行入目内眦，与足太阳经相交，向下沿鼻柱外侧，入上齿中，还出夹口两旁，环绕嘴唇，在颏唇沟承浆穴处左右相交，退回沿下颌骨后下缘到大迎穴处，沿下颌角上行过耳前，经过上关穴(客主人)，沿发际，到额前。

分支：从大迎穴前方下行到人迎穴，沿喉咙向下后行至大椎穴，折向前行，入缺盆，深入体腔，下行穿过横膈，属胃，络脾。

直行者：从缺盆出体表，沿乳中线下行，夹脐两旁，下行至腹股沟处的气街穴。

分支：从胃下口幽门处分出，沿腹腔内下行到气街穴，与直行之脉会合，尔后下行大腿前侧，至膝膑，沿下肢胫骨前缘下行至足背，入足第二趾外侧端（厉兑穴）。

分支：从膝下3寸处（足三里穴）分出，下行入中趾外侧端。

分支：从足背上冲阳穴分出，前行入足大趾内侧端（隐白穴），交于足太阴脾经（图5-6）。

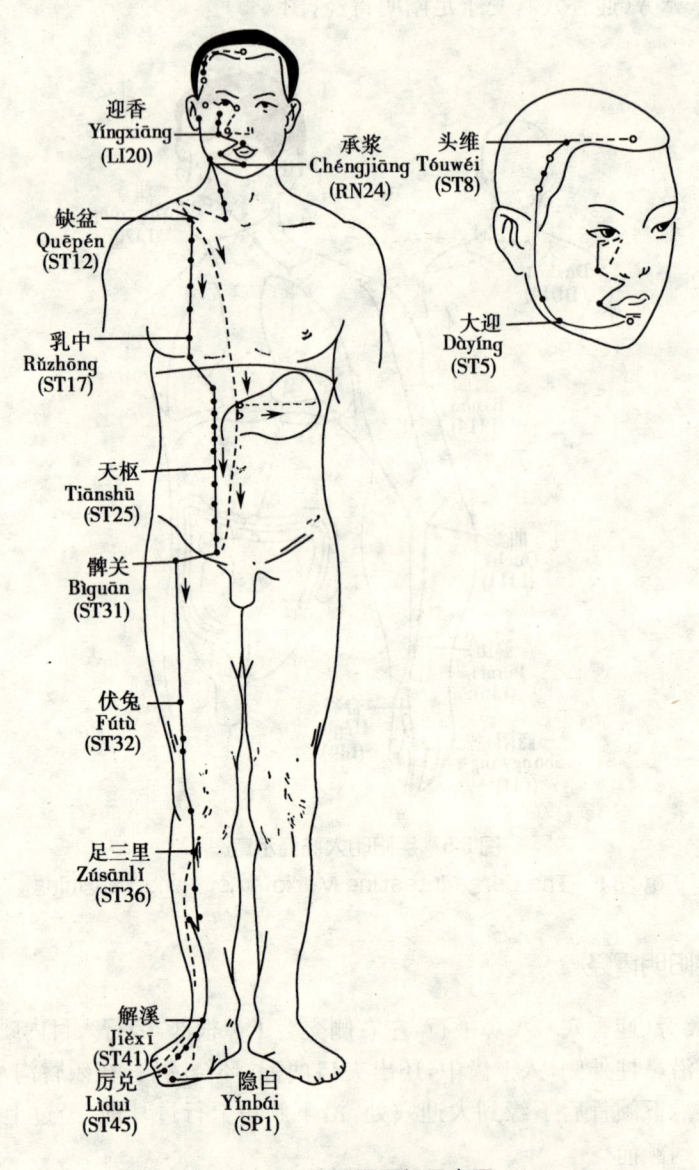

图 5-6 足阳明胃经示意图

Fig. 5-6 The Stomach Meridian of foot Yangming

5.2.3.4 足太阴脾经

起于足大趾内侧端(隐白穴),沿内侧赤白肉际,上行过内踝的前缘,沿小腿内侧正中线上行,在内踝上8寸处,交出足厥阴肝经之前,上行沿大腿内侧前缘,进入腹部,属脾,络胃。向上穿过横膈,沿食道两旁,连舌本,散舌下。

分支:从胃别出,上行通过横膈,注入心中,交于手少阴心经(图5-7)。

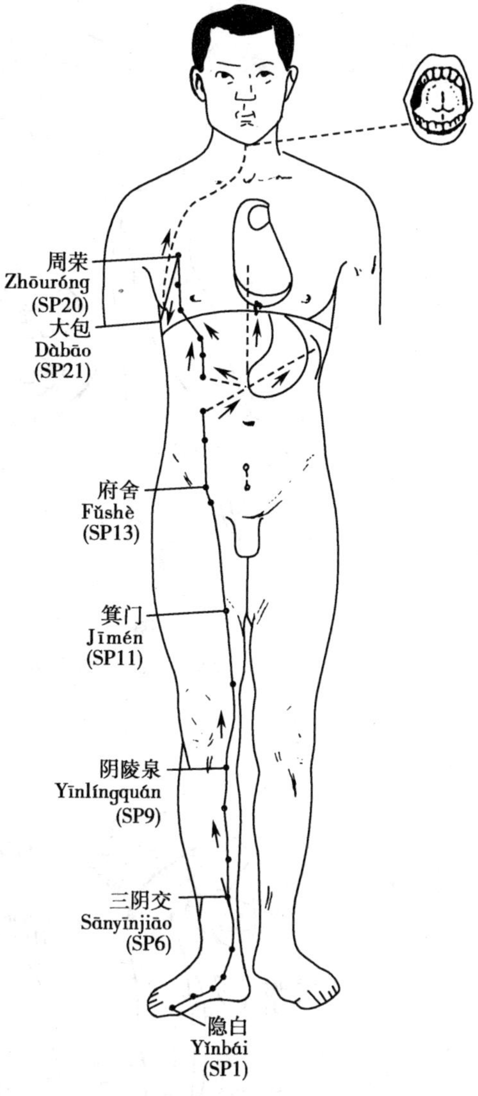

5.2.3.5 手少阴心经

起于心中,走出后属心系,向下穿过横膈,络小肠。

分支:从心系分出,夹食道上行,连于目系。

直行者:从心系出来,退回上行经过肺,向下浅出腋下(极泉穴)沿上肢内侧后缘,过肘中,经掌后锐骨端,进入掌中,沿小指桡侧,出小指桡侧端(少冲穴),交于手太阳小肠经(图5-8)。

5.2.3.6 手太阳小肠经

起于小指外侧端(少泽穴),沿手背、上肢外侧后缘,过肘部,到肩关节后面,绕肩胛部,交肩上,前行入缺盆,深入体腔,络心,沿食道,穿过横膈,到达胃部,下行,属小肠。

分支:从缺盆出来,沿颈部上行到面颊,至目外眦后,退行进入至听宫穴。

分支:从面颊部分出,上向颧骨,至目内眦(睛明穴),交于足太阳膀胱经(图5-9)。

5.2.3.7 足太阳膀胱经

起于目内眦(睛明穴),向上到达额部,左右交会于头顶部(百会穴)。

分支:从头顶部(百会穴)分出,到耳上角部。

直行者:从头顶部分别向后行至枕骨处,进入颅腔,络脑,回出分别下行到项部(天

图 5-7 足太阴脾经示意图
Fig. 5-7 The Spleen Meridian of Foot Taiyin

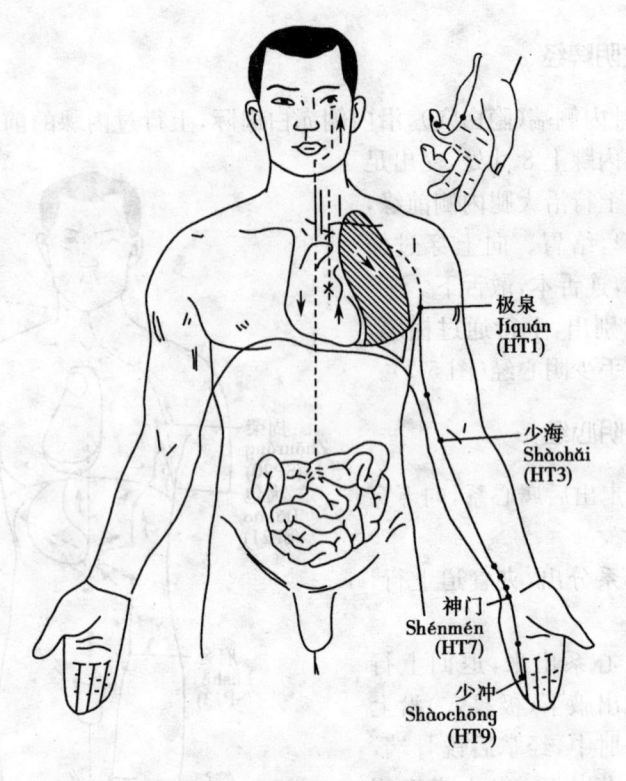

图 5-8 手少阴心经示意图
Fig. 5-8 The Heart Meridian of Hand Shaoyin

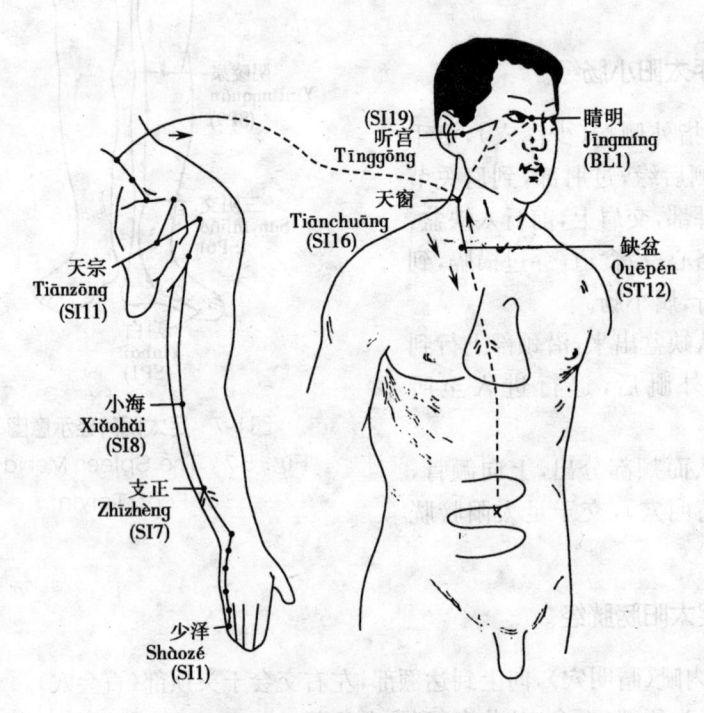

图 5-9 手太阳小肠经示意图
Fig. 5-9 The Small Intestine Meridian of Hand Taiyang

柱穴),下行交会于大椎穴,再分左右沿肩胛内侧,脊柱两旁(1.5寸),到达腰部(肾俞穴),进入脊柱两旁的肌肉(膂),深入体腔,络肾,属膀胱。

分支:从腰部分出,沿脊柱两旁下行,穿过臀部,从大腿后侧外缘下行至腘窝中(委中穴)。

分支:从项分出下行,经肩胛内侧,从附分穴夹脊(3寸)下行至髀枢,经大腿后侧至腘窝中与前一支脉会合,然后下行穿过腓肠肌,出走于足外踝后,沿足背外侧缘至小趾外侧端(至阴穴),交于足少阴肾经(图5-10)。

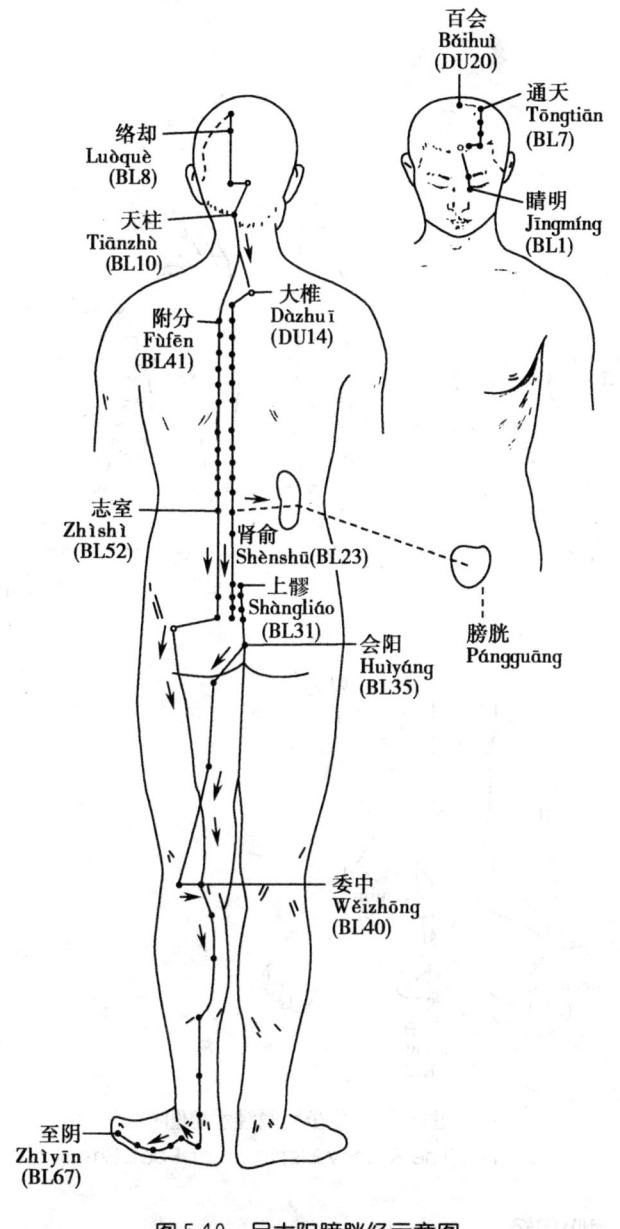

图 5-10　足太阳膀胱经示意图

Fig. 5-10　The Bladder Meridian of Foot Taiyang

5.2.3.8 足少阴肾经

起于足小趾下,斜行于足心(涌泉穴),出行于舟骨粗隆之下,沿内踝后,分出进入足跟,向上沿小腿内侧后缘,至腘内侧,上股内侧后缘入脊内(长强穴),穿过脊柱,属肾,络膀胱。

直行者:从肾上行,穿过肝和横膈,进入肺,沿喉咙,到舌根两旁。

分支:从肺中分出,络心,注于胸中,交于手厥阴心包经(图5-11)。

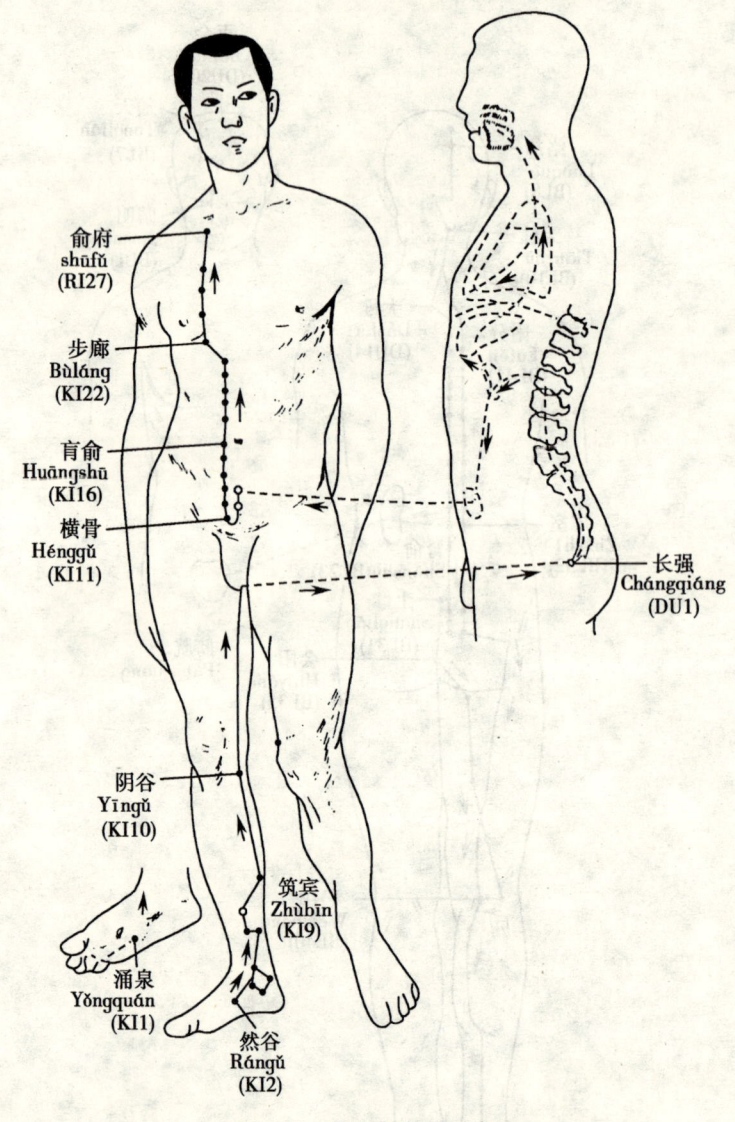

图 5-11 足少阴肾经示意图

Fig. 5-11 The Kidney Meridian of Foot Shaoyin

5.2.3.9 手厥阴心包经

起于胸中,出属心包络,向下穿过横膈,依次络于上、中、下三焦。

分支:从胸中分出,沿胸浅出胁部当腋下3寸处(天池穴),向上至腋窝下,沿上肢内侧中线入肘,过腕部,入掌中(劳宫穴),沿中指桡侧,出中指桡侧端(中冲穴)。

分支:从掌中分出,沿无名指出其尺侧端(关冲穴)。交于手少阳三焦经(图5-12)。

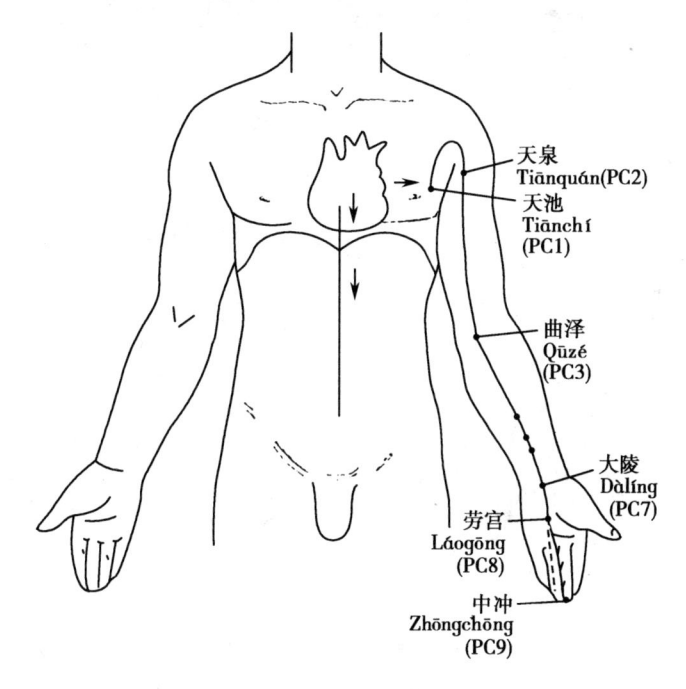

图 5-12　手厥阴心包经示意图
Fig. 5-12　The Pericardium Meridian of Hand Jueyin

5.2.3.10　手少阳三焦经

起于无名指尺侧端(关冲穴),向上沿无名指尺侧至手腕背面,上行尺骨、桡骨之间,通过肘尖,沿上臂外侧向上至肩部,向前行入缺盆,布于膻中,散络心包,穿过横膈,依次属上、中、下三焦。

分支:从膻中分出,上行出缺盆,至肩部,左右交会于大椎穴,上行到项,沿耳后(翳风穴),直上出耳上角,然后屈曲向下经面颊部至目眶下。

分支:从耳后分出,进入耳中,出走耳前,经上关穴前,在面颊部与前一分支相交,至目外眦(瞳子髎穴),交于足少阳胆经(图5-13)。

5.2.3.11　足少阳胆经

起于目外眦(瞳子髎穴),上至头角(颔厌穴)。再向下到耳后(完骨穴),再折向上行,经额部至眉上(阳白穴),又向后折至风池穴,沿颈下行至肩上,左右交会于大椎穴,前行入缺盆。

分支:从耳后进入耳中,出走于耳前,至目外眦后方。

分支:从目外眦(瞳子髎穴)分出,下行至大迎穴,与手少阳经分布于面颊部的支

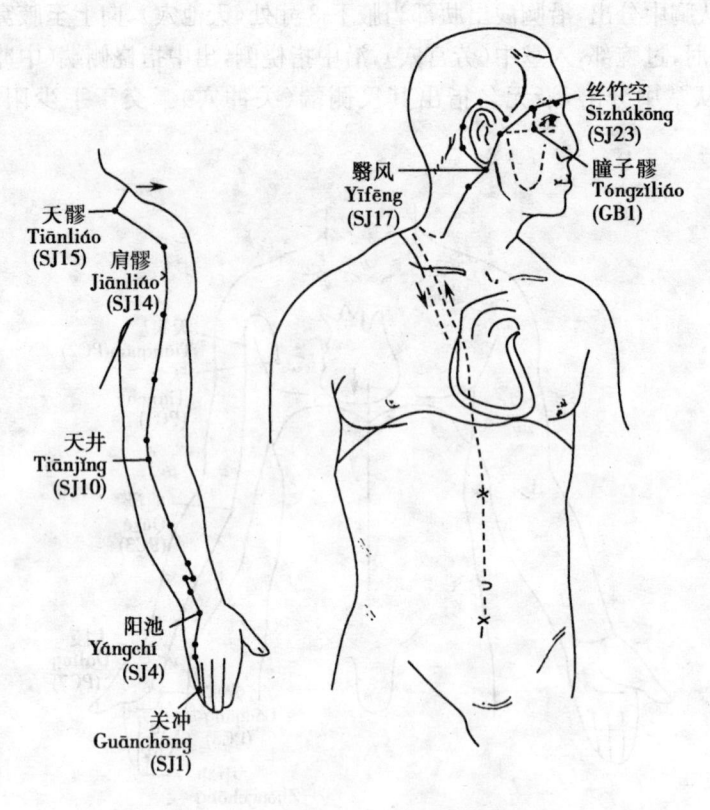

图5-13 手少阳三焦经示意图
Fig. 5-13 The Tri-Jiao Meridian of Hand Shaoyang

脉相合,行至目眶下,向下经过下颌角部下行至颈部,与前脉会合于缺盆后,进入体腔,穿过横膈,络肝,属胆,沿胁里浅出气街,绕毛际,横向至环跳穴处。

直行者:从缺盆下行至腋,沿胸侧,过季肋,下行至环跳穴处与前脉会合,再向下沿大腿外侧、膝关节外缘,行于腓骨前面,直下至腓骨下端,浅出外踝之前,沿足背行出于足第四趾外侧端(足窍阴穴)。

分支:从足背(足临泣穴)分出,前行出足大趾外侧端,折回穿过爪甲,分布于足大趾爪甲后丛毛处,交于足厥阴肝经(图5-14)。

5.2.3.12 足厥阴肝经

起于足大趾爪甲后丛毛处,向上沿足背至内踝前1寸处(中封穴),向上沿胫骨内缘,在内踝上8寸处交出足太阴脾经之后,上行过膝内侧,沿大腿内侧中线进入阴毛中,绕阴器,至小腹,夹胃两旁,属肝,络胆,向上穿过横膈,分布于胁肋部,沿喉咙的后边,向上进入鼻咽部,上行连接目系,出于额,上行与督脉会于头项部。

分支:从目系分出,下行于颊里,环绕在口唇的里边。

分支:从肝分出,穿过横膈,向上注入肺,交于手太阴肺经(图5-15)。

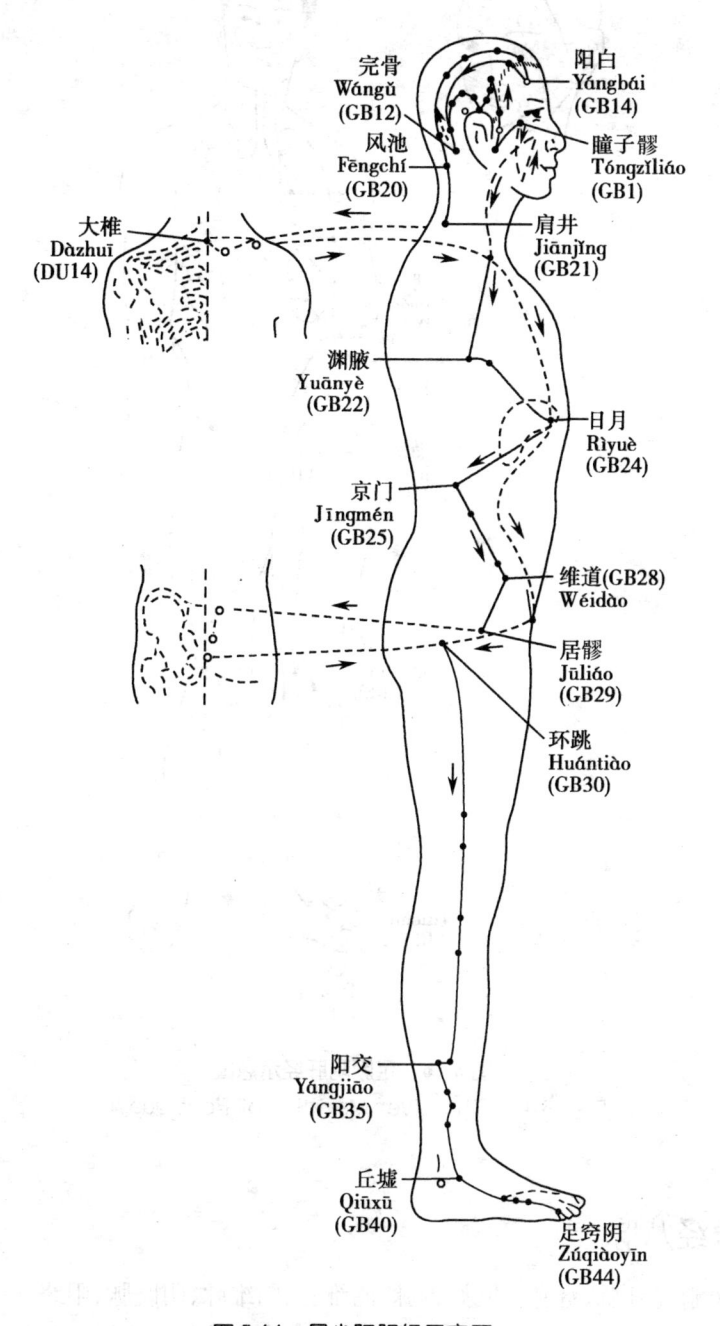

图 5-14 足少阳胆经示意图

Fig. 5-14 The Callbladder Meridian of Foot Shaoyang

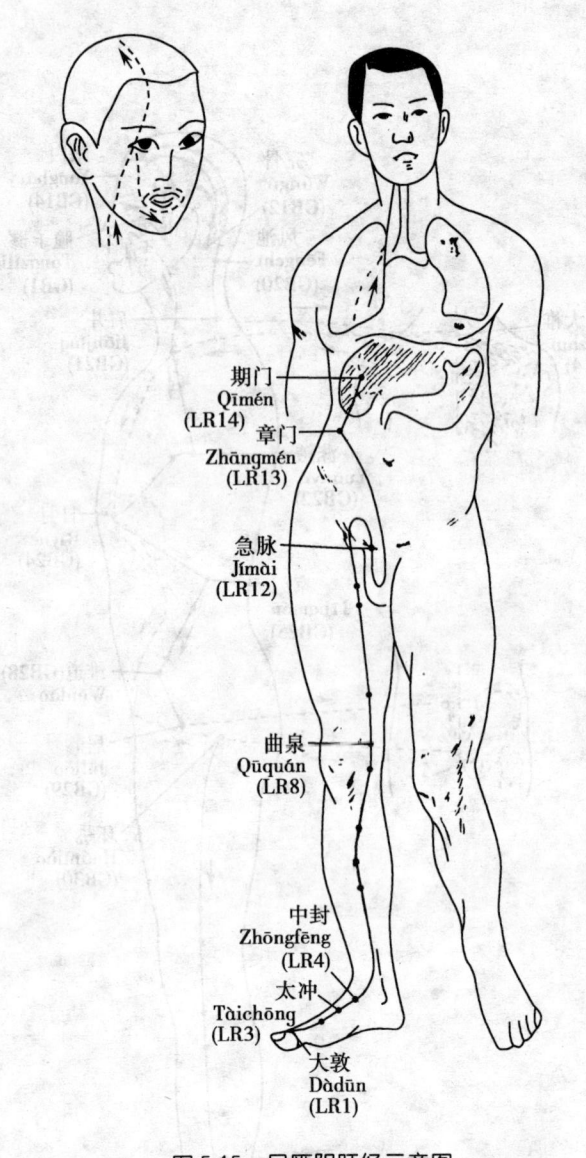

图 5-15　足厥阴肝经示意图
Fig. 5-15　The Liver Meridian of Foot Jueyin

5.3 奇经八脉

奇经八脉是任脉、督脉、冲脉、带脉、阴维脉、阳维脉、阴跷脉、阳跷脉的总称,由于它们的分布不像十二经脉那样规则,与脏腑没有直接的相互络属,相互之间也没有表里关系,与十二正经不同,故称奇经。又因其数有八,故曰"奇经八脉"。

八脉中,任脉行于人体前正中线;督脉行于人体后正中线;冲脉行腹部、下肢及脊柱前;带脉横行腰部;阴维脉行于下肢内侧、腹部和颈部;阳维脉行于下肢外侧、肩和头项;阴跷脉行于下肢内侧、腹胸及头目;阳跷脉行于下肢外侧、腹部、胸后及肩、头部。其中除带脉外,多自下而上行,上肢没有奇经的分布,对内与脏腑没有直接的属络关系,但与脑、女子胞等联系较为密切。此外,八脉之间不存在表里关系,每一条脉的循行不像十二正经那样存在必然的左右对称关系。其中,任脉、督脉、带脉都只有一条而单行。

奇经八脉纵横交叉于十二经脉之间,具有加强经脉之间的联系、调节正经气血的作用。奇经八脉的功能主要表现于以下几方面:

——密切十二经脉的联系:奇经八脉在循行分布过程中,不但与十二经脉交叉相接,加强十二经脉间的联系,补充十二经脉在循行分布上的不足,而且对十二经脉的联系还起到分类组合的作用。如督脉与手足六阳经交会于大椎穴而称"阳脉之海";任脉与足三阴经交会于关元穴,而足三阴又接手三阴经,故任脉因联系手足六阴经而称"阴脉之海";冲脉通行上下前后,渗灌三阴三阳,有"十二经脉之海"之称;带脉约束纵行诸经,沟通腰腹部的经脉;阳维脉维络诸阳,联络所有阳经而与督脉相合,阴维脉维络诸阴,联络所有阴经而与任脉相会;阳跷脉与阴跷脉左右成对,有"分主一身左右阴阳"之说。

——调节十二经脉气血:奇经八脉虽然除任、督外不参与十四经气血循环,但具有涵蓄和调节十二经气血的功能。当十二经脉气血满溢时,就会流入奇经八脉,蓄以备用;当十二经脉气血不足时,奇经中所涵蓄的气血则溢出给予补充,以保持十二经脉气血的相对恒定状态,有利于维持机体生理功能的需要。这正是古人将正经比作"沟渠",将奇经比作"湖泽"的涵义。可见,奇经八脉对十二经气血的涵蓄和调节是双向性的,既能蓄入也能溢出。

——与某此脏腑关系密切:奇经八脉虽然不似十二经脉那样与脏腑有直接的属络关系,但它在循行分布过程中与脑、髓、女子胞以及肾等有较为密切的联系。如督脉的"入颅络脑"、"行脊中"以及"属肾";任、督、冲三脉,同起于胞中,相互交通等。

5.3.1 督脉

(1) 循行部位:起于胞中,下出会阴,沿脊柱里面上行,至项后风府穴处进入颅内,络脑,并由项沿头部正中线,经头顶、额部、鼻部、上唇,到上唇系带处。

分支:从脊柱里面分出,属肾。

分支:从小腹内部直上,贯脐中央,上贯心,到喉部,再向上到下颌部,环绕口唇。向上至两眼下部的中央(图5-16)。

(2) 功能:督脉的"督"字,有总督、督促的含义。督脉循身之背,背为阳,说明督脉对全身阳经脉气有统率、督促的作用。故有"总督诸阳"和"阳脉之海"的说法。因为督脉循行于背部正中线,它的脉气多与手足三阳经相交会,大椎是其集中点。另外,带脉出于第二腰椎,阳维脉交会于风府、哑门,所以,督脉的脉气与各阳经都有联系。又因为督脉行于脊里,入络于脑,与脑和脊髓有密切的关系。经脉的神气活动与脑有密切关系。体腔内的脏腑通过足太阳膀胱经背部的腧穴受督脉经气的支配,因此,脏腑的功能活动均与督脉有关。而且,督脉又"属肾",故与肾也有密切关系。肾为先天之本,主生殖,所以历代医家多认为精冷不育等生殖系统疾患与督脉有关,常以补督脉之法治之。

图 5-16　督脉示意图

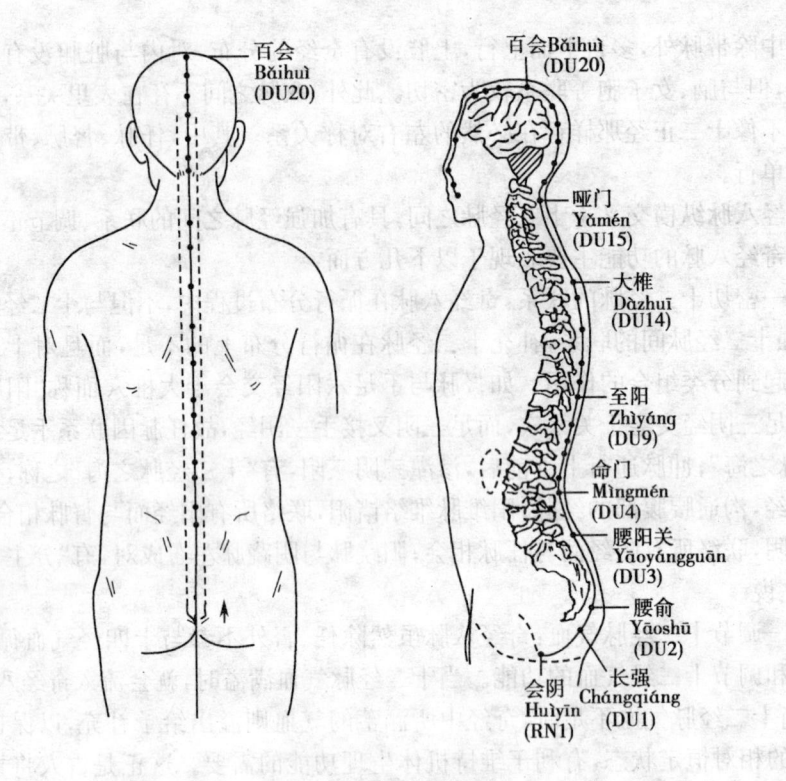

Fig. 5-16　Du Meridian

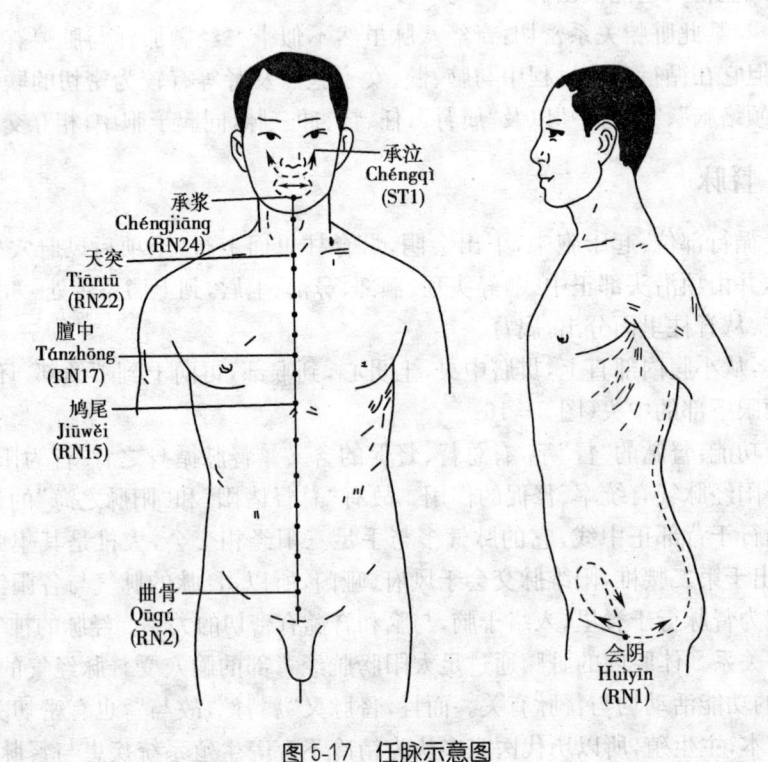

图 5-17　任脉示意图

Fig. 5-17　Ren Meridian

5.3.2 任脉

(1) 循行部位:起于胞中,下出会阴,经阴阜,沿腹部和胸部正中线上行,至咽喉,上行至下颌部,环绕口唇,沿面颊,分行至目眶下。

分支:由胞中别出,与冲脉相并,行于脊柱前。(图5-17)

(2) 功能:任脉的"任"字,有担任,妊养的含义。任脉循行于腹部正中,腹为阴,说明任脉对全身阴经脉气有总揽、总任的作用,故有"总任诸阴"和"阴脉之海"的说法。其脉气与手足各阴经相交会。足三阴经与任脉交会于中极、关元,阴维脉与任脉交会于天突、廉泉,又冲脉与任脉交会于阴交。足三阴脉上交于手三阴经。因此,任脉联系了所有阴经。任脉起于胞中,与女子月经来潮及生殖功能有关,称"任主胞胎"。

5.3.3 冲脉

(1) 循行部位:起于胞中,下出会阴后,从气街部起与足少阴经相并,夹脐上行,散布于胸中,再向上行,经喉,环绕口唇,到目眶下。

分支:从气街部浅出体表,沿大腿内侧进入腘窝,再沿胫骨内缘,下行到足底;又有支脉从内踝后分出,向前斜入足背,进入大足趾。

分支:从胞中分出,向后与督脉相通,上行于脊柱内。

(2) 功能:冲脉的"冲"字,含有要冲、要道的意思。冲脉上至于头,下至于足,后行于背,前布于胸腹,贯穿全身,成为气血的要冲,能调节十二经气血。且上行者,行于脊内渗之于阳;下行者,行于下肢渗之于阴,能容纳和调节十二经脉及五脏六腑之气血,故有"十二经脉之海"和"五脏六腑之海"之称。另一方面,女子月经来潮及孕育功能,皆以血为基础。冲脉起于胞中,分布广泛,为"血海",因此女子月经来潮及妊娠与冲脉盛衰密切相关。只有当冲任二脉通畅、气血旺盛时,其血才能下注于胞中,或泻出为月经,或妊娠时以养胚胎。若冲任气血不足或通行不利,则会发生月经不调、绝经或不孕。因此,临床上治月经病及不孕症,多以调理冲任二脉为要。

5.3.4 带脉

(1) 循行部位 起于季胁,斜向下行到带脉穴,绕身一周。在腹面的带脉下垂到少腹。

(2) 功能 带脉的"带"字,含有束带的意思。因其横行于腰腹之间,统束经过腰腹间的纵行经脉,状如束带,故称带脉。十二正经与奇经八脉多为上下纵行,唯有带脉环腰一周,有总束诸脉的功能。带脉约束相关经脉,以调节脉气,使之通畅。另一方面,带脉又主司妇女带下,因带脉亏虚,不能约束经脉,多见妇女带下量多、腰酸无力等症。

5.3.5 阴跷脉、阳跷脉

(1) 循行部位:跷脉左右成对。阴跷脉、阳跷脉均起于足踝下。

阴跷脉从内踝下照海穴分出,沿内踝后直上下肢内侧,沿前阴,沿腹、胸进入缺盆,出行于人迎穴之前,经鼻旁,到目内眦,与手足太阳经、阳跷脉会合。

阳跷脉从外踝下申脉穴分出,沿外踝后上行,经腹部,沿胸部后外侧,经肩部、颈外侧,上夹口角,到达目内眦,与手足太阳经、阴跷脉会合,再上行进入发际,向下到达耳后,与足少阳胆经会于项后。

(2) 功能:跷脉的"跷"字有足跟和矫捷的含意。因跷脉起于足踝下,从下肢内、外侧上行头面,具有交通一身阴阳之气和调节肢体肌肉运动的功能,故能使下肢灵活矫捷。又由于阴阳跷脉交会于目内眦,入属于脑,阳跷主一身左右之阳,阴跷主一身左右之阴,故还有濡养眼目、司眼睑开合和下肢运动的功能。

5.3.6 阴维脉、阳维脉

(1) 循行部位:阴维脉起于小腿内侧足三阴经交会之处,沿下肢内侧上行,至腹部,与足太阴脾经同行,到胁部,与足厥阴经相合,然后上行至咽喉,与任脉相会。

阳维脉起于外踝下,与足少阳胆经并行,沿下肢外侧向上,经躯干部后外侧,从腋后上肩,经颈部、耳后,前行到额部,分布于头侧及项后,与督脉会合。

(2) 功能:维脉的"维"字,含有维系、维络的意思。维脉的主要功能是维系全身经脉。由于阴维脉在循行过程中与足三阴经相交会,并最后合于任脉,故有维系、联络全身阴经的作用;阳维脉在循行过程中与手足三阳经相交,并最后合于督脉,故有维系、联络全身阳经的作用。在正常情况下,阴阳维脉互相维系,对气血盛衰起调节溢蓄的作用,而不参与环流。

附:经别、别络、经筋、皮部

(1) 经别:经别是别行的正经。十二经别是从十二正经别出,循行于胸腹及头部的重要支脉。

分部规律 十二经别各自从同名正经在四肢肘膝以上别出(称"离")后,深入胸腹(称"入"),然后在头项部浅出体表(称"出"),阳经经别合于同名正经;阴经经别合于相表里的阳经(称"合")。每一对相为表里的经别组成"一合",共为"六合"。

生理功能 十二经别加强了十二经脉中相为表里两经在体内的联系,加强了脏腑之间的联系,使十二经脉与人体各部分的联系更趋周密,扩大了十二经脉腧穴的主治范围。

(2) 别络:别络是络脉中较大者。十二经脉和任督二脉各别出一络,加上脾的一条大络,共计十五条,称"十五别络"(若再加胃之大络,则称"十六别络")。别络统摄、主导着浮于表浅的"浮络"和细小的"孙络"。

分布规律 十二经脉的别络在本经四肢肘膝关节以下等部位分出后,均走向与其相为表里的相应正经,与其络通。任脉的别络从鸠尾穴分出后,散布于腹部;督脉别络从长强穴分出后,散布头部;脾之大络从大包穴分出后,散布于胸胁。

生理功能 十二正经的别络,加强了互为表里两经之间在体表的联系;在所有别络的参与下,加强了人的前后、侧面等的联系,使人成为一个密切关联的整体;统率所有络脉,形成密布的网络,以渗灌气血,濡养全身组织。

(3) 经筋:经筋是十二经脉连属于经筋(肌腱、韧带)、肌肉和关节的体系,是十二经脉与外周联系的部分。其功能有赖于经络气血的濡养和调节。

分布规律 十二经筋的分布与十二经脉的体表循行基本一致,其循行分布一般都在浅部,从四肢末端走向头身,行于体表,结聚于关节、骨骼部。通常不入内脏。

生理功能 经筋能约束骨骼,有利于关节屈伸运动。

(4) 皮部:皮部是十二经脉功能反映于体表的部位,也是该正经及所属络脉之气散布的区域。

分布规律 皮部的分布,是以十二经脉在体表的循行路线分布区域范围的。

生理功能 皮部的功能同于皮肤。具有保护机体,抵御外邪的功能。皮部可用于诊断,并且是实施治疗的部位所在。

5.4 经络的生理功能

经络的功能活动,称为"经气"。其生理功能对于维持人体正常的生命活动起着非常重要的作用,现分述如下:

5.4.1 沟通上下表里,联系全身各部

人体是由五脏六腑、四肢百骸、五官九窍、皮肉筋骨等组成的,它们虽各有不同的生理功能,但又共同进行着有机的整体活动,使机体内外、上下保持协调统一,构成一个有机的整体。这种有机配合、相互联系,主要是依靠经络的沟通、联络而实现的。由于十二经脉及其分支的纵横交错,入里出表,通上达下,相互属络于脏腑;奇经八脉联系沟通于十二正经;十二经筋、十二皮部联络筋脉皮肉,从而使人体的各个脏腑组织器官有机的联系起来,构成了一个表里、上下彼此间紧密联系,协调共济的统一体。经络在人体内所发挥的沟通联系作用是多方位、多层次的,主要表现为以下几个方面:

脏腑与体表肢节的联系,主要是通过十二经脉的沟通作用来实现的。十二经脉对内与脏腑发生特定的属络关系,对外联络筋肉、关节和皮肤,即十二经筋与十二皮部。十二经脉的内属外连把外周体表的筋肉、皮肤组织及肢节等与内在脏腑相互沟通。

脏腑与官窍之间的联系,也是通过经络的沟通作用而实现的。十二经脉内属于脏腑,在循行分布过程中,又经过口眼耳鼻舌及二阴等官窍。十二经脉与耳、目、舌等官窍有非常密切的联系。又如手阳明"夹口",足阳明"夹口环唇",足厥阴"环唇内",手阳明"夹鼻孔"等,使得内在脏腑通过经络与官窍相互沟通而成为一个整体。

脏腑之间的联系,也与经络的沟通联系密切相关。十二经脉中,每一经都分别属络一脏和一腑,这是脏腑相合理论的主要结构基础。如手太阴经属肺络大肠,手阳明经属大肠络肺等。某些经脉除属络特定内脏外,还联系多个脏腑。如足少阴肾经,不但属肾络膀胱,还贯肝,入肺,络心,注胸中接心包;此外,还有经别补正经之不足,如足阳明、足少阳及足太阳的经别都通过心。这样,就构成了脏腑之间的多种联系。

经络系统各部分之间,也存在着密切联系。十二经脉有一定的衔接和流注规律,除了依次首尾相接如环无端外,还有许多交叉和交会。如手足阳经与督脉会于大椎,手少阴经与足厥阴经皆连目系等。十二经脉之中,无论表里经、同名经和异名经之间,都存在着经脉相互贯通,内部气血相互交流的关系,尤以表里经更为突出。十二

经别、十二别络也从内外加强了表里经之间的联系,十二经脉和奇经八脉之间也是纵横交错相互联系的。奇经八脉除与十二经脉多处交叉相连外,其本身也自有联系。如阴维脉与冲脉会于任脉,冲脉与任脉并于胸中,又向后与督脉通等,都体现出奇经间的关联。

5.4.2 运行气血,濡养全身

人体的各个脏腑组织器官均需要气血的温养濡润,以发挥其正常作用。气血是人体生命活动的物质基础,必须依赖经络的传注,才能输布周身,以温养濡润全身各脏腑组织器官,维持机体的正常功能,如营气之和调于五脏,洒陈于六腑,为五脏藏精、六腑传化的功能活动提供了物质条件。所以说经脉具有运行气血,调节阴阳和濡养全身的作用。

5.4.3 感应传导

人的生命活动是一个极其复杂的过程,机体中每时每刻都有许多生命信息的发出、交换和传递。这就必须依赖经络系统的感应传导作用,进行生命信息的传递,沟通各部分之间的联系。当人体的某一部位受到刺激时,这个刺激就可沿着经脉传入体内有关脏腑,使其发生相应的生理或病理变化。而这些变化,又可通过经络反映于体表。针刺中的"得气"、"行气",就是经络感应、传导功能的具体体现。内脏功能活动或病理变化的信息,亦可由经络系统传达于体表,反映出不同的症状和体征。

5.4.4 调节机体平衡

经络在正常情况下能运行气血和协调阴阳,在疾病情况下,出现气血不和及阴阳偏胜偏衰时,即可运用针灸等治法以激发经络的调节作用,以泻其有余,补其不足,调节机体,维持平衡。实验证明,针刺有关经脉穴位,可以对脏腑功能产生调整作用,而且在病理情况下尤为明显。如针刺足阳明胃经的足三里穴,可调节胃的蠕动与分泌功能。当胃的功能低下时给予轻刺激,可使胃的收缩加强,胃液浓度增加;当胃处于亢奋状态时给予重刺激,则可引起抑制性效应。又如针刺手厥阴心包经的内关穴,既可使心动加速,在某些情况下,又可抑制心动,故该穴在临床上既可治心动过缓,又可治心动过速。可见,经络的调节作用可表现出"适应原样效应",即原来亢奋的,可通过它的调节使之抑制;原来抑制的,又可通过它的调节而使之兴奋。这是一种良性的双向调节作用,在针灸、推拿等疗法中具有重要意义。

5.5 经络学说在中医学中的应用

5.5.1 说明病理变化

在正常生理情况下,经络有运行气血和感应传导的作用。而在发生病变时,经络就成为传递病邪和反映病变的途径。

由于经络内属于脏腑,外布于肌表,因此当体表受到病邪侵袭时,可通过经络由表入里,由浅及深,逐次向里传变甚至波及脏腑。经络是外邪从皮毛腠理内传于脏腑的途径。如外邪侵袭肌表,初见发热恶寒、头身疼痛等,因肺合皮毛,表邪不解,久之则内传于肺,出现咳嗽、胸闷、胸痛等症状。肺经和大肠经相互络属,故而又可伴有腹痛、腹泻或大便燥结等大肠病变。

由于内在脏腑与外在形体、官窍之间,通过经络密切相连,故脏腑病变可通过经络的传导反映于外。临床上可用经络学说阐释五脏六腑病变所出现的体表特定部位或相应官窍的症状和体征,并可用"以表知里"的思维方法诊察疾病。如足厥阴肝经绕阴器,抵小腹,布胁肋,上连目系,故肝气郁结可见两胁及少腹痛,肝火上炎易见两目红赤,肝经湿热多见阴部潮湿、瘙痒等。

脏腑病变的相互传变,亦可用经络理论来解释。由于脏腑之间有经脉相互联系,所以某一脏腑的病变可以通过经络影响到另一脏腑。如足厥阴肝经属肝,夹胃,故肝病可以影响到胃,又"注肺中",所以肝火又可犯肺;足少阴肾经"入肺"、"络心",所以肾水泛滥,可以"凌心"、"射肺";足太阴脾经"注心中",脾失健运则心血不充。

5.5.2 指导疾病的诊断和治疗

5.5.2.1 指导辨证归经

由于经络有一定的循行路线和脏腑络属,它可以反映所属脏腑的病证,因而在临床上,就可以根据疾病所出现的症状,结合经络循行的路线及所联系的脏腑,作为辨证归经的依据。例如,两胁疼痛,多为肝胆疾病;缺盆中痛,常是肺的病变。又如头痛一症,痛在前额者,多与阳明经有关;痛在两侧者,多与少阳经有关;痛在后头部及项部者,多与太阳经有关;痛在巅顶者,多与厥阴经有关。此外,某些疾病的过程中常发现在经络循行路线上,或在经气聚集的某些穴位上,有明显的压痛、结节、条索状等反应物和皮肤形态变化、皮肤温度、电阻改变等,也有助于对疾病的诊断。如肠痈患者,有时在足阳明胃经的上巨虚穴出现压痛;真心痛发生时往往在胸前左乳下有疼痛,甚至痛连左手臂及小指;脾胃病变时脾俞穴往往有异常变化;月经不调或遗精时多有横骨压痛;长期消化不良的病人,有时可在脾俞穴见到异常变化。临床上采用循经诊察,扪穴诊察,经络电测定等方法检查有关经络、腧穴的变化,可作诊断参考。

经络学说在疾病诊断中还有多方面的应用,如络脉诊察,观察小儿指纹、耳壳视诊等,均以经络学说为其理论基础。通过经络诊察,还有助于判断疾病的寒热虚实性质。

5.5.2.2 指导临床治疗

经络学说被广泛用于指导临床各科疾病的治疗,是针灸、推拿、药物疗法、针刺麻醉以及耳针的理论基础。经络能够通行气血,联系五脏六腑四肢百骸,传导信息,同时也是病邪转移的通道。我们可以利用经络的这些特性,用针灸、药物、激光、超声波等多种方式刺激腧穴,以达到调理经络、脏腑气血阴阳,达到驱邪扶正的治疗目的。

腧穴是人体气血转输交会的地方，又是病邪侵入脏腑经络的门户。所以刺激穴位可以治疗脏腑经络的疾病，因而可以认为，经络是发挥药物性能，感受机械、声、光、电、磁等刺激的通路。针灸作用大多不是直接针对致病因子、病变组织，主要是通过调节体内失衡的阴阳等功能而实现的，是一种既可纠正异常的功能状态，又不会干扰正常的生理功能的治疗方式。

针灸治病是通过刺灸腧穴，以疏通经气，恢复调节人体脏腑气血的功能，从而达到治病的目的。根据经络在人体分布上呈密切联系的网状结构，所以针灸在治疗学中也呈整体性特点。即刺灸腧穴可在不同水平上同时对机体多个器官、系统的正常或异常的功能产生影响。例如在采用针刺麻醉下的手术过程中，针刺在产生镇痛效应的同时，还具有对有关系统的功能实施多方面的调节，因而术中血压、脉搏等可维持稳定，同时术后切口疼痛程度减轻、感染等并发症减少、术后恢复加快。针灸的调节作用也呈现出双向性特征，即在刺灸相同腧穴施用相同术式的条件下，可望对相反方向偏离的功能产生反向性的调节作用。例如糖尿病性膀胱病变导致的尿潴留和压力性尿失禁均出现膀胱逼尿肌与尿道括约肌之间协调功能失常，前者由于高血糖引起支配膀胱逼尿肌的副交感神经受损，导致膀胱逼尿肌收缩无力，尿道括约肌功能相对亢进；后者则相反，系各种原因导致盆底肌肉松弛，尿道括约肌收缩功能减弱，膀胱逼尿肌功能相对亢进。针灸治疗一般能有效地纠正膀胱逼尿肌与尿道括约肌间协调功能的失调，使收缩无力者得到增强，同时使亢进者受到抑制。这些都是经络学说在针灸治疗方面的体现。

药物治疗也是以经络为渠道，通过经络的传导转输，才能使药到病除，发挥其治疗作用。通过长期、反复的实践，医家们发现药物的四气五味、升降浮沉等理论，与经络学说的关系也是十分密切，某一种中药对某一经脉及其所属的脏腑的病证，具有选择性的治疗作用，从而创立了"药物归经"理论。十二经病候，按经脉脏腑对寒热虚实证候做了提示性归纳，使四气的运用有章可循，五味理论也是在经络、脏腑理论的指导下，通过临床实践，对药物治疗规律的一种概括。另外经络理论也是药物升降浮沉理论形成的主要依据。

在临床中，仅用四气五味、升降浮沉的药物理论还不能详细地指导临床用药。各个脏腑经络的疾病，对药物还有特殊的要求和选择。比如同样是寒证，但有肺寒、胃寒等不同；同样是热证，也有肺热、胃热等不同。能祛肺寒的药物不一定能祛胃寒，能清肺热的药物不一定能清胃热。利用归经理论就能把药物的特殊功效更加细微地反应出来，从而更准确地指导临床上对复杂多变的疾病进行治疗。如黄连泻心火，黄芩泻肺火、大肠火，柴胡泻肝胆火、三焦火，白芍泻脾火，知母泻肾火，木通泻小肠火，石膏泻胃火。归经理论的产生促使引经报使药的实际应用。引经，即某些药物能引其他药物选择性地治疗某种脏腑经络的病证。报使则略同药引，因方剂不同而分别选用。常用药引如以酒为引者，取其活血引经；以姜为引者，取其发表祛寒；以大枣为引者，取其补血健脾；以龙眼肉为引者，取其宁心；以灯心草为引者，取其安睡宁神；以葱白为引者，取其发散诸邪；以莲子心为引者，取其清心养胃和脾。归经理论使得药物运用更为灵活多变，总结了临床用药的一些特殊规律。

经络学说是指导方剂组成的主要理论之一。如交泰丸，由黄连、肉桂组成，如仅从药性分析,黄连苦寒,属清热泻火药,主要功效是泻火解毒,清热燥湿;肉桂性味辛甘,大热,属祛寒药,主要功效是温肾壮阳,温中祛寒。但由于黄连入心、脾、胃经,能清心以泻上亢之火,肉桂入肾、肝、脾经,配之能引火归原,故黄连、肉桂合用能交通心肾,治疗心肾不交的失眠证。又如治疗水肿,因肺、脾、肾三脏发生病变时均能产生水肿,根据水肿的病因病机,分别选用归脾经的白术,归肾经的猪苓,归肺经的通草,正确地指明了对同一病证病因病机不同的用药方法。又如,同是脾(气)虚下陷的脱肛、子宫下垂、胃下垂等不同疾病,则均可以选用归脾经的人参、白术、黄芪、升麻等药,按方剂组方原则配伍成方进行治疗。方剂的临证加减,经络学说也起着指导性作用,如在治疗头痛的方剂中,可按经络分布部位而随证加减。太阳头痛则用羌活,少阴头痛则用细辛,阳明头痛则用白芷,厥阴头痛则用川芎、吴茱萸,少阳头痛则用柴胡。总之,不论是药物配伍的变化,或药物、药量的加减,都要按病情的需要来加减化裁,又必须以经络理论为指导,才能变化得当,执简驭繁地治疗复杂的病证。

思考题

- 经络系统是由哪几部分组成的?
- 十二经脉的走向交接规律如何?
- 十二经脉的流注次序如何?
- 经络的生理功能表现在哪些方面?
- 何谓奇经八脉?其生理功能如何?

6 体质学说

体质是指人类个体在生命过程中,由遗传性和获得性因素所决定的,形态结构、生理功能以及心理活动等方面相对稳定的综合特性。体质学说是以中医基本理论为指导,研究人类体质的含义、形成、特征、类型、差异规律,及其对疾病发生、发展和演变过程的影响,并用以指导临床诊断和疾病防治的学说。体质学说认为,体质不仅是在生理状态下对外界刺激的反应和适应上的某些差异性,而且还是机体发病的内部要因,它不仅决定着对于某些致病因素的易感性,而且决定着某些疾病的证候类型。因此,重视对体质的研究,不但有助于从整体上把握个体生命特征,而且有助于分析疾病的发生、发展和演变规律,对于诊断、治疗及养生、预防和康复等均具有重要的指导意义。

6.1 体质的形成

6.1.1 体质的生理基础

人体有脏腑经络、形体官窍等组织器官,由精、气、血、津液等基本物质构成并维持正常的生命活动。通过人体组织器官所体现出来的体质差异,实际上是内在脏腑气血阴阳之偏倾和功能活动之差异的反映。换言之,脏腑经络及精气血津液是体质形成的生理学基础。研究体质,实际上就是从差异性方面研究人体的脏腑经络及精气血津液。脏腑是构成人体并维持人体生命活动的中心,人的各项生理活动均离不开脏腑,所以,体质的差异是以脏腑为中心反映出构成人体诸要素的某些或全部素质特征的。

(1) 体质与脏腑经络:脏腑形态和功能特点是构成并决定体质差异的最根本因素。在个体先天遗传因素与后天环境因素相互作用下,不同个体常表现出某一藏象系统的相对优势或劣势化的倾向。

五脏之中以肾、脾两脏在决定人的体质方面所起的作用较为明显。在先天禀赋基础上,体质的强弱取决于肾的盛衰。先天肾精充足,是出生后能够健康成长,获得较强生命活力的先决条件。若先天肾精不足,不但生长发育迟缓,而且容易罹患疾病。人的生长发育及衰老过程,实际上是以肾中精气为基本物质激发推动脏腑活动的演变过程。人在生命过程各个阶段的表现,即充分体现了不同年龄阶段所形成的体质差异,这些差异实际上就是肾中精气盛衰变化的结果。肾的盛衰会导致其他内脏也随之而产生变化,从而出现相应的形体、功能和心理的改变。

在体质形成的后天因素中,以脾胃最为关键。饮食是否相宜,直接影响脾胃的功能。同样,脾胃运纳功能是否协调,更关系到人体营养的优劣,因而对体质的影响极大。所以体质的强弱,往往与脾胃功能的盛衰相一致。其有先天禀赋不足者,得后天水谷之补养,尚可弥补;反之,虽有先天的基础,而无后天的充养,则形体也难以康健。

经络内属于脏腑,外络于肢节,是体内气血运行的通路。体质不仅取决于脏腑功能活动的强弱,还有赖于脏腑功能活动的协调,经络正是这种沟通并协调脏腑功能的结构基础。脏居于内,形现于外。体质主要通过外部形态特征表现出来,不同个体的脏腑阴阳的盛衰及经络气血的多少不同,表现于外的征象也呈现出了差异性。

(2)体质与精气血津液:精气血津液是决定体质特征的重要物质基础。精气血津液是脏腑生理活动的产物,通过经络的传输而布散周身,作为脏腑官窍功能活动的物质基础,维持着正常的生命活动。精气的盛衰、气血的多少、津液的盈亏以及布散运行状况等决定着体质的强弱,并影响着体质的类型。津液亏耗者易表现为"瘦削燥红质";体内水液代谢迟滞者多表现为"形胖湿腻质"。精之盈亏还多与年龄有关,老年体质的共性即为精的虚衰。

总之,脏腑经络的结构变化和功能盛衰,以及精气血津液的盈亏和布运都是决定体质的重要因素。体质将脏腑精气阴阳之偏倾通过形态、功能、心理的差异性表现出来,实际上就是脏腑经络、形体官窍固有素质的综合体现。

6.1.2 体质的构成要素

体质的构成要素主要包括形态结构、生理功能以及心理特征三个方面,其中形态结构和生理功能的决定性尤为突出。

6.1.2.1 形态结构

在形态结构上的差异性是个体体质特征的重要组成部分,包括外部形态结构和内部形态结构。根据"司外揣内"的认知方法,内部形态结构与外观形象之间是有机的整体,外部形态结构是体质的外在表现,内部形态结构是体质的内在基础。形态结构在内部结构完好、协调的基础上,主要通过外部形态表现出来,以躯体形态为基础,并与内部脏器结构有密切的关系,所以体质特征首先表现为外部形态的差异。

外部形态亦即体表形态,是个体外观形态的特征,包括体格、体型、体重、性征、体姿、面色、毛发、舌象、脉象等。体格是指反映人体生长发育水平、营养状况和锻炼程度的状态。一般通过观察和测量身体各部分的大小、形状、匀称程度,以及体重、肩宽、胸围、骨盆宽度和皮肤与皮下软组织情况来判断,是反映体质的基本标志。体型是指身体各部位大小比例的形态特征,又称身体类型,是衡量体格的重要指标。体型观察包括形体的肥瘦高矮、皮肉的厚薄坚松、肤色的黑白苍嫩的差异等。其中尤以肥瘦最有代表性,一般而言,肥瘦与病态体质的关系是:"肥人湿多,瘦人火多。"

形态结构是生理功能的基础,个体不同的形态结构特点决定着机体生理功能及对刺激反应的差异,而机体生理功能的个性特征,又会影响其形态结构,引起一系列相应的改变。因此,生理功能上的差异也是个体体质特征的组成部分。

6.1.2.2 生理功能

人的生理功能是其内部形态结构完整性和协调性的反映,是脏腑经络及精气血津液功能正常的体现。因此,人体生理功能的差异反映着脏腑功能的偏盛与偏衰,涉及到消化、呼吸、血液循环、代谢、生长发育、生殖、感觉、运动、意识、思维等各方面功能的强弱差异。机体的防病抗病能力、新陈代谢情况、自我调节能力,以及或偏于兴奋或偏于抑制的基本状态,诸如心率、心律、面色、唇色、呼吸状况、语声的高低、食欲、口味、体温、脉象、舌象、对寒热的喜恶、二便情况、生殖功能、女子月经情况、形体的动态及活动能力、睡眠状况、视觉、听觉、触觉、嗅觉、耐痛的程度、皮肤肌肉的弹性、须发的多少和光泽等,均是脏腑经络及精气血津液生理功能的反映,是了解体质状况的重要渠道。

6.1.2.3 心理特征

心理是客观事物在大脑中的反映,包括感觉、知觉、情感、记忆、思维、性格等,属于中医学"神"的范畴。中医学认为神由形而生,依附于形而存在,形是神的物质基础和所舍之处,同时也认为神对形体具有主宰作用。因此,形神合一的人体观、生命观和医学观决定了体质之"体"包括形和神两方面的内容。体质是特定的形态结构、生理功能与相关心理状况的综合体,形态、功能、心理之间具有内在的相关性。某种特定的形态结构常表现为某种特定的心理倾向。不同的功能活动总是表现为某种特定的情感、情绪反应与认知活动。由于脏腑精气及其功能各有所别,故个体所表现的情志活动也有差异,如有人善怒,有人善悲,有人胆怯等。但应当指出的是,人的心理特征不仅与形态、功能有关,而且与个体的生活经历以及所处的社会文化环境有着重要的关系。所以即便为同种形态结构和生理功能者,也可以表现为完全不同的心理特征。一定的形态结构与生理功能是心理特征产生的基础,使个体容易表现出某种心理特征,而心理特征又反作用于形态结构与生理功能,并表现出相应的行为特征。可见,在体质构成因素中,结构、功能、心理之间有着密切的关系。

心理特征的差异性主要表现为人格、气质、性格等的差异。人格是指个体独特的、持久的心理或行为特征的综合,常决定整个心理面貌,是个体心理行为差异性、个体化的核心因素和标志。气质则有现代心理学的和中医学的区别。现代心理学中的气质是指人在进行心理活动时或在行为方式上表现出来的强度、速度、稳定性、指向性和灵活性等动态的人格心理特征。中医学中的气质是指个体出生后,随着身体的发育、生理的成熟逐渐形成的心理特征。性格在现代心理学中是指个体对现实的稳定态度和习惯化了的行为方式。

6.1.3 影响体质的因素

体质特征取决于脏腑经络、精气血津液的强弱盛衰,因此,凡能影响脏腑经络、精气血津液功能活动的因素,均可影响体质。

6.1.3.1 禀赋因素

体质的先天因素主要取决于父母。人之始生与父母的精、神、气、血密切相关,子代的一切均由父母所赋予。子代承袭了父母的某些特质,构成了自身在体质方面的基础。子代出生以前从父母所获得的一切可统称为先天禀赋。先天禀赋的状况与父母生殖之精的质量密切相关,而父母生殖之精的优劣又与父母自身的体质、父母血缘关系的远近、父母生育时的年龄、母亲妊娠以及养胎状况等诸多因素有关。

(1) 父母体质:父母体质是子代生命产生的基础。一般而言,父母体质强壮,则子代体质也多强壮;反之,父母体质羸弱,则子代也多羸弱。子代的生命来源于父母肾中精气,只有父母肾中精气充盛,子代才能获得较强的生命力,才会有较好的体质。父母肾中精气强弱与否,又是由他们的整体脏腑功能活动是否健旺决定的。若父母体质强健,脏腑气血充盛,肾精充足,此时受胎生子,其子代体质也多健壮;反之,若父母体质衰劣,脏腑气血虚少,肾精不足,即使受胎,其子代体质也多虚弱。某些遗传性疾病可由父母传给子代,在一定后天因素的诱发下,子代会发生与父母相同的疾病,如癫痫、哮喘等。

(2) 父母的血缘关系:父母血缘关系的远近也是影响子代体质的因素之一。近亲结婚的父母将会对后代产生严重的不良影响。其中一部分表现为怪胎、畸胎,另一部分则使子代出现严重的体质缺陷,或痴呆愚钝,或体弱多病。

(3) 父母的婚育年龄:父母的婚育年龄也是影响子代体质的一个因素。父母体质状况如何与其年龄有关。人体随着年龄的变化,体质也会随之发生变化,这是体质具有动态性的一个特点。因此,若要子代体质强壮,亲代应当在最佳年龄内结婚生子。一般情况下,人在青壮年时期肾中精气充盛,精力旺盛,此时生子体多健壮。若过早或过晚生育,则肾中精气不足,其子多不强壮;年老精衰,虽育但弱。

(4) 养胎及妊娠疾病:养胎是指母体自受孕至分娩期间在饮食起居、心理、劳逸等方面的调养。父母肾中精气的盛衰虽然已经决定了子代的基本遗传因素,但胎儿的发育情况则关系到父母体质优势能否得到充分体现。同时,孕期母体的健康状况不但直接影响着胎儿的生长发育,并且可能会影响其出生后的体质。

母体在妊娠期间患病,将影响胎儿的发育和子代的体质。因此,孕妇应尽量避免疾病的发生,外避六淫,不使邪气入伤胞胎,内避七情内伤及饮食失宜,使气血充盛,经脉流畅,胞胎得养。

先天因素所形成的特定体质往往是根深蒂固的,在同等后天培育条件下,人的体质强弱主要取决于先天禀赋。在小儿,先天禀赋不足,往往影响其生长发育。先天因素不足还可能会影响人的寿命。

6.1.3.2 饮食因素

饮食是人体后天营养物质的来源,对于生命活动十分重要。合理而科学的饮食习惯是维护和增强体质的重要保证。然而人们的生活条件并非一致,饮食习惯也各有差别,因而可逐渐形成不同的体质。

(1) 饥饱失常:饥饱失常是指饮食的摄入量不均衡。饮食充足者,营养良好,体多丰腴,体质较好;而饮食不足或刻意限食者,营养较差,体多羸瘦,体质偏弱。但饱食无度,过食肥甘,体虽肥硕,往往多痰,形盛气虚,体质反差;虽粗茶淡饭,尚未至饥馁,痰湿不生,气血流畅,体质反而较好。

(2) 饮食偏嗜:饮食偏嗜是指饮食的结构不合理,过分嗜好某类食物,或五味偏嗜,或寒热偏嗜,或嗜食肥甘,或贪恋醇酒。脏腑之气血阴阳依靠饮食五味阴阳和合而生。若饮食长期偏嗜,则可造成脏腑气血阴阳的偏盛偏衰,进一步可导致脏腑功能失调。在日常生活中,有人偏嗜甘甜,有人偏嗜辛辣,有人偏嗜咸酸,更有久食温热或寒凉者。嗜食甘甜者助湿生痰,易形成痰湿体质;嗜食辛辣者易化火灼津,而形成阴虚火热体质;过咸则胜血伤心,易形成心气虚弱体质。久食温热易致阴虚阳盛;常进寒凉易致阴盛阳虚;嗜食肥腻,体虽肥白,但易痰湿内盛,或化热生火;贪恋醇酒佳酿,色虽红润,湿热在中,易伤肝脾。由此可见,饮食与人的体质有很大关系。

6.1.3.3 年龄因素

人的生命进程是一个机体生长壮老已的发展变化过程。这一过程的不同阶段,人体的内脏功能活动和气血阴阳盛衰存在差异,因而同一机体的体质也会随年龄而变化。

小儿处在生长发育的早期,其体质的特点是五脏六腑成而未充,身体柔弱,易虚易实,易寒易热。但小儿毕竟生机勃勃,蒸蒸日上,体质呈渐趋加强之势,故即使有病也容易治愈。

青壮年是人体生长发育的极盛期,其形体长成,身体盛壮,脏腑完固,气血阴阳充实,生命力旺盛,胜任劳动,体质强而少病。

衰老本身就是内脏功能活动生理性衰退的结果,故老年人的体质必然日趋下降。随着年龄的递增,正常型体质越来越少,异常型体质越来越多。同时,老年人的异常体质不像青年人那样单纯,多以某种体质为主,兼夹其他体质特征。

6.1.3.4 性别因素

由于男女在遗传性征、体形、脏腑结构等方面的差别,相应的生理功能、心理特征也就有所不同,因此体质上存在着性别差异。男为阳,女为阴。相对而言,男性多禀阳刚之气,脏腑功能较强,体魄健壮,暴发力较强,性格多外向、粗犷喜动、胸襟开阔;女性多禀阴柔之气,脏腑功能较弱,体形小巧苗条,耐久力较强,性格多内向、细腻喜静、多愁善感。男子以肾为先天,以精气为本;女子以肝为先天,以阴血为本。男子多用气,故气常亏虚;女子多用血,故血常不足。男性多病气分;女性多病血分。男子之病,多由伤精耗气;女子之病,多由伤血。此外,由于妇女有经、带、胎、产、乳等特殊生理现象,所以有月经期、妊娠期和产褥期的体质改变。当月经来潮后,体内产生明显的周期性变化。妊娠期由于胎儿生长发育的需要,产褥期由于产育、哺乳等影响,母体各系统即会产生一系列适应性反应,所以有"孕妇宜凉,产后宜温"的说法。较之女性,男性体质的不足主要表现在对于病邪更为敏感,更易罹患疾病,且病变常较严重,死亡率也较高。

6.1.3.5 劳逸因素

适度的劳作或体育锻炼,可使筋骨强壮,关节滑利,气血调和,气机通畅,脏腑功能旺盛。充分的休息有利于消除疲劳,恢复体力和脑力,维持人的正常生命活动。劳逸结合有利于身心健康,并保持良好体质。过度劳作则易于损伤筋骨,消耗气血,致使脏腑精气不足,功能减弱,形成虚性体质。而过度安逸,长期养尊处优,四体不勤,则可使气血运行不畅,筋肉松弛,脾胃功能减弱,形成形胖湿腻型体质。

6.1.3.6 情志因素

情志是人对外界客观事物刺激的正常反应,是机体对自然、社会环境变化的适应调节能力。情志活动的产生和维持有赖于内在脏腑的功能活动,以脏腑气血阴阳为物质基础。情志变化可通过影响脏腑气血的变化,进而影响人的体质。所以,精神情志贵在和调。情志和调则气血调畅,脏腑功能协调,体质强壮。反之,过于强烈或持久的情志刺激,一旦超过了人的生理调节能力,就会导致脏腑气血受损或功能紊乱,给体质造成负面影响。临床常见的气郁型体质多因此而起。气郁还可聚热化火,伤阴灼液,又能导致阳热体质或阴虚体质。气滞不畅还可形成血瘀型体质。情志变化导致的体质改变,还与某些疾病的发生有特定的关系。如郁怒不解,情绪急躁的"木火质",易患眩晕、中风等;忧愁日久,郁闷寡欢的"肝郁质",易诱发瘀血、积聚等。因此,保持良好的精神状态对体质健康十分有益。

6.1.3.7 地理因素

防治疾病要"因地制宜",即考虑到不同地域人的体质是不同的。地域不同决定着水土性质、气候类型以及人们生活习惯等多方面不同。常言道:"一方水土养一方人"。地域无疑会对体质产生直接或间接的影响。

在地质发展过程中,地表元素分布逐渐形成了不均一性,这在一定程度上控制和影响着世界各地人类和动植物的生长,从而造成了生物生态的地区性差异。中国大陆幅员辽阔,各地的地理条件和气候特点的差异很大,这些因素使不同地区的人们对长期居住地产生了适应状态。不同地区的人们具有不同的生活习惯,其中尤以饮食习惯的影响力最大。不同地理区域的人群,体质结构具有明显的差异,如北方人群阳虚体质者多于南方,南方阴虚体质者多于北方,痰瘀体质则以青藏高原和东南沿海等地多见。

6.1.3.8 社会因素

一般而言,个人对社会环境是无能为力的,因而人们往往是无奈地承受着社会的某些影响。随着科学技术和工商业的发展,社会生活的城市化、个性化,人们的生活节奏相应加快,人际关系进一步复杂化,生活事件相应增多,这些都可能成为影响体质的社会因素。

(1) 经济生活:在经济生活中,过于富裕或过于贫穷都可使人们的体质下降。现代化工业飞速发展带来的严重环境污染和越来越快的生活节奏,加之丰富的物质生活伴随的不良生活方式,从身心两个方面损害着人类的健康,使人们的体质不断下降。

(2) 社会地位:由于特定的人生观和价值观,促使人们看重自己的社会地位。由于各种原因所导致的社会地位变迁,会明显影响个体的体质。

(3) 职业:不同职业决定着相应的工作环境、劳动强度、经济收入、社会地位和经济地位等,也可成为影响各种体质类型的因素之一。

(4) 战争:由战争引起的环境破坏、疾病流行和心理压力等因素常造成战区人群整体体质下降。

6.1.3.9 疾病针药和其他因素

疾病可加速体质的改变。如某些疾病所致损伤不易迅速康复,气血阴阳的损伤即可形成影响体质的因素。尤其是一些慢性消耗性和营养障碍性疾病,对体质的影响尤其明显。

一般情况下,疾病改变体质多是向不利的方向发展,如大病、久病之后,常致体质虚弱;某些慢性疾病迁延日久,易使体质表现出一定的特异性。但感染某些疾病之后,反而会使机体具有相应的免疫力,使其终生不再罹患此病。此外,疾病损害所形成的体质改变,其体质类型还会随疾病发展而转化,如慢性肝病,早期多为气滞型体质,中后期则会转化为瘀血型或阴虚型等不同类型的体质。可见,体质与疾病因素常常互为因果。

药物的性味或针灸的补泻均能调整脏腑气血阴阳的盛衰及经络气血的偏颇。用之得当可收到补偏救弊的功效;但用之不当,将会加重体质损害,形成气血阴阳的盛衰偏倾。

除以上因素外,其他可影响体质的因素还有婚育、体育锻炼等。婚育本是人类正常的生理活动,但房事和孕育均应有所节制。纵欲、多产均可损伤精气,造成体质下降或早衰而影响寿命。体育锻炼是人类主动改造体质的活动,有利于提高身体素质,促进身心健康,所以长期缺乏体育锻炼会使体质下降。

6.2 体质的分类

中医学对体质的分类,主要是根据中医基本理论来确定人群中不同个体的体质差异性。体质分类法有多种,本节分为介绍传统分类法和现代分类法予以介绍。

6.2.1 传统分类法

传统分类法有多种,这里主要介绍阴阳分类法和五行分类法。

6.2.1.1 阴阳分类法

从总体上看,健康人群应当是保持着阴阳相对平衡状态的。但就具体人来说,不同个体之间则是存在差异的。有的人体质偏阳(阳多阴少),有的人体质偏阴(阴多阳少),另有一部分人接近于阴阳平衡。体质类型的阴阳,主要是指以对立制约为主而多表现为寒热、动静偏倾的阴阳二气,其他体质常是在阴、阳偏倾体质的基础上派生、发展而成。人体正常体质大致可分为阴阳平和质、偏阳质和偏阴质三种类型。

(1)阴阳平和质:阴阳平和质是身心较为协调的体质类型。体质特征为:身体强壮,胖瘦适中;寒热皆宜;皮肤光泽,面色明润含蓄,目光有神;性格开朗、豁达宽容;食量适中,二便通调;睡眠安和,精力充沛,反应灵活,思维敏捷,工作潜力大;自我调节和适应能力较强;舌色淡红润泽,脉象和缓均匀有神。

符合阴阳平和质特征的人,不易感受外邪,较少生病。即使患病,也多为表证、实证,且病情较轻,易于治愈,康复也快,常会不治自愈。如果后天调养得宜,无意外伤害及不良嗜好,其体质稳定,不易改变,多能长寿。

(2)偏阳质:偏阳质是指具有亢奋、偏热、多动等特性的体质类型。体质特征为:形体适中或偏瘦,但较结实;面色偏红或微苍黑,或皮肤油亮;性格外向,喜动好强,容易急躁,自制力偏差;食量较大,消化吸收健旺;大便易干,小便易赤;平时畏热喜凉,或体温偏高,动则易汗,喜饮凉水;精力充沛,动作敏捷,反应灵敏,性欲旺盛;唇舌偏红,舌苔薄黄,脉多偏数。

符合偏阳质特征的人,对风、暑、燥、热等阳邪有较强的易感性。感邪后常形成热证、实证,且易化燥伤阴;内伤多见火旺、阳亢或兼阴虚之证,如眩晕、头痛、心悸、失眠以及出血等;皮肉易生痤痱、痈疽、疔疖、热疮等。由于偏阳质者阳气偏亢,多动少静,所以日久会有耗阴之虞。若调养不当,操劳过度,思虑不节,纵欲失精,嗜食烟酒或辛辣炙煿,则必将加速阴伤,发展为阳亢、阴虚、痰火等病理性体质。

(3)偏阴质:偏阴质是指具有抑制、偏寒、沉静等特性的体质类型。体质特征为:形体适中或偏胖,但较虚弱,容易疲劳;面色偏白而少华;性格内向,喜静少动,或胆小易惊;食量偏少,消化吸收一般或较弱;平时畏寒喜暖,或体温偏低;精力不足,动作迟缓,反应较慢,性欲冷淡;唇舌色淡,舌胖齿痕,脉多迟弱。

符合偏阴质特征的人,对寒、湿等阴邪有较强的易感性。受邪后多表现为寒证、虚证,表邪易传里或寒邪直中脏腑;内伤多见阴盛、阳虚之证,如湿滞、水肿、泄泻、痰饮、瘀血等;冬季易生冻疮。由于偏阴质者阳气偏弱,长期发展易致阳气虚弱,脏腑功能偏弱,水湿内生,从而形成阳虚、痰湿、水饮等病理性体质。

应当指出,在体质分类上所使用的偏阳、偏阴、阳亢、阴盛以及痰饮、瘀血等术语,与证候名称既有区别又有联系。证候是对疾病某一阶段或某一类型的病变本质的分析和概括,而体质反映的是一种在生理范围内存在的个体特异性。由于体质是疾病发生和演变的内部因素,所以体质类型与其证候类型又具有内在的相关性。

6.2.1.2 五行分类法

五行分类法是根据人的肤色、体形、禀性、态度以及适应能力等方面的特征,归纳总结出木、火、土、金、水五种不同的体质类型。

(1)木型之人:木型之人的体质特征为:皮肤色苍,头小脸长,肩部宽阔,腰背挺直,身材弱小,手脚灵活;干练有才,好用心机,体力不强,多忧善虑,做事勤勉;对季节变化,比较喜欢春夏的温暖,难于忍受秋冬的寒冷,如感受寒湿之邪则容易生病。

(2)火型之人:火型之人的体质特征为:皮肤色赤,头小脸尖,脊背宽厚,身材匀称,手足小,步履稳重,行走摇肩,背肌丰满;洞察力强,思维敏捷,重义轻财,缺乏自信,多虑喜忧,爱好漂亮,性情急躁;对季节变化,比较喜欢春夏的温暖,难于忍受秋冬的寒冷,如感受寒湿之邪则容易生病。

（3）土型之人:土型之人的体质特征为:皮肤色黄,头大脸圆,肩背丰厚,腹大,从大腿到足胫健壮结实,手足小,肌肉丰满,身材匀称,步履稳重,走路轻盈;内心宁静,乐于助人,喜交朋友;对季节变化,比较喜欢秋冬的凉爽,难于忍受春夏的炎热,如感受温热之邪则容易生病。

（4）金型之人:金型之人的体质特征为:皮肤色白,头小脸方,肩背窄小,腹小,手足小,足跟厚壮而大,好像骨头在足跟外面似的,行动轻快,禀性清廉,性情急躁刚强,办事严肃,果断利落,善于决断;对季节变化,比较喜欢秋冬的寒冷,难于忍受春夏的炎热,如感受温热之邪则容易生病。

（5）水型之人:水型之人的体质特征为:皮肤色黑,头大面皱,颊腮清瘦,肩部窄小,腹大,手足喜动,行走身摇,上身较长,下身较短;禀性既不恭敬又无所畏惧,聪明伶俐,缺乏诚信;对季节变化,比较喜欢秋冬的凉爽,难于忍受春夏的炎热,如感受温热之邪则容易生病。

6.2.2 现代分类法

借助流行病学调研和数理统计等手段,近年来获得了较为现代的体质分类方法。该方法将现代人群的体质现状归纳为以下七种类型。

6.2.2.1 形壮亢奋质

形壮亢奋质的特征为形体较常人壮实,功能亢奋。具体表现是活泼好动,敏捷有力,身体温暖,不畏寒凉,喜冷饮食;面部易生痤疮,油性皮肤,容易脱发;性欲亢进,自制力差;代谢旺盛,消耗过多,有耗阴伤正之势,日久易演变为"身热虚亢质"。

6.2.2.2 身萎疲乏质

身萎疲乏质的特征为形体较常人虚弱,功能低下。具体表现是精神不振,不喜多动,不欲多言,易于疲乏,稍劳即倦;面色无华或萎黄,毛发少泽,既畏寒又怕热,经常感冒,病后虽少高热,但却迁延难愈;代谢低下,日久易演变为"形寒迟呆质"。

6.2.2.3 身热虚亢质

身热虚亢质的特征为形体较常人清瘦,功能虚性亢奋。具体表现是经常手足心热,手常汗出,时有阵阵升火,面部烘热潮红,口干喜冷饮;心烦易怒,急躁焦虑,情绪不宁,经常失眠,时有便秘,尿色偏深;易感受阳热病邪,患病后易于阴伤化燥,日久易演变为"瘦削燥红质"。

6.2.2.4 形寒迟呆质

形寒迟呆质的特征为形体胖瘦适中或较常人肥胖而白,功能低下。具体表现是体温偏低,四肢不温,畏寒怕冷,喜食热物,行动和反应迟缓,甚至呆顿;心率偏缓,面色苍白,唇舌紫黯,甚至灰紫,大便恒溏,极易腹痛作泻;代谢明显偏低,易感寒湿等阴邪,病后也极易寒化湿化,日久易与"身萎疲乏质"、"形胖湿腻质"和"晦黯瘀滞质"等相互转化。

6.2.2.5 形胖湿腻质

形胖湿腻质的特征为形体较常人肥白胖嫩,功能紊乱。具体表现是肢体困重,懒于活动,虽能胜任一般劳作,但反应呆顿,中年可见大腹便便;脘腹痞满,口中甜黏,不欲饮水,舌苔厚腻,易患水肿、泄泻、胸痹、中风等病;中青年妇女还常见月经不调,白带较多,甚至不孕等;易于感受寒湿之邪,患病后易损伤阳气,且从寒化湿化,日久易与"形寒迟呆质"相互转化。

6.2.2.6 瘦削燥红质

瘦削燥红质的特征是形体较常人明显瘦削,功能或偏低或虚性亢奋,液亏阴少。具体表现是肤色苍老,呈黯褐色,皮肤干涩粗糙,缺少弹性;口虽干渴,但不欲饮水;体力较差,虽欲活动却难以持久;大便艰难,数日一行,状如羊屎;唇舌黯红,少苔或无苔。此体质多由身热虚亢质发展而来。

6.2.2.7 晦黯瘀滞质

晦黯瘀滞质的特征是形体如常人或偏瘦,功能紊乱,气血瘀滞。具体表现为面色灰滞晦黯,眼眶黧黑,唇舌黯紫,指端粗大青紫;皮肤粗糙,甚至鳞状脱屑,或有红缕斑痕;常有疼痛,冬季尤甚。代谢明显障碍,患病后多迁延难愈,日久易患积聚癥瘕之类的病证。

在调查中发现上述类型以身萎疲乏质、形寒迟呆质、身热虚亢质和形胖湿腻质较为多见,尤其是年老体弱者占有较大的比例。最为普遍的是身萎疲乏质,城镇居民尤其是东部沿海城镇,形胖湿腻质居多。瘦削燥红质和晦黯瘀滞质虽较少见,但对健康的威胁反而更大。

思 考 题

- 为什么说脏腑经络及精气血津液是体质形成的生理学基础?
- 小儿、青壮年和老年人的体质特点分别是什么?
- 男女在体质上有何不同?
- 不良的饮食习惯会引起哪些体质变化?
- 劳逸和情志会对体质产生哪些影响?
- 阴阳平和质的体质特点和发病特点如何?

7 病因病机学说

人体各脏腑组织之间,以及人体与外界环境之间,它们在不断地产生矛盾而又解决矛盾的过程中,既对立又统一。维持着相对的动态平衡,从而保持着人体正常的生理活动。当这种动态平衡因某些原因而遭到破坏,又不能立即自行调节恢复时,人体就会发生疾病。

破坏人体相对平衡状态而引起疾病的原因就是病因。致病因素是多种多样的,诸如气候异常、疫疠传染、情志刺激、饮食劳倦、持重努伤、跌仆金刃外伤,以及虫兽所伤等等,均可导致疾病的发生。此外,在疾病过程中,原因和结果是相互作用的,在某一病理阶段中是病理的结果,在另一阶段中则可能成为原因,如痰饮和瘀血等,即是脏腑气血功能失调形成的病理产物,反过来又能成为造成某些病变的致病因素。

各种致病因素作用于人体,引起病变的机理就是病机,即疾病发生、发展与变化的机理。疾病是多种多样的,病变机理变化也是较为复杂的。不同的疾病,均有其相应的病理变化,如不同脏腑的病证、内伤与外感、气病与血病以及各种具体的病证,它们在病理上各有自己的特殊性,但在许多不同的致病因素引起的千差万别的各种疾病的病理变化中,却存在着共同的一般性的规律。研究并掌握这些规律,可以更深刻地把握疾病的本质,从而有效地指导辨证与治疗。

7.1 病因

导致疾病发生的原因是多种多样的,主要有六淫、疠气、七情以及饮食、劳逸等,在一定条件下都能使人发生疾病。为了说明致病因素的性质和致病特点,古代医家曾对病因做过分类。如《内经》将其分为阴阳两类。宋代陈无择提出了"三因学说",即六淫邪气外袭为外因,情志内伤为内因,饮食劳倦、跌仆金刃以及虫兽所伤等为不内外因。可以看出,这种把致病因素和发病途径相结合的分类方法,对临床辨别病证,确有一定的指导意义。

中医学认为,任何证候都是在某种因素或多种因素的影响和作用下,患病机体产生的病态反映。中医认识病因,除了解可能作为致病因素的客观条件外,主要是以病症的临床表现为依据,通过分析疾病的症状、体征来推求病因,为治疗用药提供依据,这种方法称为"审证求因"。所以,中医学的病因学,不但研究病因的性质和致病特点,同时也探讨各种致病因素所致病证的临床表现,以便更好地指导临床诊断和治疗。本章根据病因的发病途径、形成过程,将病因分为外感病因、内伤病因、病理产物以及其他病因四大类。

7.1.1 外感病因

外感病因,是指由外而入,或从肌表,或从口鼻侵入机体,引起外感疾病的致病因素。外感病是由外感病因而引起的一类疾病,一般发病较急,病初多见恶寒、发热、脉浮、骨节酸痛等。外感病因大致分为六淫和疠气两类。

7.1.1.1 六淫

六淫,即风、寒、暑、湿、燥、火六种外感病邪的统称。风、寒、暑、湿、燥、火,在正常的情况下称为"六气",是自然界六种不同的气候变化。正常的六气不至于使人生病,只有气候异常急骤的变化或人体的抵抗力下降时,六气才能成为致病因素,侵犯人体发生疾病,这种情况下的六气就称为"六淫"。淫,有太过和浸淫之意。由于六淫是不正之气,所以又称"六邪",属于发生外感病的一类病因。

六淫致病,一般具有下列几个特点:①六淫致病多与季节气候、居住环境有关。如春季多风病,夏季多暑病,长夏多湿病,秋季多燥病,冬季多寒病等。另外,久居潮湿之地常有湿邪为病,高温环境作业又常有燥热或火邪为病等等。②六淫邪气既可单独侵袭人体,又可两三种同时侵犯人体而致病。如风寒感冒,湿热泄泻,风寒湿痹等。③六淫在发病过程中,在一定条件下其证候性质可发生转化。如寒邪入里可以化热,暑湿日久可以化燥伤阴等。④六淫致病,其发病途径多侵犯肌表,或从口鼻而入,或两者同时受邪,故称之为"外感病"。

从临床实践看,除了气候因素外,六淫致病,还包括了生物(细菌、病毒等)、物理、化学等多种致病因素作用于人体所引起的病理变化。

(1) 风:风为春季的主气,但四季皆有风。故风邪致病虽春季多见,但不限于春季,其他季节亦均可发生。风邪外袭多从皮毛肌腠而入,从而产生外风病证。中医学认为风邪为外感发病的一种极为重要的致病因素。

风邪的性质和致病特点如下:①风为阳邪,其性开泄。风邪善动不居,具有升发、向上、向外的特性,故属于阳邪。其性开泄,是指易使腠理疏泄开张。正因其能升发,并善于向上向外,所以风邪侵袭常伤害人体的上部(头面)和肌表,使皮毛腠理开泄,常出现头痛、汗出、恶风等症状。②风性善行而数变。善行,是指风邪致病具有病位行无定处的特性而言。如风寒湿三气杂至而引起的"痹证",若见游走性关节疼痛,痛无定处,即属于风气偏盛的表现,故又称谓"风痹"或"行痹"。数变,是指风邪致病具有变幻无常和发病迅速的特性而言。如风疹就有皮肤瘙痒、发无定处、此起彼伏的特点。同时,由风邪为先导的外感疾病,一般发病多急,传变也较快。③风为百病之长。风邪为六淫病邪中主要的致病因素,是外邪致病的先导,其他病邪多依附于风而侵犯人体。如外感风寒、风热、风湿等。

(2) 寒:寒为冬季的主气。寒邪为病有外寒、内寒之分,外寒是指寒邪外袭,其致病又有伤寒、中寒之别。寒邪伤于肌表,郁遏卫阳,称为"伤寒",寒邪直中于里,伤及脏腑阳气,则为"中寒"。内寒则是机体阳气不足,失却温煦的病理反映。外寒与内寒虽有区别,但它们又是互相联系,互相影响的。阳虚内寒之体,容易感受外寒;而外来寒邪侵入人体,积久不散,又常能损及人体阳气,导致内寒。

寒邪的性质及致病特点如下：①寒为阴邪，易伤阳气。寒为阴气盛的表现，其性属阴，故寒邪致病，最易损伤人体阳气。如寒邪袭表，卫阳被遏，可见恶寒；寒邪直中脾胃，脾阳受损，可见脘腹冷痛、呕吐、腹泻等症。②寒性凝滞。凝滞，即凝结阻滞之意。寒邪伤人可使人之经脉气血运行不畅而出现种种疼痛。③寒性收引。收引，即收缩牵引之意。寒邪侵入人体，可使气机收敛，腠理、经络、筋脉收缩而挛急。如寒邪侵袭肌表，毛窍腠理闭塞，卫阳被郁，不得宣泄，可见恶寒、发热、无汗；寒客血脉，则气血凝滞，血脉挛缩，可见头身疼痛，脉紧；寒客经络关节，筋脉拘急收引，则见肢节屈伸不利，拘挛作痛。

（3）暑：暑为夏季的主气，乃火热所化。暑邪有明显的季节性，独见于夏季。暑邪纯属外邪，无内暑之说。

暑邪的性质及致病特点如下：①暑为阳邪，其性炎热。暑为夏季的火热之气所化，火热属阳，故暑为阳邪。暑邪伤人，多出现壮热、烦渴、面赤、脉洪等症。②暑性升散，伤津耗气。升散，即上升发散之意。暑邪伤人，易使腠理开泄而多汗。出汗过多则耗伤津液，津液亏损，即可出现口渴喜饮、尿赤短少等。在大量汗出的同时，往往气随津泄而致气虚，出现气短乏力，甚则突然昏倒、不省人事。③暑多夹湿。暑季多雨而潮湿，热蒸湿动，使空气的湿度增加，故暑邪为病，常兼夹湿邪以侵犯人体，在发热烦渴的同时，常兼见四肢困倦，胸闷呕恶，大便溏泻不爽等症。

（4）湿：湿为长夏的主气，夏秋之交，为一年中湿气最盛的季节。湿邪为病有外湿、内湿之分。外湿多由于气候潮湿、涉水淋雨、居处潮湿等外在湿邪侵袭人体所致。内湿多由于脾失健运、水湿停聚而生。外湿和内湿虽有不同，但在发病中又常相互影响。伤于外湿，湿邪困脾，脾失健运，则湿从内生；而脾阳虚损，水湿不化，亦易招致外湿的侵袭。

湿邪的性质及致病特点如下：①湿为阴邪，易伤阳气，阻遏气机。湿性重浊，其性类水，故为阴邪。其侵犯人体，最易损伤阳气。湿邪困脾，脾阳不振，运化无权，水湿停聚，发为泄泻、尿少、水肿等症。湿邪侵及人体，留滞于脏腑经络，最易阻遏气机，使其升降失常，经络阻滞不畅，出现胸闷脘痞，小便短涩，大便不爽等症。②湿性重浊趋下。重，即沉重或重着之意。常指湿邪为病，多见头身困重，四肢酸懒沉重等症状。浊，即秽浊，多指分泌物或排泄物秽浊不清而言。如面垢眵多，大便溏泻，小便浑浊，妇女白带过多，湿疹流水等病。趋下，是指湿邪为病，其症状多见于下部，如带下、淋浊、泄利等症。③湿性黏滞。黏，即黏腻；滞，即停滞。湿性黏滞主要表现在两方面：一是湿病症状多黏腻不爽，如分泌物及排泄物多滞涩而不畅；二是湿邪为病多缠绵难愈，病程较长或反复发作，如湿痹、湿疹、湿温病等。

（5）燥：燥为秋季的主气。此时气候干燥，水分亏乏，故多燥病。燥邪感染途径，多从口鼻而入，侵犯肺卫。燥邪为病又有温燥、凉燥之分：初秋有夏热之余气，燥与温热结合而侵犯人体，则多见温燥病证；深秋又有近冬之寒气，燥与寒邪结合侵犯人体，故有时亦见凉燥病证。

燥邪的性质及致病特点如下：①燥为阳邪，其性干涩，易伤津液。燥邪为干涩之病邪，故外感燥邪最易耗伤人体的津液，造成阴津亏虚的病变，而出现种种津亏干涩的症状和体征，如口鼻干燥、咽干口渴、皮肤干涩甚则皲裂、毛发不荣、小便短少、大便干结等症。②燥易伤肺。肺为娇脏，喜润而恶燥。肺主气司呼吸，外合皮毛，开窍于鼻,故燥邪伤人,多从口鼻而入,伤及肺津,影响肺的宣发肃降功能,出现干咳少痰、或痰液胶黏难咯、或痰中带血以及喘息胸痛等症。

(6) 火:火热为阳盛所生,故火热常可并称。但火与温热,同中有异,热为温之渐,火为热之极,热多属外淫,如风热、暑热、湿热之类病邪;而火常由内生,如心火上炎、肝火亢盛、胆火横逆等。

火热为病亦有内外之分,属外感者,多是直接感受温热邪气之侵袭;属内生者,则常由脏腑阴阳气血失调,阳气亢盛而成。此外,感受风、寒、暑、湿、燥等各种外邪,或精神刺激,在一定条件下皆可化火,故有"五气化火"、"五志化火"之说。

火邪的性质及致病特点如下:①火为阳邪,其性炎热。阳主躁动而向上,火热之性,燔灼焚焰,升腾上炎,故属于阳邪。因此,火热伤人,多见高热、烦渴、汗出、脉洪数等症。②火性炎上。火邪致病,症状多表现在人体的上部,如头面部位。如火热阳邪常可上炎扰乱神明,出现心烦失眠,狂躁妄动,神昏谵语等症。若心火上炎,则见舌尖红、口舌生疮;胃火炽盛,可见齿龈肿痛;肝火上炎,常见目赤肿痛。③火易伤津耗气。火邪为患,最易迫津外泄,消灼津液,耗伤阴津,故常兼有口渴喜饮、咽干舌燥、小便短赤、大便秘结等津伤症状。火邪最能损伤人体的正气,故火邪致病,还可兼见少气懒言、肢倦乏力等气衰之症。④火易生风动血。火热之邪侵袭人体,往往灼伤肝经,劫耗阴液导致"热极生风",表现为高热、神昏谵语、四肢抽搐、目睛上视、项背强直、角弓反张等。同时,火热之邪,可以加速血行,灼伤脉络,甚则迫血妄行,而致各种出血,如吐血、衄血、便血、尿血、皮肤发斑及妇女月经过多、崩漏等病证。⑤火易致肿疡。火热之邪入于血分,可聚于局部,腐蚀血肉,发为痈肿疮疡,表现为红肿热痛,甚则化脓溃烂。

此外,火与心相应,心主血而藏神,故火盛除可见血热或动血症状外,尚有火邪扰心的神志不安、烦躁、谵妄发狂或昏迷等症。

7.1.1.2 疠气

疠气,是一类具有强烈传染性的外邪。在中医文献记载中,又有"瘟疫"、"疫毒"、"戾气"、"异气"、"毒气"、"乖戾之气"等名称。

疠气致病具有发病急骤、病情较重、症状相似、传染性强、易于流行等特点。疠气病邪可通过空气或接触感染,多从口鼻侵入人体。

疠气致病既可散在发生,也可形成瘟疫流行。如大头瘟、虾蟆瘟、疫痢、白喉、烂喉丹痧、天花、霍乱、鼠疫等等,这些实际包括了现代医学中的许多传染病和烈性传染病。

疠气的发生与流行多与下列因素有关:①气候因素。自然气候的反常变化,如久旱、洪涝、酷热、湿雾瘴气等以及地震等自然灾害之后。②环境与饮食。如空气、水源或食物受到污染。③社会因素。战乱、贫穷落后、社会动荡及不良卫生习惯,现代战争中的细菌战,均可导致疠气流行。④没有及时做好预防隔离工作。

7.1.2 内伤病因

7.1.2.1 七情

七情即喜、怒、忧、思、悲、恐、惊七种情志,是机体的精神情绪状态或对客观事物的不同情志反应,在正常情况下,一般不会使人致病。只有突然、强烈或长期持久的情志刺激,超过了人体的生理活动调适范围,使人体气机紊乱,脏腑阴阳气血失调,才会导致疾病的发生,由于它是造成内伤病的主要致病因素之一,故又称"内伤七情"。

(1) 七情与内脏气血的关系:人的情志活动与内脏有密切的关系,而内脏的功能活动要靠气的推动、温煦和血的濡养。中医学认为某一内脏常与某一情志活动有关,即心在志为喜,肝在志为怒,脾在志为思,肺在志为忧,肾在志为恐。喜怒思忧恐,统称为"五志"。不同的情志变化对内脏有不同的影响,而内脏气血的变化,也会影响情志的变化。

(2) 七情的致病特点:七情致病不同于六淫。六淫侵袭人体,从皮肤及口鼻而入,发病之多见表证,而七情内伤,则直接影响相应的内脏,使脏腑气机逆乱,气血失调,导致种种病变的发生。①直接伤及内脏。怒伤肝,喜伤心,思伤脾,忧伤肺,恐伤肾。由于心主神志,为五脏六腑之大主,心神受损可涉及其他脏腑。心主血藏神,肝主疏泄藏血,脾主运化而位于中焦,是气机升降的枢纽,又为气血生化之源。故情志所伤的病证,以心、肝、脾三脏和气血失调为多见。如思虑劳神过度,常损伤心脾,导致心脾气血两虚,出现神志异常和脾失健运等证。郁怒伤肝,怒则气上,血随气逆,可出现肝经气郁的两胁胀痛、善太息等症;或气滞血瘀,出现胁痛、妇女痛经、闭经或癥瘕等病证。此外,情志内伤还常会化火,即"五志化火",而致阴虚火旺等证或导致湿、食、痰诸郁为病。②影响脏腑气机。由于导致各种情志变化的刺激因素不同,脏腑气机的变化也不一样,常表现为与各种情志相关的特殊的气机变化。即:"怒则气上,喜则气缓,悲则气消,恐则气下,惊则气乱,思则气结"。

怒则气上,是指过度愤怒可使肝气上冲,血随气逆。临床可见气逆,面红目赤,或呕血,甚则昏厥猝倒。

喜则气缓,包括缓和紧张情绪和心气涣散两个方面。在正常情况下,喜能缓和精神紧张,使营卫通利,心情舒畅。但暴喜过度,又可使心气涣散,神不守舍,出现精神不集中,甚则失神狂乱等症状。

悲(忧)则气消,是指过度悲忧,使肺气抑郁耗伤,可见意志消沉、精神委顿、少气乏力等症状。

恐则气下,是指恐惧过度,使肾气失于固摄,气泄而下,临床可见二便失禁,或因恐惧不解则伤精,而发生骨酸痿厥、遗精等症。

惊则气乱,是指突然受惊,以致心无所倚、神无所归、虑无所定、惊慌失措。

思则气结,是指思虑劳神过度,伤神损脾导致气机郁结。思虑过度不但耗伤心神,也会影响脾气。阴血暗耗,心神失养则心悸、健忘、失眠、多梦;气机郁结阻滞,脾失运化,胃的受纳腐熟失职,便会出现纳呆、脘腹胀满、便溏等症。③情志异常波动,可使病情加重,或迅速恶化。在许多疾病的过程中,病情常因较剧烈的情志波动而加重,或急剧恶化。如有眩晕病史的患者,若遇事恼怒,肝阳暴张,发生头晕目眩,甚则突然昏厥,或昏仆不语、半身不遂、口眼㖞斜,也常因情志波动使病情加重或迅速恶化。

7.1.2.2 饮食失宜

饮食是摄取营养,维持人体生命活动所不可缺少的物质。但若饥饱失宜、饮食不洁及饮食偏嗜，又是导致疾病发生的重要原因。饮食物主要靠脾胃消化，故饮食不节主要伤及脾胃，而使脾胃功能失职，升降失常，并可聚湿、生痰、化热或变生它病。

（1）饥饱失常：饮食以适量为宜，过饥、过饱均可发生疾病。过饥即摄食不足，气血生化之源匮乏，气血得不到足够的补充，久则气血衰少而为病。同时，气血衰少则正气虚弱，抵抗力降低，易于感受外邪，继发其他病证。过饱即饮食摄入过量，超过了脾胃的消化、吸收和运化能力，可导致饮食阻滞，脾胃受伤，出现脘腹胀满、嗳腐泛酸、厌食呕吐、泻下臭秽等症。小儿由于脾胃尚弱，不知饥饱，更易患病。

（2）饮食不洁：进食不洁的食物，可引起多种胃肠道疾病，出现腹痛、吐泻、痢疾等。或引起寄生虫病，如蛔虫、蛲虫、绦虫等，临床见腹痛、嗜食异物、面黄肌瘦等症。若蛔虫窜入胆道，还可出现上腹部剧痛、时发时止、四肢厥冷、甚或吐蛔的蛔厥证。若进食腐败变质的有毒食物，常出现剧烈腹痛、吐泻等中毒症状，重者可出现昏迷或死亡。

（3）饮食偏嗜：饮食要适当调节，才能起到全面营养人体的作用，若任其偏嗜，则易引起部分营养物质缺乏或机体阴阳的偏盛偏衰，从而发生疾病，如佝偻病、夜盲症等就是某些营养物质缺乏的表现。过食生冷，则易损伤脾阳，寒湿内生，发生腹痛、泄泻等症。过食肥甘厚味，或嗜酒无度，以致湿热痰浊内生，气血壅滞，常可发生痔疮下血，以及痈疽等病。

7.1.2.3 劳逸失度

劳逸，包括过度劳累和过度安逸两个方面。正常的劳动和体育锻炼，有利于气血流通，增强体质；必要的休息可以消除疲劳，恢复体力和脑力，不会使人发生疾病。只有比较长时间的过度劳累，或过度安逸，劳逸失常才作为致病因素而使人发病。

（1）过劳：过劳是指过度劳累。包括劳力过度、劳神过度和房劳过度三个方面。

劳力过度，是指较长时间的体力劳动过度而积劳成疾。劳力过度则伤气，久则气少力衰。表现为四肢困倦、懒于言语、少气乏力、精神疲惫、动则气喘、汗出等症。

劳神过度，是指脑力劳动过度，思虑太过，劳伤心脾而言。劳神过度，耗伤心血、损伤脾气，可出现心神失养的心悸、健忘、失眠、多梦及脾不健运的纳呆、腹胀、便溏等症。

房劳过度，是指性生活不节，房事过度而言。房事过频则肾精耗伤，出现腰膝酸软、眩晕耳鸣、精神委靡，或男子遗精、滑泄、阳痿，女子月经不调、带下等病证。

（2）过逸：过逸是指过度安逸，不参加劳动，又缺乏运动。人体每天需要适当的活动，气血才能流畅，若长期不劳动，缺乏锻炼，可使气血不畅，筋骨柔弱，脾胃呆滞，表现为精神不振、肢体软弱、食少乏力、动则心悸、气喘、汗出，或发胖臃肿，抗病能力低下，易受外邪侵袭。

7.1.3 病理产物性病因

疾病是由致病因素所引起的一种复杂而有一定形式的病理过程。在这个复杂的病理过程中，每一阶段都有其特有的病理变化和临床表现。痰饮、瘀血等都是在疾病过程中所形成的病理产物。这些病理产物形成后，又会直接或间接作用于人体某一脏腑组织,发生多种病证,故又属致病因素之一。

7.1.3.1 痰饮

(1) 痰饮的含义:痰和饮都是水液代谢障碍所形成的病理产物。一般以较稠浊的称为痰,较清稀的称为饮。

痰不仅是指咯吐出来的有形可见的痰液,还包括瘰疬、痰核和停滞在脏腑经络等组织中而不能排出的痰浊,临床上可通过其所表现的证候来确定,这种痰称为"无形之痰"。

饮即水液停留于人体局部者,因其所停的部位和症状不同而有不同的名称。有"痰饮"、"悬饮"、"溢饮"、"支饮"的区分。

(2) 痰饮的形成:痰饮多由外感六淫,或饮食及七情内伤等,使肺、脾、肾及三焦等脏腑气化功能失常,水液代谢障碍,以致水津停滞而成。水湿内停,受阳气煎熬则为痰,得阴气凝聚则为饮。痰饮形成后,饮多留积于肠胃、胸胁及肌肤,而痰则随气升降流行,内而脏腑,外至筋骨皮肉,形成多种病证。

(3) 痰饮的致病特点:①阻滞气血运行:痰饮为有形之邪,若滞于经络,可致气血运行失畅;若停滞于脏腑,可使脏腑气机升降失常。②影响水液代谢:痰饮停滞于脏腑,可影响脏腑气机,导致脏腑功能失调,气化不利,水液代谢障碍。③易蒙蔽心神:心神以清明为要。痰饮为浊物,随气上逆,易蒙蔽清窍,扰乱心神。④致病广泛,变幻多端:痰饮可随气流行,内至脏腑,外至肌肤,产生各种不同的病变。痰饮不仅致病广泛,而且变幻多端,从而产生错综复杂的病证。

7.1.3.2 瘀血

(1) 瘀血的含义:瘀血,指体内有血液停滞,包括逸出脉外尚未消散之血,或血行不畅所致的瘀滞之血。瘀血是在疾病过程中形成的病理产物,又是某些疾病的致病因素。

(2) 瘀血的形成:瘀血的形成,主要有两方面:一是由于气虚、气滞、血寒、血热等原因,使血行不畅所致。气为血帅,气虚或气滞,不能推动血液的正常运行;或寒邪客于血脉,使经脉蜷缩拘急,血液凝滞不畅;或热入营血,血热搏结等,均可形成瘀血。二是因内外伤、气虚失摄或血热妄行等原因造成离经之血,未能及时消散而停留体内,形成瘀血。

(3) 瘀血的致病特点:①阻碍气血运行:血能载气,瘀血形成后,必定导致气机失畅;气能行血,气机失畅,进而引起血行不畅。②影响新血生成:瘀血内阻,气血运行失畅,脏腑失于濡养,功能失常,可影响新血的生成。③病位固定,病证繁多:瘀血常停留在人体某一部位,不易及时消散,表现出病位相对固定的特征。瘀血停留的部位不同,形成的原因各异,则其病理表现也不相同,从而表现出病证繁多的临床特点。

7.1.4 其他病因

导致疾病发生的原因,除外感病因、内伤病因和病理产物之外,还有胎传、寄生虫、外伤等。

7.1.4.1 胎传

胎传,是指在胎儿发育过程中形成或由父母遗传胎儿,导致出生后发病的因素。又可称先天性病因。

胎传可由于父母精气不足,或在母妊之时,因情志、饮食、起居调摄失常,影响胎儿的正常生长发育,导致出生以后发生的各种疾病。常见有五软(头项软、口软、手软、足软、肌肉软)、五迟(立迟、行迟、齿迟、发迟、语迟),解颅(囟门迟闭),梅疮,胎搐,胎寒,胎热等。

7.1.4.2 寄生虫

进食被寄生虫卵污染的食物,或接触疫水、疫土等,寄生虫(或卵)侵入人体,内聚寄生于脏腑,即可导致多种疾病发生。因此寄生虫也可归属病因范围。常见的寄生虫有蛔虫、钩虫、蛲虫、绦虫、血吸虫等。

寄生虫大都寄生于肠道之中,发病一般常见腹痛、嗜食异物、面黄肌瘦等,但由于感染的途径、虫体寄生的部位各有不同,故临床表现也不完全一样,如蛔虫病常见脘腹疼痛,胆道蛔虫病发作时上腹部剧痛,四肢厥冷;蛲虫病多见肛门瘙痒等。此外,钩虫、血吸虫则是直接从皮肤侵入人体,内聚脏腑,导致脏腑功能失调而发病。

7.1.4.3 外伤

外伤指金创伤、烧烫伤、冻伤、雷电击伤、溺水、虫兽伤等直接侵害人体的损伤。

金创伤包括枪弹伤、金刃伤、跌打损伤、持重努伤、压轧撞击伤等。这些外伤,均能直接损伤人体的皮肤、肌肉、筋脉、骨骼以及内脏。

烧烫伤主要由高温物品、火焰、火器所引起的灼伤。烧烫伤属火毒致病,机体受到火毒伤害,受伤部位立即可以出现水泡、皮焦、疼痛等症状。

冻伤是指人体遭受低温侵袭引起的全身性或局部性损伤。一般来说,温度越低,冻伤时间越长,则冻伤程度越重。冻伤可分全身和局部两种,局部冻伤多发生在手、足、耳廓、鼻尖和面颊部位。

雷电击伤是指雷电对人体造成的伤害。

溺水,由于各种原因沉溺水中,可导致人体窒息,甚则死亡。

虫兽伤包括毒蛇、猛兽、疯狗咬伤,或蝎、蜂蜇伤等。机体被虫兽所伤,轻则损伤皮肉,重则损伤内脏,或导致死亡。

7.2 病机

病机,即是疾病发生、发展与变化的机理。疾病的发生、发展与变化,和患病机体的体质强弱和致病因素的性质相关。病机包括发病原理、发病类型和基本病机三个方面。

7.2.1 发病原理

在正常的情况下,人体脏腑经络的生理功能正常,气血阴阳协调平衡,即所谓"阴平阳秘"。在致病因素的作用下,人体的脏腑、经络的生理功能失常,气血阴阳协调平衡关系被破坏,导致"阴阳失调",出现种种临床症状,也就导致了疾病的发生。

7.2.1.1 疾病的发生关系到正气和邪气两个方面

正气,是指人体的功能活动(包括脏腑、经络、气血等功能)和抗病、康复能力,简称为"正"。邪气,泛指各种致病因素,简称为"邪"。疾病的发生与变化,就是在一定条件下邪正斗争的反映。

(1) 正气不足是疾病发生的内在根据:中医学很重视人体的正气。在一般情况下,人体的正气旺盛,气血充盈,卫外固密,邪气就不易侵入,人体就不会得病。只有人体的正气相对虚弱,卫外不固,抗邪无力,邪气才会乘虚而侵犯人体,发生疾病。

(2) 邪气是发病的重要条件:中医学在重视正气,强调正气在发病中的主导地位的同时,并不排除邪气对疾病发生的重要作用。邪气是发病条件,在一定的条件下,甚至起着主导作用,例如疠气、外伤致病就是如此。所以《素问遗篇·刺法论》在谈到预防各种传染病时,就提出了不仅要保持机体正气的旺盛,还要做好"避其毒气"的预防工作。

7.2.1.2 邪正斗争的胜负决定发病与否

邪正斗争,是指病邪与正气的斗争。这种斗争不仅关系着疾病的发生,而且影响疾病的发展与转归。

(1) 正能胜邪则不发病:在邪正斗争过程中,若正气强盛,抗邪有力,则病邪难于侵入,或侵入后即被正气及时消除,不产生病理反映,就不会发生疾病。如自然界中经常存在着各种各样的致病因素,但并不是所有接触的人都会发病,此即正能胜邪的结果。

(2) 邪胜正负则发病:在正邪斗争过程中,若邪气偏胜,正气相对不足,邪胜正负,使脏腑阴阳气血失调,气机逆乱,而导致疾病的发生。

发病以后,由于正气强弱的差异、病邪性质的不同和感邪的轻重以及所在部位的浅深,而产生不同的病证。如:

疾病与正气强弱的关系:正气强,邪正斗争剧烈,多表现为实证;正气虚,抗邪无力,多表现为虚证,或虚实错杂证。

疾病与感邪性质的关系:一般来说,感受阳邪,易导致阳偏盛而伤阴,出现实热证;感受阴邪,易导致阴偏盛而伤阳,出现寒实证。

疾病与感邪轻重的关系:一般来说,邪轻则病轻,邪重则病重。

疾病与病邪所中部位的关系:病邪侵犯人体,有在筋骨经脉者,有在脏腑者,病位不同,病证各异。

7.2.1.3 影响正气的各种因素

中医学认为致病因素(邪)是发病的重要条件,正气不足或相对不足是发病的内在根据。影响正气的主要因素是体质和精神状态。

(1) 体质与正气的关系:体质强壮,则脏腑功能活动旺盛;体质虚弱,则脏腑功能活动减退,精、气、血、津液不足,其正气虚弱。

体质与先天禀赋、饮食调养、身体锻炼有关。一般来说,禀赋充实,体质多壮实;禀赋不足,体质多虚弱。合理的饮食和充足的营养是保证人体生长发育的必要条件。饮食不足,缺少必要的营养,影响气血的生成,则可致体质虚弱。暴饮暴食,则损伤脾胃;饮食偏嗜,营养不均衡,也影响体质。体育锻炼和体力劳动,可使气血畅通,体质增强。而过度安逸,则不利气血的流畅,脾胃功能减退,使人的体质虚弱。

(2) 精神状态与正气的关系:精神状态受情志因素的直接影响。情志舒畅,精神愉快,则气机畅通,气血调和,脏腑功能协调,正气旺盛;若情志不畅,精神抑郁,则使气机逆乱,阴阳气血失调,脏腑功能失常,正气减弱。因此,平时要注意调摄精神,保持思想上清静安定,惔淡虚无,从而使真气调和,精神内守。

总之,正气不足是发病的内在根据。体质和精神状态影响着正气的强弱。体质强壮,情志舒畅,则正气充足,抗病力强,邪气难于侵入,即使受邪,病邪易被祛除,也难于发展。若体质虚弱,情志不畅,则正气不足,抗病力弱,邪气易于侵入而发病。

7.2.2 发病类型

由于致病邪气的性质、感邪的轻重和致病途径等的不同,以及人体体质和正气强弱的差异,因此发病类型上各不相同,主要有感而即发、伏而后发、徐发、继发、复发等不同发病类型。

7.2.2.1 感而即发

感而即发,又称"猝发"或"顿发",是指机体感邪后立即发病。这是一种常见的发病类型。感而即发者多见于以下几种情况:一是新感外邪。外感六淫病邪致病,大多是感而即发的外感病。二是疫疠邪气致病。某些疫疠邪气,其致病性和传染性强,病多猝发,而且所致病情也较危重。三是情志骤变,如暴怒、大悲等剧烈的情志波动,可致气血逆乱而猝发病变。四是中毒,如误食误服有毒的食品、药物或吸入秽毒之气,或毒虫、毒蛇咬伤,可迅速引起中毒反应而发病,甚者致人死亡。五是急性外伤,如金刃、枪弹、坠落、跌打、烧烫伤、冻伤、电击等,均直接迅速致病。

7.2.2.2 徐发

徐发,又称缓发,指徐缓发病。徐发是与感而即发相对而言的。疾病徐发与致病邪气的性质,以及体质因素等密切相关。如外感病中的湿邪致病,因湿性黏滞,故湿邪为病,多发病缓,病程长。某些年高体弱之人,正气较虚,虽感外邪,但由于机体反应能力低下,常可徐缓发病。在内伤性病变中,也有徐缓发病者。如思虑过度,忧愁不释,房事不节,嗜酒成癖,嗜食膏粱厚味等致病,往往是积时日久,经渐进性病理变化过程,方可表现出明显的病变特征。

7.2.2.3 伏而后发

伏而后发,又称伏邪发病,是指机体感受某些病邪后,病邪潜伏于体内某些部位,经过一段时间之后,或在一定的诱因作用下发病,如破伤风、狂犬病、艾滋病及中医

"伏气温病"等。对于伏邪致病的机理,古代医家大都认为感邪轻浅,正气不足,因而病不猝发,但邪气可乘虚潜藏伏匿,以致其病逾时而发。在内伤性病变中,伏邪致病者也不少见,如痰饮内伏,日久不去,可在情志波动等因素诱发下致风痰阻络发为中风、偏瘫等。

7.2.2.4 继发

继发是指在原有疾病的基础上继发新的病变。继发病变必然以原发病为前提,二者之间有着密切的病理联系。如肝病胁痛、黄疸,若失治或久治不愈,日久可继发"癥积"、"臌胀"。又如疟疾反复发作,日久可继发"疟母"(脾脏肿大);小儿脾胃虚弱,消化不良或虫积日久,则可继发"疳积"病等。

7.2.2.5 复发

疾病的复发是指原病再度发作或反复发作。这是一种特殊的发病形式,也是一定条件下邪正斗争的反映。

(1) 复发的特点:疾病的复发是指原有病变通过治疗或自身修复,经过一段相对静止过程后的再度发作。疾病复发的主要特点:一是任何疾病的复发,应是原有疾病的基本病理变化和主要病理特征的重现;二是疾病的复发,大多较原病有所加重,且复发次数越多,病情越复杂;三是疾病的复发大都与一定的诱发因素有关。

(2) 复发的因素:导致疾病复发的因素主要有以下几方面:①食复:疾病初愈,合理的饮食调养则有助于身体康复。若进食过多,或进食不易消化的食物,既不利于正气恢复,又可因宿食、酒热等而助余邪之势,以致疾病复发。②劳复:凡病初愈,适当的休息、调养,有利于机体正气的恢复。若过早操劳,动形耗气,或房事不节,精气更伤;或劳神思虑,损及气血,均可致阴阳不和,气血失调,正气损伤,使余邪再度猖獗而疾病复发。如水肿、痰饮、哮喘等内伤杂病,常可因劳伤正气或复感邪气而反复发作。③药复:疾病将愈,辅以药物调理,只要使用得当,亦是促进正气恢复的重要手段。用药一般以扶正不助邪,祛邪不伤正为原则。如果病后药物调理不当,或滥施补药,或补之过早、过急,则易导致邪留不去,引起疾病复发。④重感致复:疾病将愈而未愈之际,复感外邪亦是导致原病复发的因素之一。如原病经过一个发展阶段之后,病变虽已进入静止期,但余邪并未尽除,而正气损伤未复,抗病能力低下,此时最易复感新邪而诱使原病复发。⑤其他因素致复:疾病的复发还与精神因素、地域环境、护理不当等有关。若情绪波动过大,或猝然遭受强烈的精神刺激,不仅直接影响病后正气的恢复,还可使人体气血逆乱而导致原病复发。⑥自复:指疾病初愈,不因劳损、饮食、药物、情志所致复发,亦不因外感新邪引发,而自行复发者。多由余邪在里,正气亏虚,无力驱邪,致使邪气暗长,旧病复发。

7.2.3 基本病机

基本病机,是指在疾病过程中病理变化的一般规律及其基本原理。

疾病的发生、发展及变化,与患病机体的体质强弱和致病因素的性质有关。病邪作用于人体,正气奋起抗邪,引起正邪斗争,破坏了人体的阴阳相对平衡,导致脏腑气机升降失常,气血功能紊乱,从而产生一系列的病理变化。所以,疾病虽然错综复杂,千变万化,但就其病理过程来讲,总不外乎正邪斗争、阴阳失调等病机变化的一般规律。

7.2.3.1 邪正盛衰

正气与病邪的斗争不仅关系着疾病的发生,而且影响着疾病的发展与转归,同时还直接影响着病证的虚实变化。因此,从某种意义上来说,许多疾病的过程,也就是正邪斗争,邪正盛衰的过程。

(1) 正邪斗争与虚实变化:正邪双方在斗争过程中是互为消长的。一般来说,正气增长则邪气消退,而邪气增长则正气消减。随着邪正的消长,患病机体就反映出虚实两种不同的病机与证候,即如《素问·通评虚实论》所说:"邪气盛则实,精气夺则虚。"

实,主要指邪气亢盛,是以邪气盛为矛盾主要方面的一种病理反映。其病理特点是:邪气亢盛而正气未衰,正气足以与邪气抗争,故正邪斗争激烈,临床表现为反应剧烈的实证。常见于外感病的初、中期以及痰、食、血、水等滞留所引起的病证。如临床所见壮热、狂躁、声高气粗、腹痛拒按、二便不通、脉实有力等,都属于实证。

虚,主要指正气不足,是以正气虚为矛盾主要方面的一种病理反映。其病理特点是:正气已虚,无力与邪气抗争,病理反应不剧烈,临床可出现一系列虚弱、不足的证候。虚证多见于素体虚弱或疾病后期以及多种慢性病中。如大病久病,消耗精气,或大汗、吐、利、大出血等耗伤人体气血津液,均会导致正气虚弱,功能衰退,表现为神疲体倦、面容憔悴、心悸、气短、自汗、盗汗,或五心烦热,或畏寒肢冷、脉虚无力等病证。

正邪的斗争消长,不仅决定着虚或实的病理变化,而且在某些长期的、复杂的疾病中,由于病邪久留,损伤正气,或正气本虚,无力驱邪而致痰食血水凝结阻滞而成虚实错杂的病变,以致实邪结聚,阻滞经络,气血不能畅达,或脏腑气血不足,运化无力而致的真实假虚,真虚假实的病变,也是临床常见的。

(2) 邪正盛衰与疾病转归:在疾病过程中,正气与邪气不断进行斗争的结果或为正胜邪退,疾病趋于好转而痊愈,或为邪胜正衰,疾病趋于恶化甚或死亡。若正邪斗争势均力敌,任何一方都不能即刻取得胜利,便会在一定的时间内出现正邪相持。

正胜邪退 在正邪斗争中,若正气充实,抵抗力强,邪气难于发展进而促使病邪对机体的损害消失或终止,机体的脏腑、经络等组织的病理性损害逐渐得到修复,精、气、血、津液等的耗伤也逐渐得到恢复,机体阴阳两方面在新的基础上又获得新的动态平稳,疾病即可痊愈。例如由六淫所致的外感病,邪气经皮毛或口鼻侵入人体,若正气充足,抗邪有力,不仅使病变局限在肌表或经络,且可在正气的抵御下,迅速驱邪外出,一经发汗解表,则邪祛表解,营卫和调,疾病痊愈。

邪胜正衰 在正邪斗争中,若邪气强盛,正气虚衰,机体抗病能力日趋低下,不能制止邪气的发展,机体受到病理性损害日趋加剧,病情就会趋向恶化。若正气衰竭,邪气独盛,气血、脏腑、经络等生理功能衰惫,阴阳离决,生命活动亦告终止而死亡。例如,在外感热病过程中,"亡阴"、"亡阳"等证候的出现,即是正不敌邪,邪胜正衰的表现。

此外,在正邪斗争过程中,若正邪双方力量对比势均力敌,出现正邪相持或正虚邪恋,邪去而正气不复的情况,则常常是许多疾病由急性转为慢性,或留下某些后遗症,或慢性病经久不愈的主要原因之一。

7.2.3.2 阴阳失调

阴阳失调,是指机体在病因的作用下,所发生的阴阳双方失去相对平衡,从而形成阴阳偏胜、偏衰,或阴不制阳、阳不制阴的病理状态。同时,阴阳失调又是脏腑、经络、气血、营卫等相互关系失调,以及表里出入、上下升降等气机运动失常的概括。由于六淫、七情、饮食劳倦等各种致病因素作用于人体,导致机体内部的阴阳失调,进而形成疾病。所以,阴阳失调又是疾病发生、发展的内在根据。

阴阳失调的病理变化非常复杂,但其表现,不外阴阳的偏胜、阴阳的偏衰、阴阳的互损、阴阳的格拒,以及阴阳的亡失等几个方面。

(1) 阴阳偏胜:阴或阳的偏胜,主要是指"邪气盛则实"的实证。病邪侵入人体,必从其类,即阳邪侵入人体,可形成阳偏胜;阴邪侵入人体,会形成阴偏胜。

阴和阳是相互制约的,阳长则阴消,阴长则阳消。阳偏胜必然会制阴,而导致阴偏衰,阴偏胜也必然会制阳,而导致阳偏衰。

阳偏胜是指机体在疾病过程中,所出现的阳气偏胜、功能亢奋、热量过剩的病理状态。其病机特点多表现为阳盛而阴未虚的实热证。阳偏胜形成的主要原因,多由于感受温热阳邪,或虽感受阴邪,但从阳化热;也可由于情志内伤,五志过极化火;或因气滞、血瘀、食积等郁而化热所致。阳以热、动、躁为特点,阳偏胜,表现为壮热、面红、目赤、烦躁不安、舌红、苔黄燥,或腹部胀满、腹痛拒按、潮热、谵语等实热证。由于阳胜则阴病,故阳偏胜还可兼见口渴、喜冷饮、大便秘结、小便短少等阴伤症状。

阴偏胜是指机体在疾病过程中,所出现的阴气偏胜、功能障碍或减退、产热不足,以及病理性代谢产物积聚的病理状态。其病机特点多表现为阴盛而阳未虚的寒实证。阴偏胜多由感受寒湿阴邪,或过食生冷,寒滞中阻,阳不制阴而致阴寒内盛。阴以寒、静、湿为特点,阴偏胜多表现为形寒、肢冷、舌淡、脘腹冷痛拒按、大便溏泻等寒实证。由于阴胜则阳病,故阴偏胜还可兼见畏寒、神疲蜷卧等阳虚症状。

(2) 阴阳偏衰:阴或阳的偏衰,是指"精气夺则虚"的虚证。由于某些原因,出现阴或阳的某一方面物质减少或功能减退时,必然不能制约对方而引起对方的相对亢奋,形成阳虚则阴盛、阳虚则寒(虚寒);阴虚则阳盛、阴虚则热(虚热)的病理现象。

阳偏衰是指机体在疾病过程中所出现的阳气虚损、功能减退或衰弱,温煦不足的病理状态。其病机特点多表现为机体阳气不足,阳不制阴,阴相对亢盛的虚寒证。阳偏衰多由于先天禀赋不足,或后天饮食失养和劳倦内伤,或久病损伤阳气所致。阳虚则寒,故临床多表现为畏寒肢冷、神疲蜷卧、腹痛喜温喜按、大便稀溏、小便清长、脉迟无力等虚寒证。

阴偏衰是指机体在疾病过程中所出现的精、血、津液等物质亏耗,以及阴不制阳,导致阳相对亢盛,功能虚性兴奋的病理状态。其病机特点多表现为阴液不足,滋养、宁静和制约阳热的功能减退,阳气相对偏盛的虚热证。阴偏衰多由于阳邪伤阴,或因五志过极,化火伤阴,或因久病耗伤阴液所致。阴虚则热,故临床表现为五心烦热、骨蒸潮热、面红、消瘦、盗汗、咽干口燥、舌红少苔、脉细数无力等虚热证。

（3）阴阳互损：阴阳互损，是指在阴或阳任何一方虚损的前提下，病变发展影响到相对的另一方，形成阴阳两虚的病理状态。

阴损及阳 是指由于阴液亏损，累及阳气生化不足或无所依附而耗散，从而在阴虚的基础上又导致的阳虚，形成了以阴虚为主的阴阳两虚病理状态。如肾阴不足，出现头晕目眩、腰膝酸软，一旦累及肾阳的化生，会同时兼见阳痿、肢冷等肾阳虚的症状，转化为阴损及阳的阴阳两虚证。

阳损及阴 是指由于阳气虚损，累及阴液的生化不足，从而在阳虚的基础上又导致的阴虚，形成了以阳虚为主的阴阳两虚的病理状态。如阳虚水泛的水肿，一旦累及阴精的生成，可同时兼见消瘦、心烦，甚则瘈疭等阴虚症状，转化为阳损及阴的阴阳两虚证。

（4）阴阳格拒：阴阳格拒，是阴阳失调中比较特殊的一类病机，包括阴盛格阳和阳盛格阴两方面。形成阴阳格拒的机理，主要是由于某些原因引起阴或阳的一方偏盛至极，因而壅遏于内，将另一方排斥格拒于外，使阴阳之间不相维系，出现真寒假热或真热假寒等复杂的病理现象。

阴盛格阳 是指阴寒之邪壅盛于内，逼迫阳气浮越于外，使阴阳之气不相顺接，相互格拒的一种病理状态。阴寒内盛是疾病的本质，但由于格阳于外，在临床上会出现面红、烦热、口渴、脉大等假热之象，故称之为真寒假热证。

阳盛格阴 是指阳热内盛，深伏于里，阳气被遏，郁闭于内，不能外达于肢体而格阴于外的一种病理状态。阳热内盛是疾病的本质，但由于格阴于外，在临床上会出现四肢厥冷、脉象沉伏等假寒之象，故称之为真热假寒证。

（5）阴阳亡失：阴阳亡失包括亡阴和亡阳两大类。是指机体阴液或阳气突然大量地亡失，导致生命垂危的病理状态。

亡阳 是指机体的阳气发生突然性脱失，而致全身功能突然衰竭的病理状态。亡阳多由于邪盛，正不敌邪，阳气突然脱失所致；或素体阳虚，正气不足，疲劳过度，耗气过甚；或误用、过用汗、吐、下，阳随津泄；或慢性消耗性疾病而致亡阳等，使虚阳外越所致，临床表现为大汗淋漓、肌肤手足逆冷、蜷卧、神疲、脉微欲绝等危重证候。

亡阴 是指由于机体阴液发生突然性大量消耗或丢失，而致全身功能严重衰竭的病理状态。亡阴多由于热邪炽盛，或邪热久留，煎灼阴液所致。也可由其他因素大量耗损阴液而致亡阴。临床表现为喘渴烦躁、手足虽温而汗多欲脱的危重证候。

亡阴、亡阳虽病机不同，表现各异，但由于阴阳互根互用，阴亡，则阳无所依附而耗散；阳亡，则阴无以化生而耗竭。故亡阴可迅速导致亡阳，亡阳亦可继而出现亡阴，最终导致"阴阳离决"而死亡。

7.2.3.3 气血失常

气血失常是指在疾病过程中，由于正邪斗争的盛衰，或脏腑功能的失调，导致气或血的不足、运行失常和各自生理功能及其相互关系的失常而产生的病理状态。

（1）气的失常：是指气的生化不足或耗散过多而致气的不足，或气的功能减退，以及气机失调的病理状态。

气虚 是指在疾病过程中,气的生化不足或耗散太过而致气的亏损,从而使脏腑组织功能活动减退,抗病能力下降的病理状态。气虚的形成多因先天禀赋不足,元气衰少;或后天失养,生化不足;或久病劳损,耗气过多;或肺、脾、肾等脏腑的功能失调,以致气的生成减少。

由于气具有推动、固摄、气化等作用,所以气虚的病变,常表现为推动无力,固摄失职,气化不足等异常改变,如精神疲乏、全身乏力、自汗、易于感冒等。气虚的进一步发展,还可导致精、血、津液的生成不足,运行迟缓,或失于固摄而流失等。

气机失调 是指在疾病过程中,由于致病邪气的干扰,或脏腑功能失调,导致气的升降出入运动失常所引起的病理变化。气机失调可以概括为气滞、气逆、气陷、气闭、气脱五个方面。

气滞:气滞是指气运行不畅而郁滞的病理状态。主要是由于情志郁结不舒,或痰湿、食积、瘀血等有形实邪阻滞,或因外邪困阻气机,或因脏腑功能障碍,影响气的正常流通,引起局部或全身的气机不畅或阻滞所致。不同部位的气机阻滞,其具体病机和临床表现各不相同,如外邪犯肺,则肺失宣降,上焦气机壅滞,多见喘咳胸闷;饮食所伤,胃肠气滞,则通降失职,多见腹胀而痛,时轻时重,得矢气、嗳气则舒等。但气机郁滞不畅是其共同的病机特点。因此闷、胀、痛是气滞病变最常见的临床表现。

气逆:气逆是指气的升降运动失常,升之太过,降之不及,以致气逆于上的病理状态。多由情志所伤,或因饮食寒温不适,或因外邪侵犯,或因痰浊壅滞所致。气逆病变以肺、胃、肝等脏腑最多见,如外邪犯肺,或痰浊阻肺,可致肺失肃降而气机上逆,出现气喘、短息等症;饮食寒温不适,或饮食积滞不化,可致胃失和降而气机上逆,出现恶心、呕吐、嗳气、呃逆等症;情志所伤,怒则气上,或肝郁化火,可致肝气升动太过,气血冲逆于上,出现面红目赤、头胀头痛、急躁易怒,甚至吐血、昏厥等病症。

气陷:气陷是在气虚的基础上表现以气的升举无力为主要特征的病理状态,也属于气的升降失常。由于脾胃居于中焦,为气血生化之源,脾气主升,胃气主降,为全身气机升降之枢纽,所以气陷病变与脾胃气虚关系密切,通常称气陷为"中气下陷"或"脾气下陷"。主要是由于久病体虚,或年老体衰,或泄泻日久,或妇女产育过多等,气虚较甚,升举无力所致。因脾气亏虚,升清不足,无力将水谷精气充分上输至头目等,则上气不足,头目失养,常表现为头晕眼花、耳鸣耳聋等。由于脾虚升举无力,则气陷不举,甚至引起内脏下垂,常表现有小腹坠胀、便意频频,或见脱肛、子宫脱垂、胃下垂等病变。

气闭:气闭是气机郁闭,外出受阻的病理变化。主要是指气机郁闭,气不外达、出现突然闭厥的病理状态。多因情绪过极,肝失疏泄,阳气内郁,不得外达,气郁心胸;或外邪闭郁,痰浊壅滞,肺气闭塞,气道不通等所致。所以气闭病变大都病情较急,常表现为突然昏厥、不省人事、四肢欠温、呼吸困难、面唇青紫等。

气脱:气脱是气虚之极而有脱失消亡之危的病理变化。主要是正不敌邪,或正气持续衰弱,气虚至极,气失内守而外脱,出现全身性功能衰竭的病理状态。气脱是各种虚脱性病变的主要病机。多因疾病过程中邪气过盛,正不敌邪;或慢性疾病,长期消耗,气虚至极;或大汗出、大出血、气随津血脱失所致。由于气的大量流失,全身严重气虚,功能活动衰竭,所以气脱者多表现为面色苍白、汗出不止、口开目闭、全身瘫软、手撒、二便失禁等危重征象。

(2) 血的失常：血的失常是指血的生化不足或耗伤太过而致血虚，或血的濡养功能减退，以及血的运行失常的病理状态。

血虚 血虚是指血液不足，或血的功能减退的病理状态。由于心主血，肝藏血，故血虚的病变以心、肝两脏最为多见。形成血虚病变的原因主要有三个方面：一是大出血等导致失血过多，新血未能及时生成补充；二是化源不足，如脾胃虚弱，运化无力，血液生化减少，或肾精亏损，精髓不充，精不化血等；三是久病不愈，日渐消耗营血等。

由于全身各脏腑组织器官，都依赖于血液的濡养，而且血能载气，血少则血中之气亦虚。血液又是神志活动的重要物质基础，所以当血虚时，血脉空虚，濡养作用减退，就会出现全身或局部的失荣失养，功能活动逐渐衰退，神志活动衰惫等一派虚弱表现，如面色、唇色、爪甲淡白无华，头晕健忘，神疲乏力，形体消瘦，心悸失眠，手足麻木，两目干涩，视物昏花等。

血行失常 血行失常是指在疾病过程中，由于某些致病邪气的影响，或脏腑功能失调，导致血液运行瘀滞不畅，或血液运行加速，甚至血液妄行，逸出脉外而出血的病理变化。

血瘀 血瘀是指血液运行迟缓或运行不畅的病理状态。导致血瘀病变的因素常见的有气滞而血行受阻；气虚而推动无力，血行迟缓；寒邪入血，血寒而凝滞不通；邪热入血，煎熬津血，血液黏稠而不行；痰浊等阻闭脉络，气血瘀阻不通，以及"久病入络"，等，影响血液正常运行而瘀滞。血瘀既可见于某一局部，又可见于全身。血液瘀滞于脏腑、经络等某一局部，不通则痛，可出现局部疼痛，固定不移，甚至形成癥积肿块等。如果全身血行不畅，则可出现面、唇、舌、爪甲、皮肤青紫色黯等症。

血行迫疾 血行迫疾是指在某些致病因素的作用下，血液被迫运行加速，失于宁静的病理变化。血行迫疾的形成多是外感阳热邪气，或情志郁结化火，或痰湿等阴邪郁久化热，热入血分所致；也可因脏腑阳气亢奋如肝阳上亢，血气躁动等所致。血液失于宁静而躁动，必然会引起血行迫疾，甚至损伤脉络，迫血妄行。同时因血液与神志关系十分密切，血躁则神亦躁，易致神志不宁。所以血行迫疾，常表现为面赤舌红、脉数、心烦，甚至出血、神昏等病症。

出血 出血是指在疾病过程中，血液运行不循常道，逸出脉外的病理变化。导致出血的原因颇多，常见的有外感阳热邪气入血，迫使血液妄行和损伤脉络；气虚固摄无力，血液不循常道而外逸；各种外伤，破损脉络；脏腑阳气亢奋，气血冲逆，或痰血阻滞，以致脉络破损等。出血，主要有吐血、咳血、便血、尿血、月经过多，以及鼻衄、齿衄、肌衄等。由于导致出血的原因不同，其出血的表现亦各异。火热迫血妄行，或外伤破损脉络者，其出血较急，且血色鲜红、血量较多；气虚固摄无力的出血，其病程较长，且出血色淡、量少，大多出现在人体的下部；瘀血阻滞，脉络破损的出血，多是血色紫黯或有血块等。

(3) 气血关系失调：气血关系失调是指气与血相互依存、相互为用的关系破坏，而产生的病理状态。

气滞血瘀 气滞血瘀是指气滞和血瘀同时存在的病理状态。气的运行阻滞，可以导致血液运行的障碍,而血液瘀滞又必将进一步加重气滞。由于肝主疏泄而藏血,肝的疏泄在气机调畅中起着关键性作用,关系到全身气血的运行,因而气滞血瘀多与肝的功能密切相关。由于心主行血,肺朝百脉,主司全身之气,所以心、肺两脏的功能失调也可形成气滞血瘀病变。

气不摄血 气不摄血是指因气的不足,固摄血液的功能减弱,血不循经,逸出脉外,导致各种出血的病理状态。由于脾主统血,若脾气亏虚,统血无力,则易致血不循常道而外逸,甚至中气不举,血随气陷于下。气不摄血的病变多与脾气亏虚有关。

气虚血瘀 气虚血瘀是指气虚无力推动血行,致使血液瘀滞的病理状态。气虚血瘀是以气虚为基础的。

气血两虚 气血两虚是气虚与血虚同时存在的病理状态。多因久病消耗,渐致气血两伤;或先因气虚,血液生化无源而日渐衰少等所致。

气随血脱 气随血脱是指在大量出血的同时,气也随着血的流失而耗脱的病理状态。气随血脱是以大量出血为前提的,如外伤出血、妇女崩漏、产后大失血等。由于血为气母,血能载气,大量出血,则气无所依附,气也随之耗散而亡失。

气血不荣经脉 是指因气血虚衰或气血失和,以致对经脉、筋肉、皮肤的濡养作用减弱,从而产生肢体筋肉等运动失常或感觉异常的病理状态。

7.2.3.4 津液代谢失常

津液代谢失常是指津液的生成、输布、排泄失常,引起体内津液不足,或在体内滞留的病理变化。

(1) 津液不足:津液不足是指津液的亏少,导致脏腑、组织官窍失于濡润滋养而干燥枯涩的病理状态。多由外感阳热病邪,或五志化火,消灼津液;或多汗、剧烈吐泻、多尿、失血,或过用辛燥之物等引起津液耗伤所致。

由于津和液在性状、分布、生理功能等方面均有所不同,因而津和液亏损不足的病机及表现,也存在着一定的差异。津较稀薄,流动性较大。内则充润血脉、濡养脏腑,外则润泽皮毛和孔窍,易于耗散,也易于补充。如炎夏季节而多汗尿少,或高热而口渴引饮,或气候干燥而口、鼻、皮肤干燥等,均以伤津为主。液较稠厚,流动性较小,可濡润脏腑,充养骨髓、脑髓、脊髓和滑利关节,一般不易耗损,一旦亏损则又不易迅速补充。如外感热性病后期,或久病耗阴,症见形瘦肉脱、舌光红无苔、手足震颤等,均以脱液为主。虽然伤津和脱液,在病机和表现上有所区别,但津和液本为一体,二者之间在生理上互生互用,在病理上也相互影响。伤津时不一定脱液,脱液时则必兼伤津。

(2) 水液停聚:水液停聚是对津液的输布、排泄障碍,导致水湿痰饮积聚的病理概括。津液的输布和排泄障碍主要与肺、脾、肾、膀胱、三焦的功能失常有关,并受肝失疏泄病变的影响。如脾失健运,则津液运行迟缓,清气不升,水湿内生;肺失宣降,则水道失于通调,津液不行;肾阳不足,气化失职,则清者不升,浊者不降,水液内停;三焦气机不利,则水道不畅,津液输布障碍;膀胱气化失司,浊气不降,则水液不行;肝失疏泄,则气机不畅,气滞则水停,影响三焦水液运行等。

汗和尿是体内津液代谢后排泄的重要途径,所以汗、尿的排泄障碍,虽是内脏功能失调的表现,但也是最易导致津液停蓄而内生水湿的环节。津液化为汗液,主要是肺的宣发布散作用;津液化为尿液,并排出体外,主要是肾阳的蒸腾气化功能和膀胱的开合作用。因此肺、肾、膀胱的生理功能衰退,不仅影响到津液的输布,还明显地影响着津液的排泄过程。其中肾阳的蒸腾气化功能贯穿于整个津液代谢的始终,在津液排泄过程中同样起着主要作用。当肺气失于宣发布散,腠理闭塞,汗液排泄障碍时,津液代谢后的废液,仍可化为尿液而排出体外。但是如果肾阳的气化功能减退,尿液的生成和排泄障碍,则必致水液停留而为病。

（3）津液与气血关系失调：津液的生成、输布和排泄,依赖于脏腑的气化和气的升降出入,而气之循行亦以津液为载体,通达上下内外遍布全身。津液与气血的功能协调是保证人体生理活动正常的重要方面。一旦关系失调,可出现如下几种病理变化：

水停气阻 指津液代谢障碍。水液停聚于体内,导致气机阻滞的病理状态。其病理表现因津气阻滞部位不同而异,如痰饮阻肺,则肺气壅滞,宣降不利,可见胸满咳嗽、痰多、喘促不能平卧等病症；水湿停留中焦,则阻遏脾胃气机,导致清气不升,浊气不降,可见脘腹胀满、嗳气食少症；水饮泛溢四肢,则可阻滞经脉气机,而见肢体沉重、胀痛不适等症。

气随津脱 指由于津液大量亡失,气随津液外泄,致使阳气暴脱的病理状态。多由高热伤津,或大汗出,或严重吐泻、多尿等,耗伤津液,气随津脱所致。如暑热邪气致病,迫使津液外泄而大汗出,不仅表现有口渴饮水、尿少而黄、大便干结等津伤症状,而且常伴有疲倦乏力、少气懒言等耗气的表现。由于津能载气,所以凡在吐下等大量亡失津液的同时,必然导致不同程度伤气的表现,轻者津气两虚,重者津气俱脱。

津枯血燥 津枯血燥是指津液和血同时出现亏损不足的病理状态。由于津血同源,津液是血液的重要组成部分,所以津伤可致血亏,失血可致津少。如高热大汗、大吐、大泻等大量耗伤津液的同时,可导致不同程度的血液亏少,形成津枯血燥的病变,常表现有心烦、肌肤甲错、皮肤瘙痒等症。

津亏血瘀 津亏血瘀是指因津液亏损而导致血液运行瘀滞不畅的病理状态。由于津液是血液的重要组成部分,因此津液充足则血行滑利。如因高热、大面积烧烫伤,或大吐、大泻、大汗出等,引起津液大量耗伤,则可致血量减少,血液浓稠而运行涩滞不畅,可在津液耗损的基础上,发生血瘀病变。其临床表现除津液不足的症状外,还可见到面质紫黯、皮肤紫斑、舌体紫黯,或有瘀点、瘀斑等血瘀表现。

7.2.3.5 内生五邪

"内生五邪",或称"内生五气"是指在疾病的发展过程中,由于脏腑阴阳失调,气、血、津液代谢异常所产生的类似风、寒、湿、燥、火（热）五种外邪致病特征的病理变化。由于病起于内,所以分别称为"内风"、"内寒"、"内湿"、"内燥"、"内火（热）"。"内生五邪"不是致病邪气,而是脏腑阴阳失调,气、血、津液失常所形成的综合性病理变化。

（1）风气内动：风气内动简称"内风",是指机体阳气亢逆变动而形成的一种病理状态。由于风气内动多是肝失调畅出现的一系列病理现象,故又称为肝风或肝风内动。根据其成因和临床特点不同,分为肝阳化风、热极生风、阴虚风动、血虚风动四类。

肝阳化风 多是情志所伤,操劳太过等耗伤肝肾之阴,筋脉失养,阴虚阳亢,水不涵木所形成的病理状态。其临床表现,轻则肢体麻木、震颤、眩晕欲仆,或为口眼㖞斜,或为半身不遂。甚则血随气逆于上,出现猝然昏倒、不省人事等。

热极生风 又称热甚动风。多见于外感热性病的热盛阶段,是因邪热炽盛,煎灼津液,伤及营血,燔灼肝经,使筋脉失养,阳热亢盛而化风的病理状态。热极生风的主要病机是邪热亢盛,属实性病变。故其临床表现以高热、神昏谵语、四肢抽搐、目睛上吊、角弓反张等症。

阴虚风动 是指机体阴液枯竭,无以濡养筋脉,筋脉失养而变生内风的病理状态。多由热性病后期,阴津亏损,或慢性久病阴液耗伤所致。由于其病变本质属虚,所以其动风之状多较轻、较缓,常表现为手足蠕动等症。

血虚生风 是指血液亏虚,筋脉失养,或血不荣络而变生内风的病理状态。多是出于失血过多,或血液生化减少,或久病耗伤阴血,或年老精血亏少,以致肝血不足所引起。病变本质属虚,其动风之状亦较轻、较缓。多表现为肢体麻木、筋肉跳动、手足拘挛等。

(2) 寒从中生:寒从中生即是内寒,是指机体阳气虚衰,温煦气化功能减退,虚寒内生,或阴寒之邪弥漫的病理状态。内寒的形成多与脾肾阳气虚衰有关。

阳气不足,虚寒内生,其病理变化主要表现在三个方面:一是阳气不足,机体失于温煦,如畏寒肢冷等;二是气化功能减退,津液代谢障碍导致病理产物在体内聚积,如痰饮、水湿等;三是阳不化阴,蒸化无权,津液不化,如尿频清长、痰涎清稀等。

寒从中生与外感寒邪之间既有区别,又有联系。"内寒"主要是体内阳虚阴盛而寒,以正虚为主,属虚寒;"外寒"主要是外感寒邪为病,虽然也有寒邪伤阳的病理变化,但以邪实为主,属实寒。两者之间的主要联系是寒邪侵犯人体,必然会损伤机体的阳气情况出现,病变发展可以导致阳虚;而阳气亏虚之体,因抗御外邪能力低下,则又易感寒邪而致病。

(3) 湿浊内生:湿浊内生,即是"内湿",是指因体内津液输布、排泄障碍,导致水湿痰饮内生并蓄积停滞的病理状态。内湿病理的形成多主要以脾的运化功能失常为病机关键。

湿浊内生的病理变化主要表现在两个方面:一是由于湿性重浊黏滞,多易阻滞气机,出现胸闷、腹胀、大便不爽等症;二是湿为阴浊之物,湿邪内阻,可进一步影响肺、脾、肾等脏腑的功能活动。如湿阻于肺,则肺失宣降,可见胸闷、咳嗽、吐痰等症;若湿浊内困日久,进一步损伤脾、肾阳气,则可致阳虚湿盛的病理改变。湿浊虽可阻滞于机体上、中、下三焦的任何部位,但以湿阻中焦,脾虚湿困最为常见。

外感湿邪与湿邪内生之间,既有区别,又有联系。"外湿"是从外感受湿邪为病,以湿邪伤于肌表、筋骨关节为主;"内湿"是由肺、脾、肾等脏腑的功能失调,尤其是脾失健运,水津不布,留而生湿所致。两者之间的联系是湿邪外袭每易伤脾,若湿邪困脾伤阳,则易致脾失健运而滋生内湿;脾虚失运,内湿素盛者,又每易招致外湿入侵而致病。

(4) 津伤化燥:津伤化燥,即是"内燥",是指体内津液不足,导致人体各组织器官失于濡润而出现一系列干燥枯涩症状的病理状态。

内燥病变的形成多由久病耗伤阴津,或大汗、大吐、大下,或亡血、失精等导致阴液亏少,或某些外感热性病过程中热盛伤津等所致。由于津液亏少,内不足以灌溉脏腑,外不足以润泽肌肤官窍,则出现一系列干燥失润的症状,如肌肤干燥、口燥咽干、大便燥结等。由于内燥的本质是体内津液亏损,故内燥病变可发生于各脏腑组织,但以肺、胃、大肠最为多见。

(5) 火热内生:火热内生,即是"内火",又称"内热",是指由于阳盛有余,或阴虚阳亢,或五志化火等而致的火自内扰,功能亢奋的病理状态。火热内生有虚实之别,其病机如下:

阳气过盛化火　人身的阳气在正常情况下,有温煦脏腑组织的作用,称为"少火"。但在病理状态下,若阳气过于亢奋,则亢烈化火,可使功能活动异常兴奋,这种病理性的阳亢,则称为"壮火"。

邪郁化火　邪郁化火包括两个方面。一是外感风、寒、湿、燥等病邪,在病理过程中,郁久而化热化火,如寒邪化热、湿郁化火等;二是体内的病理性产物,如痰湿、瘀血、饮食积滞等,郁久而化火。

五志过极化火　是指由于精神情志刺激,影响脏腑气血阴阳,导致脏腑阳盛,或气机郁结,气郁日久而从阳化火所形成的病理状态。

阴虚火旺　是指阴液大伤,阴不制阳,阴虚阳亢,虚热内生的病理状态。多见于慢性久病之人,如阴虚而引起的牙龈肿痛、咽喉疼痛、骨蒸颧红等均为虚火上炎所致。

思 考 题

- 试述风、寒、暑、湿、燥、火的性质及致病特点。
- 试述七情致病的特点。
- 瘀血病证的共同特点是什么?
- 试述阴阳失调的病机。
- 寒从中生的病机及临床表现如何?

8 防治原则

8.1 预防

预防是指采取一定的措施防止疾病的发生和发展。

预防在《内经》中称为"治未病",这里指的是在预防疾病和治疗疾病时,强调防患于未然。"治未病"包括未病先防和既病防变两个方面。

8.1.1 未病先防

未病先防是指在疾病发生以前,采取各种措施以防止疾病的发生。

疾病的发生与"正气"和"邪气"关系密切。正气是指人体的功能活动(包括脏腑、经络、气血等功能)和抗病、康复能力。邪气是指引发疾病的各种原因。人体正气充足,则抗病能力强盛,就不会受到邪气的侵害,即使受到邪气侵犯,也能抗邪外出,而不致发病,所以,正气不足是疾病发生的根本原因。在特殊情况下,邪气常常会成为疾病发生的决定性因素,因此,邪气是引起疾病发生的重要条件。预防疾病就应一方面提高正气,增强机体的抗病能力,一方面避免邪气的侵害。

8.1.1.1 提高正气的抗邪能力

(1) 调养形体:调养形体,是增强人体健康,提高防病能力,减少疾病发生的重要环节。保持身体健康,精神充沛,益寿延年,应当认识自然界的变化规律,并能适应自然环境的变化。对于饮食起居和劳逸要进行适当的节制与安排,即生活规律要正常,饮食要有节制,劳而不妄,则可维持正气之充盛,从而减少疾病的发生。反之,若生活起居没有规律,饮食劳逸没有节制,就会削弱机体的抗病能力,影响身体健康,从而导致疾病的发生。

生命在于运动,健康在于锻炼。生命是物质运动的最高形式,而形体的健康也正是反映了生命活动的正常进行。实践证明,充沛的精力必须寓于健壮的身体,而健壮的体魄,又常来源于适当的劳动和经常不懈的体育锻炼。因此,加强身体锻炼,也是增强体质,减少或防止疾病发生的一项重要措施。

汉代著名医学家华佗,根据"流水不腐,户枢不蠹"的道理,创造了"五禽戏"健身运动,其中以"虎戏"的动作刚猛,有助于增强体力;以"鹿戏"的心静体松,柔刚共济,有利于舒展筋骨;以"熊戏"的步态沉稳,以缓解上实下虚之证;以"猿戏"的轻健敏捷,有利于疏通关节;以"鹤戏"的轻柔亮翅,有利于增强呼吸功能,并调达气血,疏通经络。人体通过运动和适当的劳动,不仅能促进血脉流通,使关节灵活,且可使气机调畅,从而增强机体的抗病能力,提高健康水平,防止和减少疾病的发生。同时,对于某些疾病也有一定的治疗作用。

(2) 调摄精神:中医学不仅重视形体的调养,而且还特别注意精神的调养,使之饱满乐观,充沛而不涣散。尽量减少不良的精神刺激和过度的情志变动,防止或减少情志疾病的发生,无疑具有十分重要的意义。

人的精神活动的正常与否,对于机体生理活动和病理变化,具有十分重要的影响。因为精神情志活动是以精、气、血、津液为物质基础,与脏腑的功能活动密切相关。精神、意识、思维活动对于机体既可起到积极的或增强的作用,也可起到消极的或减弱的作用。而积极的、增力的作用,可以提高人体的活动能力,如愉快的情绪,可以使人体的气血畅达,功能旺盛;而消极的、减力的作用,则可能降低人的活动能力,如抑郁的情绪可以导致人体气滞血瘀,功能紊乱,抗病能力下降,从而导致疾病的发生。

古人强调对内在精神的调养,是既要注意意志的锻炼、情绪的稳定,树立起战胜病痛的意志和决心,又要心胸开朗,清心寡欲,方能防止和减少情志的刺激,从而达到却病延年长寿的目的。因此,强调精神调养,必须做到"恬惔虚无,真气从之",才能够达到"精神内守,病安从来"的养生目的。

(3) 饮食有节:饮食是人类生存不可缺少的条件之一,饮食的适宜、规律与否,直接影响着人的健康。饮食所化生的水谷精微是生成气血的物质基础,是维持人体生长发育,完成各种生理功能,保证生存和健康的必要条件。饮食有节是指饮食要适宜、规律。若饮食不节,食饮无度,则会引起疾病的发生。所以要养成良好的饮食习惯,定时适量,不可过饥,也不要过饱,尤其不宜过食肥甘厚味。二要注意调剂饮食性味,使寒热调和,五味均衡。此外,还应注意饮食卫生,防止"病从口入"。

(4) 药物预防:《素问遗篇·刺法论》有运用"小金丹"预防疫病传染的记载。我国于16世纪或更早一些时候所发明的"人痘接种法",用于预防天花,是世界免疫学的先驱。此外,中医还有用苍术、雄黄等药物烟熏以消毒的方法等。近年来,运用中草药预防疾病,已经越来越引起医学界的重视,并得到很大的发展。如用贯众、板蓝根或大青叶等预防流感;用茵陈、栀子预防肝炎;用马齿苋预防痢疾等,都获得了较好的效果。

8.1.1.2 避免邪气侵害

邪气是疾病发生的重要条件,在某些特殊的情况下,邪气还会起主导作用。如高温、高压电流、化学毒剂、枪弹杀伤、虫兽咬伤等,即使正气强盛,机体也难免被伤害而发病。疠气在特殊情况下,常常会成为疾病发生的决定性因素。所以,避免邪气的侵害,也是防止疾病发生的一项重要措施。

8.1.2 既病防变

防病于未然,是最理想的愿望和目的,但若疾病已然发生,则应争取早期诊断、早期治疗,以防止疾病的发展与传变。在防治疾病的过程中,一定要掌握疾病发生发展的规律及其传变的途径,从而进行有效的治疗,才能控制其传变。所以,根据此传变规律和防治原则,中医临床常于治肝的同时,配用健脾和胃的方药,这就是既病防变思想的具体体现。清代著名医家叶天士,根据温热病伤及胃阴之后,病势进一步发展,往往耗及肾阴的病变规律,主张在甘寒养胃治疗胃阴虚的方药中加入咸寒滋肾之品,以滋补肾阴,防止胃阴不足日久波及肾阴,并提出了"务在先安未受邪之地"的防治原则,这就是既病防变在临床上具体运用之范例。

8.2 治则

中医临床学在长期的医疗实践过程中,通过历代医家丰富的临床经验的积累和总结,在深入认识疾病发生发展规律的基础上,形成了一套完整的辨证论治理论和方法。对疾病进行辨证论治,不仅在于对疾病的各种临床征象,运用中医理论去辨别分析,从而对病情做出正确的诊断,更重要的还在于根据辨证的结果,制定正确的治疗原则,采用恰当的治疗方法,给予合理的药物,或应用其他有效的治疗手段以治疗疾病。在论治的过程中,治疗原则的确立和治疗方法的选用,具有十分重要的意义。

治则,即治疗疾病的法则。治则是在整体观念和辨证论治精神指导下所制定的,对于临床各科病证的治法、处方及用药,具有普遍的指导意义。

治法,是指治疗疾病的具体方法。治疗法则与具体的治疗方法不同,治疗法则是针对临床病证的总的治疗原则,是用以指导治疗方法的总则,而治疗方法则是针对某一具体病证(或某一类型病证)所适用的具体方法,是治则的具体化。因此,任何具体的治疗方法,总是从属于一定的治疗法则的。例如,各种病证的本质都是正邪相争,从而表现为阴阳的消长盛衰变化,因此,扶正祛邪即为总的治疗原则,而在此指导下所采取的益气、滋阴、养血、温阳等方法,即是扶正的具体方法;而发汗、涌吐、攻下、清解等方法,则是祛邪的具体治法。可见,治则与治法既有严格的区分,又有着密切的内在联系。

由于疾病的证候表现是多种多样的,病理变化亦是极其复杂,而且病情又有轻重缓急的差异,所以,不同的时间、地点,不同的年龄和个体等因素,对病情变化亦会产生不同的影响。为此,必须善于从复杂多变的疾病现象中审症求因,把握住病变的本质,治病求本,审因论治,采取相应的措施,调整机体的阴阳,使其失调的阴阳关系,重新恢复相对平衡,方能获得满意的治疗效果。治则主要有治病求本、扶正祛邪、重视整体、协调阴阳、调整脏腑、调理气血、因异制宜等。

8.2.1 治病求本

疾病是正邪相争的复杂过程,在这个过程中,机体内部的矛盾往往不止一个,临床表现也真假参半,如多数疾病表面现象和其内在本质基本一致,而有的疾病则表面征象与其本质并不一致(如寒热真假证、虚实真假证等)。因此,透过疾病的现象,分清疾病矛盾的主次,抓住疾病的本质,方能给予恰当的治疗而解决疾病。

治病求本,是治病时必须寻求疾病的根本原因,并采取有针对性的治疗,这是辨证论治的根本原则。

"标本缓急"与"正治反治"体现了治病求本这一基本原则。

8.2.1.1 标本缓急

所谓"本"是相对于"标"而言的,任何疾病的发生、发展过程,都存在着主要矛盾和次要矛盾,"本"即是指病变的主要矛盾或矛盾的主要方面,起着主导的决定性作用;"标"是病变的次要矛盾或矛盾的次要方面,处于次要和从属的地位。因此,标本是相对的含义,有多种含义,可用以说明病变过程中各种病证矛盾双方的主次关系。如从正邪关系来说,则正气是本,邪气是标;从病因与症状来说,则病因是本,症状是标;从病变部位来说,则内脏疾病是本,体表疾病是标;从疾病先后来说,则旧病是本,新病是标;原发病是本,继发病是标等。

任何疾病的发生、发展,总是要通过若干症状显现出来,但这些症状只是疾病的现象,还不是疾病的本质,只有在充分地收集、了解疾病的各方面情况,通过综合分析,方能透过现象看本质,找出疾病的根本原因,从而选用恰当的治疗方法。例如头痛,可由外感、血虚、痰湿、瘀血、肝阳上亢等多种原因所引起,故其治疗就不能简单地采用对症止痛的方法,而应加以综合分析,找出致病的原因,分别采用解表、养血、燥湿化痰、活血化瘀、平肝潜阳等方法进行治疗,方能收到满意的效果。

关于治病求本原则的具体运用,则又有急则治其标、缓则治其本、标本兼顾等方面。

(1)急则治其标:在一般的情况下,病证的主要矛盾或矛盾的主要方面是本而不是标,治本是一个根本的原则。但是在复杂多变的病证中,常有标本主次位置的变化,因而在治疗上就又有先后缓急的区分。如在疾病的发展过程中出现了严重的并发症,标病甚急,不及时解决,则将危及患者的生命或影响本病的治疗时,则应采取"急则治其标"的法则,先治其标病,后治其本病。例如大出血的病人,不论其属于何种出血,则均应采取应急措施,先止血以治标,待血止后,病情有所缓和再治其本病。又如某些慢性病患者,原有夙疾,又复感外邪而患新病,当新病较急的时候,亦应先治外感以治其标,待新病愈后,再治夙疾以求其本。可以看出,治标只是在紧急情况下的权宜之计,而治本才是解决疾病的根本之图。急则治标缓解了病情,解除了新病,即为治本创造了更为有利的条件,其目的仍是为了更好地治本。然而,治标的方法可暂用而不宜常用,否则对正气将有所损害。

(2)缓则治其本:指在一般情况下治病必须抓住疾病的本质,解决其根本矛盾,进行针对根本原因的治疗。如肺痨病证,阴虚内热,虚火灼肺而见咳嗽、低热、口干、咽燥、五心烦热、颧红盗汗等症状时,其咳嗽等症是疾病的现象为标;阴虚内热,虚火灼肺则是疾病的本质为本。因此治疗时就不应以止咳祛痰方法来治标,而应着重于运用滋阴润肺以治本,解决其阴虚。只有提高了机体的抗病能力,方能使肺痨病获愈。

(3)标本顾治:是指在标病本病俱急并重的情况下,在治病求本的同时,亦应兼顾标病的治疗,采用标本同治的原则。如外感热病,热邪入里,由于里证实热不解而阴液大伤,表现为腹满硬痛、大便燥结、身热、口干唇裂、舌苔焦燥等正虚邪实,标本俱急的证候,就当标本兼顾,泻下与滋阴两法同用,即清泻实热以治标,滋阴增液以固本。若仅用泻下,则有进一步耗伤津液之弊,而单用滋阴,则又不足以泻在里之实热。

而两法兼用,则泻下实热即可存阴,滋阴润燥以"增水行舟"亦有利于通下,标本同治,相辅相成,即可达到邪去液复之目的。又如痢疾,可见腹痛,里急后重,泻下赤白脓血,舌苔黄腻,脉象滑数。其病因湿热为本,故其治疗应以清热利湿法以治本,还应配合"宽肠理气"的方法,以解决其腹痛,里急后重之急,此亦是标本兼治法的体现。再如本有里证,又复外感表邪而见表证,或表证尚未尽解而里证又现,表里同病而标本俱急,则应表里双解,这也属于标本同治的范畴。

应当指出,临床运用急则治标、缓则治本的原则,亦不能绝对化,急的时候也未尝不须治本,如亡阳虚脱,急用回阳救逆,就是治本;大出血后,气随血脱之时,急用益气固脱也是治本。同样,缓的时候也不是不可以治标,有时治标也更有利于治本。总之,不论标本,急则先治是一个根本的原则。而在临证时,把握住病情标本的转化,以便始终抓住疾病的主要矛盾或矛盾的主要方面,做到治病求本则是其关键。

8.2.1.2 正治与反治

《素问·至真要大论》提出"逆者正治,从者反治"两种治疗法则,但就其本质来说,都是治病求本这一根本法则的具体运用。

(1) 正治:所谓"正治",就是通过分析临床症状和体征,辨明其病变本质的寒热虚实,然后分别采用"寒者热之"、"热者寒之"、"虚则补之"、"实则泻之"等不同方法来治疗。因其是属于逆疾病本质而治的一种常用的治疗方法,所以又称为"逆治"。由于临床上大多数疾病的征象与疾病的性质相符,如寒证见寒象,热证见热象,虚证见虚象,实证见实象等,所以说正治法,乃是临床最常用的一种治疗方法。

(2) 反治:有些疾病,特别是某些复杂、严重的疾病,可表现为其某些症状与病变的本质不相符,也就是出现了某些假象。因而在治疗时就不能简单地见寒治寒、见热治热,而应透过假象辨明真伪,治其本质。所谓"反治",也称"从治",就是通过分析临床症状和体征,辨明其病变本质的寒热虚实,顺从疾病假象而治。反治法适应于本质与现象相反的证候,反治法有"寒因寒用"、"热因热用"、"塞因塞用"和"通因通用"等。

例如,某些外感热病,在其里热盛极之时,由于阳盛格阴,可见到四肢厥冷之寒象,此寒象是假,而热盛才是本质,故仍须用寒凉药物进行治疗,因此称之为"寒因寒用"。

某些亡阳虚脱病人,由于阴寒内盛,格阳于外,有时亦可见到面颊浮红、烦躁等热象,因其热象是假,而阳虚寒盛方是其本质,故仍应以温热药进行治疗,因此称之为"热因热用"。

由于脾虚不运所致的脘腹胀满,因并无水湿或食积留滞,则用健脾益气,以补开塞的方法来进行治疗,因之又叫做"塞因塞用"。

由于食积停滞,影响运化所导致的腹泻,则不仅不能用止泻药,反而应当用消导泻下药以去其积滞,方能奏效,此又称之为"通因通用"。

此外,尚有一种正治反佐之法,常用于某些大热证或大寒证服药时,由于病药格拒而出现呕吐不纳现象,在某些前人的著作中亦常把它列入反治法之一。一般用法则是在大寒剂中反佐少许温药(或寒凉药热服),或于大热剂中反佐少许凉药(或温热药冷服),以使其药与病同气相求,不发生格拒而能更好地发挥药效。关于"反佐"之法,究其实质,实为制方、服药的某些具体方法,应属于中医方剂学的范围,故不再详细论述。

8.2.2 扶正祛邪

在一定意义上,疾病的过程,可以说是正气与邪气矛盾双方相互斗争的过程。邪胜于正则病进,正胜于邪则病退。因而治疗疾病,就是要扶助正气,祛除邪气,改变邪正双方的力量对比,使之向有利于疾病向愈的方向转化。所以,扶正祛邪也是指导临床治疗的一条重要法则。

"邪气盛则实,精气夺则虚",邪正盛衰决定着病证的虚实。"虚则补之,实则泻之",所以补虚泻实就是扶正祛邪法则的具体应用。但是,正邪双方的主次关系在病变过程中不是一成不变的,而是随着病情的发展而变化。因此关于扶正与祛邪的应用,一般又有如下几种情况:

8.2.2.1 扶正以祛邪

即运用药物、营养疗法、功能锻炼等各种治疗方法以扶助正气,增强体质,提高机体抗病能力和自我修复能力,从而达到祛除邪气,恢复健康的目的。即所谓"扶正以祛邪"、"正复邪自去"。扶正的措施是补虚,主要适用于正虚而邪不盛,或虽有外邪而以正虚为矛盾主要方面的病证。临床可根据病人的具体情况,针对所表现的不同的虚证,施以不同的补法,如益气、养血、滋阴、温阳等等,从而使脏腑经络功能活动的物质基础精、气、血、津液得以恢复而旺盛。

8.2.2.2 祛邪以扶正

即运用药物、针灸、火罐或手术等各种治疗方法祛除病邪,以达到邪去正复的目的。所谓"祛邪以扶正"、"邪去正自安"也。此法主要适用于邪盛而正气不虚,或虽有正虚而仍以邪盛为矛盾主要方面的病证。

实践证明,处理正邪矛盾,应以祛邪为主,且根据临床观察,外邪致病,一般亦以实证居多,亦应以泻实攻邪为法。在药物治疗上,不同的病邪亦有不同的祛除方法,故临床所用祛邪方法较为丰富,诸如解表、清热、解毒、泻下、消痰、化湿、利水、破血、祛瘀、散结、驱虫等多种治疗方法,基本上都属于攻邪的范围,都属于消除致病因素的方法,临床即可根据不同的具体病情而适当选用。

应当指出,祛邪与扶正,是相互为用,相辅相成的。扶正可使正气加强,有助于抗御和驱除病邪;而祛邪则排除了病邪的侵犯和干扰,终止了对正气的损伤,则有利于正气的保存和恢复。

8.2.2.3 先攻后补

主要适用于病邪亢盛,急需祛邪,或正气虽虚但尚未严重到不耐攻伐的病证,特别是对由于病邪存在所直接引起正气虚者,则更应先攻后补。如外感热病过程中,热结肠胃,腹满胀痛,便闭不通,且由于邪热内结,化燥伤阴,可见舌红无津、舌苔焦燥而黑、口咽干燥,甚则谵语昏迷等症,则须先攻后补,应急下之。这是因为大便不通则热结愈甚,热结愈甚则阴津更伤,故须急下存阴,然后再以养阴生津药物进行调理。

8.2.2.4 先补后攻

主要适用于病邪虽盛,但正气虚损已严重到阳衰或阴竭的程度,由于正气已不能耐受攻伐,故应先补后攻。待正气有所恢复,再解决其病邪问题。目前临床上对于某些邪实正虚的病证,如昏厥或心阳暴脱等病证,即多根据"先补后攻"的原则进行治疗。

8.2.2.5 攻补兼施

即扶正与祛邪同时应用,主要适用于正虚与邪实并重的病证。但在具体应用时,亦要分清其是以正虚为主,还是以邪实为主。如邪盛正虚,以邪实为主,则应重在祛邪,兼以扶正;若病情迁延日久,正气大虚,余邪未尽,则应着重于扶正,兼以祛邪。总之,攻补兼施的原则,在临床上最为多用,处方用药则应根据具体病情,分清主次,灵活运用。

8.2.3 重视整体

人体是一个有机的整体,人体脏腑经络各部分之间,各部分与整体之间,是紧密相联而不可分割的。故任何一个病证或一个局部病变,无不与其整体密切相关。因此,在临床治疗中,既不能只看到病变局部,而看不到整体,又不能只着眼整体而忽视病变局部,只进行全身性的治疗,而忽略对于病灶局部的处理。正确的作法是,从整体观念出发,不但重视局部,而且更重视整体,把两者辩证地结合起来应用于临床,方能达到预想的结果。

中医临床所常用的治疗原则主要有协调阴阳、调整脏腑功能、调理气血等方面。

8.2.3.1 协调阴阳

从根本上说,疾病的发生,即是阴阳的相对平衡状态遭到破坏,出现偏盛偏衰的结果。因此,协调阴阳,补偏救弊,恢复其相对平衡的状态,促进其阴平阳秘,乃是临床治疗的根本法则之一。协调阴阳法则,又分"损其有余"及"补其不足"两个方面。

(1) 损其有余:是指对于阴阳偏盛,即阴或阳的一方过盛有余的病证,临床即可采用"损其有余"的方法治之。如阳热亢盛的实热证,则应"治热以寒",即用"热者寒之"的方法,以清泻其阳热;如阴寒内盛的寒实证,则应"治寒以热",即用"寒者热之"的方法以温散其阴寒。

在阴阳偏盛的病变中,一方的偏盛,常可导致另一方的不足,即阳热亢盛易于耗伤阴液,阴寒偏盛易于损伤阳气,故在调整阴或阳的偏盛时,还应注意是否有相应的阳或阴偏衰情况的存在,若已有相对一方的偏衰时,则当兼顾其不足,适当配合以扶阳或益阴之法。

(2) 补其不足:是指对于阴阳偏衰,即阴或阳的一方虚损不足的病证,临床即可采用"补其不足"的方法治之。如阴虚不能制阳,常表现为阴虚阳亢的虚热证,则应滋阴以制阳;因阳虚不能制阴,常表现为阳虚阴盛的虚寒证,则应补阳以制阴。但是,阴阳偏衰最终常是导致肾阴或肾阳的亏损,故肾阴亏损时,则应以"壮水之主,以制阳光"的方法治之;肾阳虚损时,则应以"益火之源,以消阴翳"的方法治之。若属阴阳两虚,则应阴阳双补。

应当指出,由于阴阳是互用的,所以阴阳偏衰亦可互损,因此在治疗阴阳偏衰病证时,还应注意"阳中求阴"或"阴中求阳"的原则,即在补阴时适当配用补阳药物,补阳时适当配用补阴药物。

此外,由于阴阳是辨证的总纲,疾病的各种病理变化,亦均可以阴阳失调加以概括,故凡表里出入的失常、上下升降的紊乱,以及寒热进退、邪正虚实、营卫不和、气血不和等等,无不属于阴阳失调的具体表现。因此,从广泛的意义来讲,诸如解表攻里、越上引下、升清降浊、温寒清热、补虚泻实,以及调和营卫、调理气血等治疗方法,亦都属于协调阴阳的范围。

8.2.3.2 调整脏腑

人体是一个有机整体,脏与脏、脏与腑、腑与腑之间在生理上是相互协调、相互促进的,在病理上也是相互影响而传变的。因此,当某一脏腑本身发生病变时,亦会影响到别的脏腑,故在治疗脏腑病变时,不能单纯考虑一个脏腑,而应注意调整各脏腑之间的关系。从而形成了间接补泻及从脏治官等原则。

(1) 间接补泻:是指某一脏或腑发生病变时,除了直接治疗该脏或腑外,还应调整与其关系较密切的其他脏腑。如肺的病变,既可因本脏受邪而发病,亦可由心、肝、脾、肾及大肠的病变所引起。如因心阳不足,心脉瘀阻,而致肺失宣降发作的喘咳,则应以温心阳为主;因肝火亢盛,气火上逆所致的咳血,则应以泻肝火为主;因脾虚湿聚,痰湿壅肺,以致肺失宣肃而成的咳嗽痰多,则应以健脾燥湿为主,因肾阴虚不能滋肺,肺失津润而致的干咳、口咽干燥,则应滋肾润肺;因肾虚不能纳气,肺气上逆所致的气喘,呼多吸少,则应温肾纳气为主;若因大肠热结,肺气不降而致的气喘,则宜通腑以泻大肠之热。又如脾病,除本脏病变外,亦可由肝、心、肾及胃等病变而引起。如肝失疏泄,而致脾运失健者,则应疏肝为主;脾虚,肝木乘克脾土,则应治以扶土抑木;命火不足,火不生土(命门火衰,心阳虚损,脾虚失运),则应补火以生土;胃失和降,而致脾失健运,则应重在和降胃气,以协调脾胃的气机升降等,其他脏腑的相互影响及治疗上的互相协调,亦是如此。

(2) 从脏治官:五脏与五官,经络相连,密切相关。五官疾病,根据中医学整体治疗观点,亦可从五脏入手来进行治疗。如肝开窍于目,眼病实证,则可以采用清肝的方药进行治疗;眼病虚证,则可以采用补肝养血的方药进行治疗;又如心开窍于舌,口舌生疮,则可以采用清心火及泻小肠热的方药治疗等。

此外,在针灸取穴方面,中医学亦常从整体观念出发,运用如下选穴原则,如上病下取(治肝阳上亢型眩晕,常取涌泉或太冲)、下病上取(治脱肛常灸百会)、以左治右、以右治左(如治疗偏瘫,常配取健侧的穴位),其他还有募俞取穴、原络取穴等,无一不体现了整体治疗的原则。

8.2.3.3 调理气血

气血是脏腑功能活动的物质基础,气血虽各有功能,但又相互为用。当气血相互为用、相互滋生的关系失常时,即会出现各种气血失调的病证。故调理气血亦是整体治疗原则的体现。调理气血主要亦是运用"有余泻之,不足补之"的法则,从而使气血关系恢复协调。如:

气能生血,气虚则生血不足可致血虚,最后导致气血两虚,其治疗则应以补气为主,兼顾补血养血,而不应单纯补血。

气能行血,气虚或气滞,则可致血行瘀滞而不畅,形成气虚血瘀或气滞血瘀,治宜补气行血或理气活血化瘀。

气机逆乱,则血行亦随之逆乱,如肝气上逆,血随气涌,则常可导致昏厥或咯血,治宜降气和血。

气能摄血,气虚则统摄失职,可导致血离经隧而出血,治宜补气摄血。

血为气母,故血虚则气亦虚,血脱者,则气随血脱,根据血脱者益其气的治疗原则,则应以补气固脱治之。

8.2.4 因异制宜

因异制宜,是指治疗疾病应根据季节、地区,以及患者的体质、性别、年龄等之不同而采用适宜的治疗方法。这是由于疾病的发生、发展和转归受到多方面因素的影响,如时令、气候、地理环境等,尤其是患者个体的体质因素,对疾病的影响则更大。因此,在治疗疾病时,必须把这些方面的因素考虑进去,对具体情况作具体分析,区别对待,方能制定出比较适宜的治疗方案。

8.2.4.1 因时制宜

四时气候的变化对于人体的生理功能、病理变化均产生一定的影响。根据不同季节气候的特点来考虑治疗用药的原则,就是"因时制宜"。一般地说,春夏季节,气候由温渐热,阳气升发,人体腠理疏松开泄,即使是患外感风寒,也不宜过用辛温发散之品,以免开泄太过,耗伤气阴;而秋冬季节,气候由凉转寒,阴盛阳衰,人体腠理致密,阳气内敛,此时若非大热之证,就当慎用寒凉之品,以防苦寒伤阳。

暑邪致病有明显的季节性,且暑多兼湿,故暑天治病,应注意清暑化湿;秋季气候干燥,若外感温燥,则宜辛凉润燥。此与春季风温、冬季外感风寒用药亦不甚相同。风温宜辛凉解表,风寒则宜辛温解表。这就说明治疗用药必须因时制宜。

8.2.4.2 因地制宜

根据不同地区的地理环境特点,来考虑治疗用药的原则,即是"因地制宜"。不同地区,由于地势高低、气候条件及生活习惯不同,人的生理活动和病变特点也不尽相同,所以治疗用药亦应有所差异,应根据当地环境及生活习惯而有所变化。如中国西北地区,地势高,气候寒冷,干燥少雨,且生活习惯多食肉类食品及乳制品,故体质较壮,患病则多外寒而里热,其治疗则应散其外寒,清其里热;东南地区,滨海傍水,地势低洼,气候温热多雨,而体质较弱,腠理疏松,其病多发痈疡或较易外感时邪。由于阳气外泄,故易生内寒。其治疗则应敛其外泄阳气并温其内寒。中医临床治病,有时同一种病而治法各不相同,且都能治好,就是因为地势不同,而治疗用药各有所宜的缘故。如外感风寒病证,西北严寒地区,使用辛温解表药量较重,且常用麻黄、桂枝;东南温热地区,用辛温解表药量较轻,且多用荆芥、防风。这也是地理气候不同之特点在治疗用药上的体现。所以治病务须因地而制宜。

8.2.4.3 因人制宜

根据病人的年龄、性别、体质及生活习惯等不同特点,来考虑其治疗用药的原则,叫做"因人制宜"。

(1) 年龄:不同年龄的生理状况和气血盈亏各不同,故其治疗用药亦应有所区别。老年人气血虚亏,生理功能减退,故患病多虚或正虚邪实,其治疗,虚证宜补,而邪实须攻者则应慎重,用药量应比青壮年较轻,以免损伤正气。小儿生机旺盛,但气血未充,脏腑娇嫩,易寒易热,易虚易实,病情变化较快。加之婴幼儿生活不能自理,多病饥饱不匀,寒温失调,故治疗小儿病证,忌投峻剂,少用补益,且用药量宜轻。总之,一般用药剂量,亦须根据年龄而加以区别,药量太小则不足以祛病,药量过大则反伤正气,不得不予注意。

(2) 性别:男女性别不同,有其生理特点,妇女有经、带、胎、产等情况,其治疗用药应加以考虑。如在妊娠期,对于峻下、破血、滑利、走窜等伤胎药物或有毒药物,则当禁用或慎用。

(3) 体质:由于每个人的先天禀赋和后天调养不同,个体素质不但有强弱,而且还有偏寒偏热之差异。一般来说,阳亢或阴虚之体,慎用温热之品;阳虚或阴盛之体,慎用寒凉之品。所以体质不同,虽患同样病证,其治疗用药亦当有所区别。

其他如患者的职业、工作条件以及情志因素、生活习惯等亦可能与某些疾病的发生有关,在诊治时亦应有所注意。

综上所述,可以看出,因人制宜是指治病时不能孤立地看待病证,而应把握人的整体和不同个体的特点;因时、因地制宜,则是强调了自然环境对人体的影响。所以,因异制宜的原则,充分体现了中医学的整体观念和在实际应用时的原则性和灵活性。只有全面地看问题,具体情况具体分析,善于因时、因地、因人制宜地处方用药,方能取得较好的疗效。

思 考 题

- 何谓"治未病"?如何做到"既病防变"?
- 如何提高正气的抗邪能力?
- 何谓正治与反治?举例说明如何应用正治与反治。
- 何谓扶正与祛邪?如何运用扶正祛邪这一治疗原则?
- 协调阴阳的治疗原则是什么?
- 何谓因人制宜、因地制宜和因时制宜?因异制宜体现了中医学什么观念?

Fundamental Theory of Traditional Chinese Medicine

1 INTRODUCTION

Chinese medicine has a long history. It is a summary of experiences of Chinese people in their struggles against diseases, being an important part of the outstanding Chinese culture. In a long period of medical practice, it had gradually formed and developed into a medicine with a unique and integral theoretical system. It has been making a great contribution to Chinese people's cause of health care and development of Chinese nation.

Chinese medicine belongs to the category of life science. It is an important part of world medicine, taking the mission to promote continual progression and creativity of life science. The unique theoretical system and feature of clinical diagnose and treatment of Chinese medicine will contribute its efforts to the development of world medicine and health cause of the human being.

1.1 Initiation and Development of Theoretical System of Chinese Medicine

The initiation of theoretical system of Chinese medicine can date back to the Warring States and the Qin and Han dynasties, undergoing a long historical process. It needs a certain basis and conditions for Chinese medicine to become a systematical medical system of knowledge, developing from knowledge of sporadic, subjective, local and folk medical practice to a medical theoretical knowledge with guiding significance.

(1) An accumulation of long period of medical experience: The social development history tells us that the medical practice begins since man takes the production activity. It is proved by textual research that as early as in the Yin dynasty there were records of disease names such as *Zheng* (concretion), *Jie* (scabies), *Gu* (tympanites and ascites), *Qu* (carious tooth), *Erming* (tinnitus), *Xiali* (diarrhea), and *Bumian* (insomnia). Viewing from the names of "diseased ear", "diseased nose" and "diseased eye" involving the human organs, the recognition of life activity by ancient Chinese is related to their observation in anatomy.

Up to the West Zhou dynasty and Spring-Autumn Warring States, the recognition of disease had been further developed. For example, in *Shān Hǎi Jīng* (*The Classic of Mountains and Seas*), a literature of Early Qin dynasty, there were records of 38 kinds of diseases. In the medical literatures from No.3 Han dynasty's grave exhumed in Mawangdui of Changsha city in 1973, besides records of formulas for 52 kinds of diseases, more than 100 names of disease were brought up. According to an incomplete statistic datum in the ancient literatures of Early Qin dynasty the number of disease names had been up to more than 180 sorts. It is sufficiently shown that the recognition of diseases at that times had been rather profound, and a richer medical experience had been accumulated, so that the direct data were given for sorting out the knowledge of medical theory, summarizing the law of medicine and establishing the frame of the theory, and a practical basis was built up.

(2) Influence of ancient philosophical thinking: Philosophy is a theory on worldview and methodology. No subject can initiate and develop without philosophy, and any subject must be governed and checked by philosophy. What is more, in the ancient time natural science was underdeveloped, so medical experts had to have the aid of ancient philosophical thought and its containing methods to sort out their medical experiences, analyze the law and sum up the characteristics.

Ancient philosophical views gave a thinking frame for research of medical theory. Especially the doctrines of qi monism, yin-yang and the five elements provided a philosophical evidence for development of theoretical system of Chinese medicine. They established a guiding thinking that the life is of material, a unity of opposites of yin-yang and in a endlessly developmental and changeable process, and also the illness can be both prevented and treated. They provided methods for Chinese medicine to adapt an integral and compound study and establish a unique theoretical system of Chinese medicine. They also built up a basis for Chinese medicine to expound the major theoretical problems such as the relationship between mean and nature, the essence of life, and health and disease. Thus they made an essential standardization and guideline in sorting out, summing up and studying the sporadic and odd medical experiences, leading to a gradual systematization and standardization of Chinese medicine, and promoting the initiation of theoretical system of Chinese medicine. Therefore there is no doubt that the ancient philosophical thinking is the thinking basis for establishment of theoretical system of Chinese medicine.

(3) Infiltration of ancient natural science: Natural science is a theoretical system on the law of material motion. Its development is never isolated, but inter-penetrating, inter-influencing and inter-promoting. Chinese medicine is of natural science, its initiation and development must obey the rule. The knowledge of some leading subjects in ancient China such as astronomy, calendar, meteorology, geography, phenology, acoustics, agronomy, mathematics and art of war, was taken by the ancient medical experts as the technique and means in researching the phenomena of human life and the prevention and treatment of disease, and some of them were even absorbed, transplanted and merged. It can be seen that the development of ancient natural science laid a scientific foundation for establishment of theoretical system of Chinese medicine.

1.1.1 Initiation of Theoretical System of Chinese Medicine

The coming out of medical classics, or *Huángdì Nèi Jīng* (*Huangdi's Inner Classic of Medicine*), *Nàn Jīng* (*Classic on Medical Problems*), *Shāng Hán Zá Bìng Lùn* (*Treatise on Cold Pathogenic and Miscellaneous Diseases*) and *Shénnóng Běn Cáo Jīng* (*Shennong's Classic of Medicinal Herbs*), symbolizes the primary formation of theoretical system of Chinese medicine.

The writing of *Huangdi's Inner Classic of Medicine* was started in the Spring-Autumn Warring States and completed in the meddle-late stage of the Western Han dynasty. It is completed by many medical experts through collection, sorting out and synchronizing, and it is the earliest medical classic extant in China. It is generally held that *Sù Wèn* (*Plain Questions*) and *Líng Shū* (*Miraculous Pivot*) are the two parts of *Huangdi's Inner Classic of Medicine*. In the book, medical contents are taken as the center, applying philosophical theory and scientific knowledge and taking the holism as the guiding line, to expound the life regularity and the integrity of man with its external surroundings, and to study the theories of human morphological structure, physiology and pathology, as well as the diagnosis, prevention and treatment of disease. Many contents in *Plain Questions* and *Miraculous Pivot* had at that times and in a longer period of time since then held a leading a place in the world. For example, in tissue structure, the records of the lengths of skeleton and the sizes and volumes of internal organs are basically consistent with those revealed in modern anatomy. The systematic recognition of blood circulation and multiple functions of human internal organs in physiology, as well as the integral relations in physiology and pathology play a decisive role in the establishment of the unique theoretical system of Chinese medicine and thinking model. In diagnostics, not only a methodological basis for four diagnostic techniques of inspection, olfaction-auscultation, inquiry and palpation is laid, but also a viewpoint of overall consideration of both exogenous and endogenous pathogenic factors in diagnosis is emphasized. All these theories have been effectively guiding the clinical practice. The coming out of *Huangdi's Inner Classic of Medicine* indicates that Chinese medicine has grown from the stage of simple accumulation of experiences to a stage of systematical summarization of theories. The book provides a theoretical guide and basis for development of Chinese medicine.

Classic on Medical Problems, originally named *Eighty-One Medical Problems* or *Eighty-One Medical Questions*, was written approximately before the East Han dynasty and, according to legend, by *Qn Yueren*. In the book a question-and-answer model is used to expound the contents of viscera, meridians, pulse lore, pathology and acupuncture technique. In the book the basic theory is taken as its main contents and, at the same time, some symptoms of diseases are also analyzed. There are some development in expounding meridians, vital gate and tri-Jiao based on *Huangdi's Inner Classic of Medicine*, so it is another classic book following *Huangdi's Inner Classic of Medicine*.

Treatise on Cold Pathogenic and Miscellaneous Diseases was written by Zhang Zhongjing at the end of East Han dynasty. In the book the rich experiences on prevention and treatment of disease before the East Han dynasty are summed up, and diagnosis and treatment of cold pathogenic and miscellaneous diseases are dealt with respectively according to the visceral syndrome differentiation and six-meridian syndrome differentiation. In the book the theory, principle, fomula and medicinal are all given, laying a basis for the development of clinical medicine in later ages. This outstanding work is well known in later ages as "the ancestor of formula". The coming out of this book indicates the establishment of system of treatment determination based on syndrome differentiation in Chinese medicine. It was later on divided into two parts of *Shāng Hán Lùn* (*Treatise on Cold Pathogenic Diseases*) and *Jīn Guì Yào Luè* (*Synopsis of Golden Chamber*). In the former cold pathogenic diseases, and in the latter miscellaneous diseases, are dealt with.

Shennong's Classic of Medicinal Herbs, called for short *Shénnóng Běn Jīng* or *Běn Căo Jīng* (*Classic of Medicinal Herbs*), was compiled approximately at the Han dynasty. It is the earliest monograph of materia medica in China. In the book, 365 kinds of medicinals are recorded, and divided into three grades of upper, meddle and lower agents. The medicinals of the upper grade are mainly used for strengthening physical health to correspond with the heaven, the ones of middle grade for culturing mental health to correspond with man, and the ones of lower grade for treating diseases to correspond with the earth, which is the first classification of medicinals in China. In the book the briefly generalized pharmaceutical theories are also four natures (cold, hot, warm and cool), five flavors (sour, bitter, sweet, acrid and salty), and seven conditions of ingredients in prescription (single effect, mutual accentuation, mutual enhancement, mutual counteraction, mutual antagonism, mutual suppression and mutual incompatibility). The coming out of this book is the important mark of establishment of theoretical system of Chinese pharmacy, laying a basis for development of Traditional Chinese pharmacy.

1.1.2 Development of Theoretical System of Chinese Medicine

Basing on *Huangdi's Inner Classic of Medicine*, *Classic on Medical Problems*, *Treatise on Cold Pathogenic and Miscellaneous Diseases,* and *Shennong's Classic of Medicinal Herbs*, medical experts in ages have enriched and developed the theoretical system from different angles.

(1) Period of the Jin, Sui and Tang dynasties: The medicine and pharmacy in this period had been developed comprehensively. Especially, there came many summing-up monographs in diagnostics, etiology, acu-moxibustion, and prescription. For example, during the Jin dynasty, *Mài Jīng* (*Pulse Classic*) written by an imperial medical official Wang Shuhe, in which the conditions of 24 pulses and their indicating syndromes are expounded, is the earliest monograph of pulse lore extant in China; *Zhēn Jīu Jiă Yĭ Jīng*

(*A-B Classic of Acupuncture and Moxibustion*), compiled by well known scholar *Huang Pumi* through sorting out the expounding of meridians, points and acupuncture methods in *Sù Wèn* (*Plain Questions*) and *Zhēn Jīng* [or *Líng Shū* (*Miraculous Pivot*)], is the earliest monograph of acupuncture; in *Zhǒu Hòu Bèi Jí Fāng* (*Handbook of Prescriptions for Emergency*), written by Ge Hong, some infectious diseases such as smallpox and measles can be diagnosed according to their pathogenic features and clinical manifestations. In the Sui dynasty, *Zhū Bìng Yuán Hòu Lùn* (*General Treatise on Causes and Manifestations of All Diseases*), known as *Bìng Yuán* (*Causes of Diseases*) or *Cáo Shì Bìng Yuán* (*Cao's Causes of Diseases*) for short, compiled by an imperial physician Cao Yuanfang and his coworks, is a representative work of studying pathogens and manifestations of diseases. In the book the pathogenic factors and manifestations of diseases in various clinical subjects are described, and the recognition and description are mostly correct. The monumental works on medicinals and prescriptions coming out in the Tang dynasty are the focus of attention. Among them, *Bèi Jí Qiān Jīn Yào Fāng* (*Essential Recipes for Emergent Use Worth a Thousand Gold*) and *Qiān Jīn Yì Fāng* (*A Supplement to Recipes Worth a Thousand Gold*) compiled by Sun Simiao, and *Wài Tái Mì Yào* (*Arcane Essentials from the Imperial Library*) written by Wang Tao are all the handed down prescription books that record the effective formulas of well-known physicians and their various therapeutic measures.

(2) Period of the Song, Ji and Yuan dynasties: In this period there comes an active atmosphere that "a hundred schools of thought content"; various schools by using their unique academic views had greatly enriched the medical theories and practice.

During the Song dynasty, Chen Wuze in his work of *Sān Yīn Jí Yī Bìng Zhèng Fāng Lùn* (*Treatise on Three Categories of Pathogenic Factors and prescriptions*) put forth the well known "theory of three categories of disease causes". He completely summarized the disease causes as three respects: Endogenous cause is endogenous injury by the seven affects; exogenous cause is exogenous contraction by six climatic pathogens; and non-endo-exogenous cause are improper died, injury of qi by loudly crying, wounds by insects and animals, poisonings, incised wounds, injuries from falls and heavy load, drowning, etc.. This classification is more consistent with clinical conditions, so it not only makes a progression for Chinese medicine etiology, but also deeply influences the thinking model of etiological recognition in later ages. Qian Yi who is respectively called "the father of pediatrics" is the forerunner in visceral diagnosis and treatment, his syndrome differentiation method taking the five *Zang*-viscera as the principle is recorded in the book of *Xiǎo ér Yào Zhèng Zhí Jué* (*Key to Therapeutics of Children's Diseases*). He also had relatively clearly recognized some eruptive diseases such as measles and smallpox, and could make differentiating diagnosis.

Many medical schools with their own features in the Jin and Yan dynasties came out, among them the most representative physicians are Liu Wansu, Zhang Congzheng, Li Dongyuan and Zhu Danxi, called respectively in late ages "four great physicians in the

Jin and Yuan dynasties".

Enlightened by theories of pathomechanism and five circuits and six climates in *Plain Questions*, Liu Wangsu raised the theory that diseases mostly arise from "fire", believing that "exogenously contracted six climatic agents would be transformed into fire" and "extremely hyperactivity of the five emotions can all lead to production of fire". Therefore he preferred to use cold and cool medicinals and prescriptions in treatment of disease, and he is later named the "school of cold medicine". Zhang Congzheng held that a person's illness is mainly caused by invasion of pathogenic qi, once the pathogenic qi was dispelled, the illness will disappear; so he advocated that elimination of pathogenic qi is the key matter in treatment of disease. His therapies are mainly diaphoresis, emesis and purgation in order to get the aim of eliminating the pathogen and safeguarding the vital, and he is known in later age as the "school of eliminating pathogen". Li Dongyuan believed that the occurrence of disease is mostly related to the endogenous injury of the spleen and stomach. He emphasized the spleen and stomach belong to the earth in the five elements that is the mother of everything, serve as the source of generation; if the spleen and stomach get disordered, many diseases will appear consequently. He also expounded a lot the theory of ascending-descending of qi dynamic of the spleen and stomach, and put first the nourishing the spleen and stomach in treatment of disease, thus he is noted as the "school of strengthening the earth". In addition, his originally created theory of "yin-fire" and the method of "removal of fever by sweet-warm remedy" had given a great impact in later ages. Zhu Danxi blended the opinions of the three schools of Liu, Zhang and Li, and he was good at diagnosis and treatment of miscellaneous diseases, with many original ideas. He gave further explanation of ministerial fire theory. He believed the basic pathological change of disease is that "yang is ever excessive while yin is ever in deficiency", and advocated the remedies of nourishing yin and reducing fire, so he is regarded in later ages as the "school of nourishing yin". Some other medical experts like Zhang Yuansu also made a great contribution to enrich and promote theoretical system of Chinese medicine.

(3) Period of the Ming and Qing dynasties: Owing to the wanton massacre of infectious diseases, in this period there emerged the school of warm diseases who study the law of occurrence and development of warm-heat diseases in four seasons and their diagnosis and treatment. This indicates that Chinese medicine had gone into a new stage in investigation of infectious diseases. Wu Youke, a physician of the Ming dynasty, in his work of *Wēn Yì Lùn* (*Treatise on Pestilence*) set forth the theory of "pestilential qi", holding that the pathogens of "pestilence" are "a noxious qi rather than wind, cold, summer-heat and dampness." The way of infection is through the mouth and nose. This is a great breakthrough in etiology of warm diseases (especially pestilential diseases). Up to the Qing dynasty, famous physicians of warm disease Yie Tianshi, Xue Shengbai, Wu Jutong and Wang Mengying systematically summarized the relative

research achievements gained formerly, broken through the traditional viewpoint of "warm diseases are not beyond the category of cold pathogenic diseases". They created the norm of treatment of warm diseases based on syndrome differentiation taking the defensive-qi-nutritive-blood levels and the three *Jiao* levels as the core, thus forming a complete theoretical system for warm diseases in their causes, pathomechanisms, pulse diagnoses, syndromes and treatments. It should be pointed out both theories of warm and cold pathogenic diseases, as two great schools of treating exogenous extraction of febrile disease, are supplemental to each other. They have been of important guiding role in clinical treatment, and up to now still of higher value for research.

In addition, Zhao Xianke and Zhang Jingyue of the Ming dynasty put forth the theory of vital gate of kidney yin and yang. Wang Qingren of the Qing dynasty advocated the theory of pathogenesis of stagnant blood and created a series of formulas with action of activating blood to resolve stasis. All these not only substantiated new contents for basic Chinese medicine theory, but also gave greater contribution to the development of Chinese medicine therapeutics.

(4) Modern times: Chinese experts in modern times, on one hand set forth to collect and sort out the forerunners' experiences, and on the other hand, in the condition of import of Western medicine, attempted to make convergence of Chinese and Western medicine from a dispute on Chinese and Western medicine, thus leading to a way of integration of traditional Chinese and Western medicine. After a long argument, Chinese medicine and Western medicine gradually communicate with each other in science. Some learnt figures firstly advocated the convergence of Chinese and Western medicine. For example, *Yī Xué Zhōng Zhōng Cān Xī Lù* (*Records of Traditional Chinese and Western Medicine in Combination*) written by Zhang Xichun is a good representative monograph in convergence of Chinese and Western medicine. With development of Chinese medicine cause, in modern standardization and research of basic Chinese medicine theory encouraging achievements have been made. Chinese medicine basic theory has become an independent essential subject, and there has been a rapid progress in systematization and experimental study. There have been heartening traces of a trend in research and exploration of the essence of some theories by using modern scientific and technical means. For example, in study on the essences of yin deficiency, yang deficiency, cold and heat syndromes; kidney essence and spleen essence; the regularity of medicinal composition in prescription, and the law of syndrome, there have all been a certain progress that arouses concern among all walks of medicine. It has been constantly proved in practice that the development of Chinese medicine theory will certainly promote the development of the whole Chinese medicine and the improvement of theoretical system of Chinese medicine, so that it will make an important contribution to the deepening and development of bioscience study.

1.2 Cardinal Characteristics of Theoretical System of Chinese Medicine

Theoretical system of Chinese medicine is mainly of two cardinal characteristics of conception of holism and treatment determination based on syndrome differentiation.

1.2.1 Conception of Holism

So called "wholeness" signifies the unity and integrity of a thing. Chinese medicine holds that the human body is an organic whole in which all constituent parts are structurally inseparable, functionally coordinative and interactive, and pathologically inter-influencing. And it also recognizes man is closely related with natural and social environments, man maintains its normal life activity in the practice of active adapting and transforming nature. This kind of thinking of the integrity of the body itself and the unity of man's internal and external environments is the conception of holism of Chinese medicine.

1.2.1.1 Human Body as an Organic Whole

The human body is composed of several viscera and tissues, each of them has its own different functions which are the constituent part of the whole activity and thus it makes the body an integral unity. The integral unity forms by taking the five *Zang*-viscera as its center, combining with the six *Fu*-viscera to link such tissues and organs of the whole body as the five body constituents, sense organs, orifices, four limbs and the bones to be an organic whole through the connection of meridian system; and to perform the unifying and coordinative functions through the actions of essence, qi, blood and body fluid. Chinese medicine classifies all organs and tissues and their relative functions into the five great systems. This conception of the five *Zang*-viscera as an integral whole has guided the research and recognition of human physiology and pathology in Chinese medicine.

The human's normal physiological activity depends on every viscus and tissue to perform their own functions, on the other hand, on the synergic actions by supplementing and complementing one another and the restricting actions by opposing and yet complimenting one another. Only in this way can the body maintain its physiological balance. Each viscus has its own different functions, however this is also a kind of dividing the work and cooperating and an organic coordination in an integral activity, being an unity of locality and whole.

Chinese medicine views a local disorder from the angle of the integral pathological reaction caused by it, believing that a local pathological change is usually related with the abundance of qi and blood of the whole body's viscera. So in examination of an illness, its internal pathological changes of the viscera and qi-blood can be understood and judged through the external changes of sense organs, orifices, body constituents, complexion, and pulse conditions. For example, the tongue connects with the five *Zang*-viscera directly or indirectly through meridian system. Therefore the hypofunction or hyperfunction of an internal viscus, the abundance of qi-blood and the exuberance of body fluid, as well as the severity and favorableness of a disease can all be reflected by the tongue picture. Then by inspecting the tongue picture one can detect the functional states internally.

As for local illness Chinese medicine usually determines the therapeutic principle and method from view point of the whole body's condition. For example, the heart opens into the tongue, and is external-internally related with the small intestine. So oral erosion may be treated by using the method of clearing heart heat and reducing small intestine fire. The other examples are treatment of eye illness based on the liver condition, treatment of deafness by focusing on the kidney. All these are the therapeutic principles established under the guidance of the holism.

To sum up, the basic standpoint of "human body as an organic whole" in Chinese medicine goes through all respects in expounding the human physiological function and pathological change, as well as in diagnosis and treatment of disease.

1.2.1.2 Close Relation of Man with Its Surroundings

Man lives in nature. As the environment changes the human body must change correspondingly. At the same time, man is closely related with social environment which inevitably gives an impact on man. Of course, man can also transform the society.

(1) Unity of man and nature: There is in nature necessary material conditions for man to live. When the natural changes directly or indirectly influence the human body, it will result in a corresponding reaction. If the reaction is within the physiological range, that is an adaptable regulation physiologically; if it is beyond physiological range, that is pathological reaction.

In a year, the general law of climatic changes is warm in spring, hot in summer, damp in late-summer, dry in autumn and cold in winter. Under the influence of climates there are adaptable changes for living things of germination in spring, growth in summer, change in late-summer, reap in autumn and storage in winter. And no exception for man, it must adapt itself to the season. For example, in spring and summer, yang qi goes outward and flourishes, qi-blood of the body trends to go and circulate superficially, marked by relaxation of the skin, more sweat and less urine. The body regulates its yin-yang balance by perspiration and heat dissipation. And during autumn and winter, yang qi goes inward and astringes, qi-blood of the body trends to go internally, manifested as compaction of the skin, less sweating and more urine. In this way the body keeps its balance of water metabolism within the body, and also avoids over consumption of yang qi. The pulse picture of a person can also have an adaptable change following the changes of seasons. For example, during the spring and summer, the pulse is often superficial and large; and during autumn and winter, it is usually deep and small, which signifies that the seasonal climate change can influence on the circulation of qi and blood.

Even during a day, the qi-blood and yin-yang of the body can also conduct an adaptable change following the changes of day and night. For example, along with the rise of the sun in the morning, human's yang qi rises to drive the functional activities of the tissues and organs. At noon, yang qi gets supreme, the function increases. At night yang qi astringes internally so as to facilitate rest and recover energy. Although not like in four seasons, the range of temperature in a day is not so obvious, its impact on the human's physiological activities has been paid more and more attention in medical field.

In addition, the geographical difference in living environment is also an important factor directly influencing the physiological function of human body. For instance, in the south of the Yangtze river in China, it is usually damp and hot, the striae of people there are porous; and in the north of China, it is dry and cold, the striae of people there are compact. Once a person changes his living area, the natural conditions change suddenly, thus he or she will get inadaptable at the beginning, and can become adaptable only through a period of time.

Besides directly influencing the physiological function, the changes of natural conditions are also closely associated with the onset of human disease. For example, the changes of four seasons are one of the important factors for living things to germinate, develop, change, reap and store; and in the long process of evolution, man has developed a set of laws in adaptable regulation. Once the climate abruptly changes and the environment gets too adverse as to beyond the limit of normal functional regulation of the body, or the regulatory function of the body gets disordered, thus the body cannot make an adaptable regulation to the changes of natural environment, there will occur disease.

There exists a unified integral relationship between man and nature. Human's physiology and pathology are restricted and influenced by nature, therefore the principles of suiting the treatment to season, locality and individual for a disease become important in Chinese medicine therapeutics.

(2) Close relation of man to society: Besides definite natural attribution, man also is of social attribution because of its mental activities. Chinese medicine has always paid close attention to man's social attribution, attached importance to the correlation between mental activities and viscera and body constituents, and subsumed this under its own theoretical system.

Social advance undoubtedly brings about many benefits for human health, with the average human lifespan becoming longer and longer. However along with rise of material conditions, some social problems unfavorable to human health are also growing with each passing day, such as environmental pollution, food safety, traffic accidents, employment difficulty, stress and anxiety, false, fake, bogus and inferior commodities, aging process of urban population, etc..

The order of society gives a great impact to man. In a stable society, people live a regulatory life, the resistance will be strong, and incidence of disease will be lower, then the lifespan of people will get longer. While in a turbulent society or with war occurring frequently, people are forced to leave home and live a vagrant's life, and cannot get regulatory diet, or over strain; what is more, there is prevalence of pestilence, thus the incidence will obviously increase.

The change of an individual status in the society will definitely bring on the rise or fall in individual material life and spiritual life, the influence of which on the health cannot be neglected. So one should avoid influence by the changes of poor or rich life condition, or noble or humble position to his physical and mental health.

In the long period of medical practice, Chinese medicine has recognized the action of social activity on mind, reaction of mind to the physical health, and mutual relationship and influence between mental activity and physiological activity. For example, great or violent anger will injure the liver, great or violent joy will injure the heart, over thinking will injure the spleen, continuous anxiety will injure the lung, and great fear will injure the kidney. Chinese medicine emphasizes the coexistence , interdependence and interaction between the body and mind. This is the basis of unity and mutual harmony between man and his social environment.

1.2.2 Treatment Determination Based on Syndrome Differentiation

So called syndrome differentiation is to analyze, differentiate and recognize the syndrome of a disease; and treatment determination is to consider and formulate the corresponding therapeutic principle and method according to the result of syndrome differentiation. Syndrome differentiation is the prerequisite and basis for determining the treatment; and treatment determination is the means and method for treating disease, and also a check for whether the conclusion from the syndrome differentiation is correct or not. The two are the mutually related and inseparable stages in diagnosing and treating a disease, being an embodiment of combination of theory and practice.

Disease, symptom and syndrome are different in meaning. So called disease means a complete morbid process including specific cause, mode of onset, typical clinical presentation, developing law and outcome, for example, common cold, dysentery, malaria, and stroke. So called symptom is a discomfort felt subjectively by the patient, for example, pain, dizziness, nausea and lassitude. Sign is the abnormal changes presented objectively by the morbid body, for example, macule and pacule, red tongue, superficial pulse. Therefore generally symptom in a broad sense includes sign. So called syndrome is a pathological summary in a given stage of a disease in its course made by the doctor, which includes the cause of disease (such as wind-cold, wind-heat, stagnant fluid, and stagnant blood), focus of disease (such as externally, internally, in a viscus, and in a meridian), nature of disease (such as cold and heat), situation of disease (such as mild, severe, chronic and acute), and relationship between the pathogenic and the vital (such as deficiency and excess). It marks the essence of pathological change at present.

The occurrence and development of any disease are ever presented by a certain symptoms and signs. Therefore symptom and sign are the basic elements for a disease to manifest externally. They are basis for diagnosis clinically, but not a conclusion of diagnosis. The conclusion that can reveal the essence of a disease is syndrome. Nevertheless, syndrome is a rational diagnosis made by the doctor for current disease essence, so the consistent degree between syndrome conclusion and disease essence depends upon the theoretical level and practical experience of the doctor.

Basing on judgment of disease, one should put the focus of attention on the differentiation of "syndrome", and then can determine the therapeutic principle and method with a definite aim. Take common cold as an example, symptoms are aversion to cold, fever, pain of the head and general body, superficial pulse, which belongs to a superficial illness; however because of different causes and body's reactivity, there are two different conditions of wind-cold and wind-heat. Only one can further clearly differentiate whether the cold belongs to wind-cold or wind-heat, can he determine to chose the method of releasing the exterior with acrid-warm or with acrid-cool. The core of treatment determination based on syndrome differentiation is to master the relation between disease essence and syndrome manifestation. It needs disease differentiation, but what is more, syndrome differentiation, so as to get the purpose of curing disease through treatment of syndrome.

Chinese medicine demands a doctor to view the relationship between disease and syndrome dialectically. One should understand that several different syndromes can be summarized in a disease, and the same syndrome can be analyzed in different diseases. Thus there come important ideas of "different treatments for the same disease" and "the same treatment for different diseases".

So called different treatments for the same disease means, for the same disease because of different times and geographic areas of attack, as well as the patient's reactions, or because of different stages of development in which the disease is, the conclusion on syndrome analyzed is different, so the therapeutic method for it is not the same. Also take common cold as an example; because the season of attack is different, the treatment is different, too. A cold in summer-heat season is mostly caused by pathogenic qi of summer-heat-dampness; the treatment for it should be resolving the turbid with aromatic agents, expelling the summer-heat and dampness. This is different from those with acrid-cool or acrid-warm in other seasons. An another example, measles at its beginning stage has rash pathogen externally, so the treatment should be relieving the exterior to promote eruption; in the meddle stage of accumulation of intense heat in the lung, the treatment should be clearing heat from the lung; in the late stage, there is residual heat with injury of yin of the lung and stomach, then the treatment should mainly be nourishing yin and clearing heat.

The same treatment for different diseases means for different diseases, because there is the same pathomechanism in their course of development, the same or similar treatment is given. For instance, gastroptosis, proctoptosis in a long standing diarrhea, and hysteroptosis are different diseases; however if they belong to the syndrome of sinking of middle qi, then they can all be treated with the method of supplementing and elevating the meddle qi.

It thus can be seen Chinese medicine pays attention to disease differentiation, and more to syndrome differentiation, or putting focus of attention to the difference of pathomechanisms. If the pahtomechanism is the same, then the treatment will be basically the same; and vise versa. So called "the same treatment for the same syndrome" and "different treatments for different syndromes" are in essence because that the meaning of "syndrome" includes pahtomechanism. This principle that contradictions of different natures occurring in the course of a disease are resolved by different measures sufficiently reflects the essence of treatment determination based on syndrome differentiation.

Briefly, Chinese medicine investigates the reactive state of man to its surroundings from the angle that the human body is an organic whole and man and its external environment are closely related, and grasps the primary contraction and the primary contradictory respect for the body's reactive state by seeing through the clinical signs to explore the essence of a disease. It takes the corresponding therapeutic means based on the dynamic balance theory so as to get the purpose of curing the disease through regulation to re-establish the dynamic balance of yin-yang harmony. Treatment determination based on syndrome differentiation is the essential principle for Chinese medicine to recognize and treat a disease. It is a special method of research and treatment of disease, and also one of the essential characteristics of Chinese medicine.

Review Questions

- How does theoretical system of Chinese medicine form and develop?
- What academic features does each of the four physicians in the Jin and Yuan dynasties? And what roles do they play in development of theoretical system of Chinese medicine?
- Please explain the unity between man and nature with examples.
- What is the conception of holism? And what is its significance in clinic?
- What is treatment determination based on syndrome differentiation?
- Please describe the essence of "different treatments for the same disease" and "the same treatment for different diseases" with examples.

2 THEORIES OF YIN-YANG AND THE FIVE ELEMENTS

Theories of yin-yang and the five elements include the theory of Yin-yang and the theory of five elements. They are the world outlook and the methodology by which our ancestors recognize and explain the nature, belonging to the category of ancient philosophy. The theories of yin-yang and five elements are used in medical field by ancient doctors to expound the physiological function and pathological changes of the human body, and to direct the clinical diagnosis and treatment. They have had a deep influence on the initiation and development of the theory of Chinese medicine. So far, they are still in an irreplaceable position in the theoretical system of Chinese medicine and practical application of clinical treatment based on syndrome differentiation.

2.1 Theory of Yin-Yang

2.1.1 The Basic meaning of Yin-Yang

Yin and yang are the summarization of the attributes of two opposite aspects of correlative things or phenomena in nature. The original meanings of yin and yang are simple, mainly referring to facing towards and away from the sunshine, or facing towards the sun belongs to yang and facing away from the sun belongs to yin. Then they are extended to mean warmth and cold of the weather; upper and lower, right and left, inner and outer in orientation, activeness and stillness in moving state. Through long term of observation of living practice, people have gradually found there generally exist two opposite aspects of yin-yang in things, and further recognized the mutual action of the two promotes the formation, development and change of things. Consequently yin and yang are used to explain all kinds of phenomena in nature, and lay the foundation for development of yin-yang theory.

The theory of yin-yang considers that all kinds of things and phenomena can be generalized as two opposite sides of yin and yang. For instance, day and night, hotness and cold, activeness and stillness. The interaction between yin and yang exist intrinsically within all kinds of things. The beginning, developing and changing of all natural things are consequences of the movements of yin-yang.

Yin and yang can stand for opposite things or phenomena, and also can be used to analyze two opposite aspects within one thing. Generally speaking, the things that bear the properties of being active, external, ascending, warm, bright, invisible and functional pertain to yang; while the things that bear properties of being static, internal, descending, cold, dim, visible and organic pertain to yin. In the terms of the heaven and earth, the heavenly qi pertains to yang for its light and clear nature, and the earthly qi to yin for its heavy and turbid nature; in terms of water and fire, water pertains to yin for its cold and moist property, while fire pertains to yang for its hot and rising property; in terms of matter movement, steaming and transforming pertain to yang, while agglomeration and formation pertain to yin.

The theory of Yin-yang is introduced into medical field as a methodology and forms a doctrine of medicine. It classifies the things that have the characters of moving warming and exciting into yang and the things that have the characters of agglomerating, moistening and restraining into yin.

2.1.2 The Basic Content of Yin-Yang Theory

The theory of Yin-yang includes basic contents of opposition and interdependence, restriction and reciprocity, wane-wax and transformation, balance and imbalance of yin and yang.

2.1.2.1 Opposition and Interdependence of Yin and Yang

The opposition of yin and yang means there exist contrary attributes of two opposite aspects in all kinds of things and phenomena in nature, such as heaven and earth, day and night, cold and heat, active and static, internal and external, ascending and descending, entering and exiting, etc.. The theory of yin and yang holds: heaven belongs to yang and earth to yin; day to yang and night to yin; warm to yang and cold to yin; rising to yang and descending to yin; exiting to yang and entering yin.

Interdependence of yin and yang indicates that yin or yang must take the existence of its counterpart as the prerequisite for the existence of its own, and no one can exist solitarily without its counterpart. For example, upper belongs to yang and lower to yin, without the lower there would be no the upper; and vice versa. Heat belongs to yang and cold to yin, without heat there would be no cold; and vice versa.. External belongs to yang and internal to yin, without external there would be no internal; and vice versa.. It is obvious that yin and yang rely on each other; each of yin-yang must take its counterpart's existence as the pre-condition of its own.

2.1.2.2 Restriction and Reciprocity of Yin and Yang

Restriction of yin and yang indicates that two opposite sides of yin and yang present with relationship of mutual restriction and control. For example, in spring, summer, autumn, winter, there are warm, hot, cool, and cold changes in climate. The warmth-hotness in spring and summer are because rising yang qi restricts the cold-cool qi. The coolness-cold in autumn and winter are because rising yin qi restricts the warm-hot qi. That is the consequence that yang qi and yin qi restrict each other in nature. The outcome of restriction of yin and yang makes a dynamic homeostasis within one thing or among the things.

Reciprocity of yin and yang means the interdependent yin and yang often express the relationship of mutual generation and promotion. Take heaven and earth, cloud and rain as examples, the water on the earth can be carried up to the heaven to form cloud and mist by rising of earthly qi; while the cloud and mist in the sky can fall onto the surface of the earth in form of rain by the descending of heavenly qi. The reciprocal process of cloud and rain is the process of reciprocity of yin and yang. Therefore, there is an old saying that "yin cannot generate without yang and yang cannot develop without yin". This generating and promoting relationship that takes the interdependence between yin and yang as the base called reciprocity of yin and yang.

The restriction and reciprocity of yin and yang are contrary, but both can exist in some relationships of yin and yang some times. For instance, the process of anabolism and catabolism in the metabolite process, excitement and inhibition in the functional activity, the two sides both restrict mutually and depend on each other.

It should be pointed out that, the restriction and reciprocity of yin and yang are of no universal, that is to say, all two sides of yin and yang do not have the relationship of restriction and reciprocity.

2.1.2.3 Wane-wax and Transformation of Yin-Yang

The two opposite and interdependent sides of yin and yang are not in a state of stillness but constant change, or in a state of yin wane with yang wax or yang wane with yin wax. This change includes forms of wane-wax quantitatively and transformation qualitatively.

(1) Wane-wax of yin-yang: Wane means decrease, and wax means increase. It concretely shows that one wanes while the other wanes, or one waxes while the other wanes, and one waxes and the other also wanes or one wanes and the other also waxes.

① One wanes while the other wanes or one waxes while the other wanes: Under the condition of mutual restriction of yin and yang, any side of yin-yang gets too declined to restrict the other side, the latter will grow, even get hyperactive. While any side of yin-yang gets too strong, it will inevitably over-restrict the other side, and thus the latter declines, even gets inferior. For example, in the change all the year round from winter to spring and summer, the weather becomes warm gradually, this is called "yin wanes and yang waxes". From summer to fall and winter, the weather becomes cold gradually; it is called "yang wanes and yin waxes". In a day, it is the same in change of temperature.

In the morning, yang qi increases and yin qi decreases; so the temperature gradually gets high. In the noon, yang qi gets to the prime and yin qi declines; so the temperature is the highest. In the evening, yang qi declines and yin qi decreases; so the temperature gradually gets lower. At the mid-night, yin qi gets to the prime and yang qi declines, so the temperature is the lowest. ② One waxes and the other also wanes or one wanes and the other also waxes: Under the condition of reciprocity of yin and yang, any side of yin-yang gets too deficient to promote its counterpart, and thus makes it weak too; and nay side of yin-yang gets abundant and can promote its counterpart, so it also gets abundant. Take the earth and heaven as example, the yang qi in spring and summer grows and gets to the prime; thus the things in the earth also germinate and get to the prime. While yang qi in fall and winter decreases and hides; and thus the things in the earth reaped and store.

(2) Transformation of yin-yang: This means one side of yin-yang under certain conditions can transform itself into the other, or yin may change into yang and yang into yin. Generally this occurs during "the extreme phase" in change of things. The wane-wax of yin-yang is a process of quantitative change, while the transformation of yin-yang is a process of qualitative change on the basis of quantitative change.

The transformation of yin-yang must need certain conditions. That is to say, if a thing does not reach to a certain extent of stage, its yin or yang attribute will not change. Take four seasons for example, yin-cold in winter develops to the extreme, it will get the condition for transformation, then the yin-cold weather will change into yang-heat weather. Yang-heat in summer develops to the extreme, it will get the conditions for transformation, and then the yang-heat weather will change into yin-cold. Here the "extreme" is the condition for transformation.

Wane-wax of yin-yang (quantitative change) and transformation of yin-yang (qualitative change) are two inseparable phases in the whole process of development and change of a thing. Wane-wax is the prerequisite for transformation and the transformation is the outcome of the wane-wax.

2.1.2.4 Balance and Imbalance of Yin-Yang

Balance of yin-yang means that a harmoniously balanced state is maintained by an appropriate change in strength during the motion of yin-yang. In other words it maintains a dynamic balance through motion of yin-yang kept in a certain range. This is the best state formed in auto-motion of a thing. Ancient people call it "sound yin and firm yang".

The motion and change of things is absolute and endless, but it is not without order or disordered. When the wane-wax of yin-yang and transformation of yin-yang can be kept within a certain range, degree and period, it will belong to the dynamic balanced state of yin-yang. And then a series of procedure and change (such as the process of germination, growth, change, reap and storage of things) will perform smoothly.

Imbalance of yin-yang means that the change in strength of yin or yang gets too much or too little, beyond the range limited, and leading a state of occurrence of various calamities. Things belonging to the category of imbalance of yin-yang include natural phenomena of flood, waterlogging, drought, hurricane and earthquake.

To sum up, yin and yang are the summary of relative attributes of things and phenomena, so there is a divide infinitely. The relationship between yin and yang is not isolated and still, but mutual relative, affective and casual.

2.1.3 Application of Yin-Yang Theory in Chinese Medicine

2.1.3.1 To Attribute Tissue Structure

Chinese medicine believes that all the tissues and organs in the body are organically related with each other; and these tissues and organs can also be signified by yin and yang. Generally speaking, the upper part of the body pertains to yang while the lower part to yin; the body surface belongs to yang while the interior of the body to yin. The back pertains to yang while the abdomen to yin; the lateral sides of the four limbs pertain to yang while the medial sides to yin. Viewing the functions of the viscera, the five *Zang*-viscera pertain to yin because they store essential and spiritual qi, but do not transport and transform foodstuffs; the six *Fu*-viscera pertain to yang because they transport and transform foodstuffs, but do not store essential and spiritual qi. Among the five *Zang*-viscera, the heart and lung are located in the upper (thorax), so they pertain to yang; while the liver, spleen and kidney are located in the lower (abdomen), so they pertain to yin. Each viscus itself can be further divided into yin and yang aspects, such as heart-yin and heart-yang, kidney-yin and kidney-yang, etc..

In brief, among every part of tissue structure of the human body superior-inferiorly, internal-externally, interior-exteriorly, and anterior-posteriorly, as well as among the inner organs may all be attributed by using yin and yang.

2.1.3.2 To Explain Physiological Function

The theory of yin-yang holds that human life activity is the outcome of keeping coordination by the two sides of yin-yang. In terms of the viscera and tissues and functional activities, the viscera and tissues pertain to yin and the functional activities to yang. In terms of nutrients and functional activities, nutrients pertain to yin and functional activities to yang. If the spleen and stomach dysfunction, the nutrients will be difficult to be digested and absorbed. Conversely, if the nutrients are short long, the function of the spleen and stomach will decline. Viewing the correlations between qi and blood, qi pertains to yang and blood to yin. Qi can produce, circulate, and control blood; so the normality of qi helps blood to produce and circulate. Blood can generate qi and convey qi; so the abundance of blood can promote qi so as to function normally.

The life activities of human beings take material metabolism as the basis, without metrical metabolism there would be no life activities; and the life activities constantly promote the material metabolism. The relation between the physiological functions of human body and the viscera and tissues is also the relationship that yin and yang are independent upon and serve each other. If yin and yang do not depend on but separate from each other, the life activities of human beings will end.

2.1.3.3 To Explain Pathological Changes

The imbalance between yin and yang is in Chinese medicine considered as the basic reason of the occurrence, development and change of disease. And it is a summarization of high degree for various diseases and pathological mechanisms.

The imbalance between yin and yang mainly expresses the superiority or inferiority of one side, and affection or implication of one side by the other. This can also be collectively called "discordance between yin and yang". If analyzing further on this basis, the occurrence and development of disease mainly involve two respects of the vital qi in the body and the invading pathogenic qi. The so-called vital qi is the normal histological structure, physiological functions, and the ability to resist, stand and repair the damage by disease. The pathogenic qi generally refers to various factors leading to disease.

The vital qi can be divided into yang qi and yin fluid, while the pathogenic qi can also be classified into two kinds of yin and yang. For example, in the six climatic pathogens pathogenic wind, summer heat, dryness and fire (heat) belong to yang, but pathogenic cold and dampness belong to yin.

The process of the occurrence, development and change of disease is a process of conflict between the vital and the pathogen with victory or defeat. The conditions reflected by the interaction and mutual conflict between the vital and the pathogen can all be briefly explained by superiority or inferiority of yin or yang, namely imbalance on wane-wax of yin and yang.

(1) Superiority of yin or yang: This means the pathological changes resulting from that any side of yin and yang is too predominant so as to damage the other side. The pathological changes generally have the following cases:

Superiority of yang results in heat: The predominance of yang refers to that the yang pathogen leads to disease or the yang belonging side in functional activities goes beyond the physiological limit and reaches the absolute exuberance degree, which all belong to superiority of yang. Most of the cases of yang superiority are an excess-heat syndrome. Predominance of yang often consumes yin-fluid within the body and leads to the pathological changes of short yin-fluid. Therefore there is a saying of "predominance of yang makes yin suffer".

Superiority of yin results in cold: The predominance of yin usually refers to that yin pathogen leads to disease, or the yin belonging side in functional activities goes beyond the physiological limit and reaches to the absolute exuberance degree, which all belong to superiority of yin. Most of the cases of yin superiority are an excess-cold syndrome. Predominance of yin often damages yang-qi within the body and leads to the pathological changes of short yang-qi. Therefore there is saying "predominance of yin makes yang suffer".

(2) Inferiority of yin or yang: This means the pathological changes resulting from that any side of yin or yang declines below the normal level. It usually has the following cases:

Deficiency of yang leads to cold: Deficiency of yang refers to pathological change that the driving and warming actions of yang are remarkably decreased because of insufficiency of yang-qi. Since deficient yang fails to restrain the yin with relative exuberance of yin-cold, so there appears the sign of deficiency-cold.

Deficiency of yin leads to heat: Deficiency of yin refers to the pathological change that the moistening and nourishing actions of yin is obviously lower because of shortage of yin-fluid. Deficient yin cannot normally moisten and nourish the viscera and tissue organs, leading to failure of yin to restrict yang, so that the yang belonging functions gets relative hyperactive, and there appears the sign of heat of deficient nature.

Mutual involvement of yin and yang: This refers to the pathological change of dual deficiency of yin and yang because that as one side of yin-yang gets deficient to a certain degree, it must affect its counterpart. There are mainly the conditions as the following.

Yang deficiency affects yin: This means that as yang gets deficient to a certain degree, it may further lead to deficiency of yin-fluid because of failure of deficient yang to produce yin-fluid.

Yin deficiency affects yang: This means that as yin gets deficient to a certain degree, it may further lead to deficiency of yang because of failure of deficient yin to nourish yang-qi.

Either involvement of yin by yang deficiency or involvement of yang by yin deficiency finally presents with dual deficiency of yin and yang because of both yin and yang are short. However, in the case of dual deficiency of yin and yang due to involvement of yin by yang deficiency, yang deficiency prevails; and in the case of dual deficiency of yin and yang due to involvement of yang by yin deficiency, yin deficiency prevails.

(3) Transformation of Yin-Yang: Yin or yang syndrome, under certain conditions, may transform itself into its opposite direction, or a yang syndrome may transform itself into yin syndrome; and a yin syndrome may transform itself into yang syndrome. For example, an exogenous heat disease, manifested by high fever, red face, panting with coarse respiration, vexation, thirst, rapid and forceful pulse, belongs to a yang pattern. Because of rampant heat-toxin, the primordial qi may be greatly damaged, thus under the condition of continuous high fever, the patient may show the critical condition of sudden collapse of yang qi such as sudden lowering of the temperature, pale complexion,

extreme cold limbs, faint pulse hard detected. This is a transformation of yang syndrome into yin one. Another example, a case of accumulation of cold-fluid in the middle, essentially belongs to a yin syndrome, because of long accumulation the cold-fluid may transform into heat. This is a transformation of yin syndrome into yang one. The above cases indicate that there must be conditional factors for transformation of yin-yang. The former is depletion of yang-qi due to extreme heat toxin; and the latter is transformation of cold-fluid into heat due to a long accumulation, which are the inner conditions for the transformation.

2.1.3.4 To Guide Clinical Diagnosis

Chinese medicine holds that imbalance between yin and yang is the root cause of onset and development of a disease. Therefore for all diseases, no matter how changeable or intricate their clinical manifestations may be, one must first distinguish yin from yang in a correct diagnosis. Thus he can grasp the essence of the disease.

In the process of the four diagnostic methods, the yin or yang attributes of the color and luster of the skin, sound of voice and breathing, and pulse condition,

The color and luster of the skin can be used to differentiate yin and yang attributes of the conditions. A bright color pertains to yang while a dark and gloomy color to yin.

In auscultation, hearing the sound of breathing and speech may also be taken to differentiate yin and yang attributes of the conditions. A case of sonorous voice with a high tone, talkativeness and restlessness pertains to yang, while a low and feeble voice, reticence and rest to yin.

Pulse condition can also be classified as yin and yang. Viewed from the location of pulse, *cun* site belongs to yang and *chi* side to yin. As for the rate of pulse, rapid belongs to yang and slow to yin. And for shape, superficial, surging, large and slippery pulse pertain to yang, while deep, thready, small and choppy pulse to yin.

To sum up, distinguishing between yin and yang is the chief work in four diagnostic methods, namely inspection, listening and smelling, inquiring, pulse taking and palpation.

A right diagnosis should first distinguish between yin and yang. Then, the essence of the disease can be examined. The clinically commonly used "eight principles for syndrome differentiation" (yin and yang, external and internal, cold and heat, deficiency and excess) are a framework for various syndrome differentiations, and among them, yin and yang are the most general and fundamental principles. According to such a gradation, external, excess and heat syndromes pertain to yang; while internal, deficiency and cold syndromes to yin. In distinguishing between yin and yang, the attribute may be differentiated either for the whole disease symptoms for the large, or for an individual pulse or symptom for the small. So, clinically the basic principle for differentiating syndrome is to differentiate a yin syndrome from a yang syndrome.

2.1.3.5 To Guide Treatment of Disease

The application of the theory of yin-yang used to guide treatment of disease is mainly to determine the therapeutic principle and to summarize medicinal property.

(1) To determine the therapeutic principle: The therapeutic principle for superiority of yin or yang may be generalized as "reducing the surplus". Superiority of yin or yang, or there is a case of excess or surplus of yin or yang, is the pattern mostly with excess of the pathogenic qi. Since predominance of yang results in heat, and makes yin suffer. Exuberance of yang-heat may easily consume yin-fluid. This is an excess-heat pattern, so it should be treated by restricting the yang with cold-cool natured medicinals, treating the hot with coldness, or "cooling what is hot". Predominance of yin results in clod, and makes yang suffer. Exuberance of yin-cold may easily damage yang-qi. This is an excess-cold pattern, so it should be treated by restricting the yin with warm and hot natured medicinals, treating cold with the hot, or "heating what is cold". In regulation of superiority of yang or yin, one should pay attention to whether there is the corresponding inferiority of yin or yang. If there is, the inferior respect needs to be considered, and the method of supporting yang or supplementing yin should be taken in combination.

The therapeutic principle for inferiority of yin or yang may be generalized as "reinforcing the deficient". Inferiority of yin or yang presents with either yin deficiency or yang deficiency. It may be directly treated by the method of either nourishing yin or warming yang. For a case of deficiency-heat pattern due to yang hyperactivity caused by failure of deficient yin to restrict yang, generally no cold-cool natured medicinals should be taken to directly reduce its heat, but a method of nourishing yin to strengthen water should be used to restrict flaring of fire due to hyperactive yang. For a case of deficiency-cold pattern due to excess of yin caused by failure of deficient yang to check yin, no dispersing medicinals of acrid and warm nature should be taken to dispel yin-cold, but a method of supporting yang and supplementing fire to expel yin-nebula is needed.

According to the theory of interdependence between yin and yang, the methods of "seeking yin from yang and seeking yang from yin" may also be considered in treatment of inferiority of yin or yang. That is to say, when using yang warming medicinals, one may prescribe yin nourishing medicinals as the subsidiary; and when using yin to nourish medicinals, one may prescribe yang supplementing medicinals as the subsidiary. Thus the generating action by reciprocity of yin-yang may play a role.

Briefly, the basic therapeutic principles are reducing the surplus and reinforcing the deficit. Purging the heat is used for a case of yang exuberance; and dispelling the cold is used for a case of yin exuberance. Supporting yang is taken for a case of yang deficiency; and nourishing yin is taken for a case of yin deficiency. As such it will make the pathological changes of superiority or inferiority of yin or yang return to normal state of balanced coordination of yin-yang.

(2) To summarize property of medicinal: The property and acting tendency of a medicinal herb can be summarized by the theory of yin-yang to be the basis of guiding clinic medication. Generally speaking, properties of drugs mainly concern the natures, flavors and acting tendencies (namely ascending, descending, sinking and floating).

The natures: These refer to cold, hot, warm, and cool natures of medicinals, being also called "four natures". Among them, cold and cool natures belong to yin while hot and warm natures pertain to yang. Generally, the medicinals that can reduce or eliminate the heat syndromes pertain mostly to cold-cool nature, such as *Huangqin* (*RadixAstragali*), *Zhizi* (*Fructus Gardeniae*). Conversely, the medicinals that can reduce or eliminate the cold syndromes pertain to warm-hot nature, such as *Fuzi* (*Radix Aconiti Praeparata*) and *Ganjiang* (*Rhizoma Zingiberis*).

The five flavors: These refer to acrid, sweet, sour, bitter, and salty flavors of medicinals. Among them, sour flavor can astringe, bitter flavor can purge, salty flavor can soften and moisten, so the sour, bitter and salty flavors pertain to yin, such as *Wumei* (*Fructus Mume*), *Dahuang* (*Radix et Rhizoma*), and *Mangxiao* (*Natrii Sulfas*). Acrid flavor can disperse, sweet flavor can nourish, so the acrid and sweet pertain to yang, such as *Guizhi* (*Ramulus Cinnamoli*) and *Gancao* (*Radix Glycyrrhizae*). Besides there are some medicinals with no distinct flavor, so they are known as bland, such as *Fuling* (*Poria*) and *Yiyiren* (*Semen Coicis*). These medicinals pertain to yang with their bland flavor. There also some other medicinals with astringent flavor pertain to yin. Although, there are more than five flavors, it is habitually called five flavors.

Ascending, descending, floating and sinking: Herbs with actions of elevating yang, relieving the exterior expelling wind and cold, emesis, and opening orifice are mostly of ascending and outward going properties; they are characterized by ascending and floating actions, so they belong to yang. While herbs with actions of purgation, clearing away heat, diauresis, tranquilizing the mind with heavy quality, subduing yang to quench wind, promoting digestion and removing food retention, lowering the rebellious qi, and astringency are mostly of descending and inward going properties; they are characterized by sinking and descending, so they belong to yin. The examples of herbs with ascending and floating are Sangye (*Folius Mori*) and Juhua (*Flos Chrysanthemi*); and those with descending and sinking are *Biejia* (*Carapax Trionycis*) and Cishi (*Magnetitum*).

2.2 The Theory of the Five Elements

2.2.1 Fundamental Meaning of the Five Elements

In Chinese, *"Wu"* refers to five categories of things in the natural world, namely wood, fire, earth, metal and water; "*Xing*" means movement and change. So *"Wu Xing"*, or the five elements refer to the movement and change of the five elements of world, namely wood, fire, earth, metal and water. Chinese ancients recognized in their long period of life practice that wood, fire, earth, metal and water are the essential materials in human life, so they are called the "five materials"

The theory of the five elements, taking the knowledge of the five materials as the basis, to extract and deduct the attributes of the five materials so as to explain the motion and changes of inter-promotion and inter-restriction among all things and phenomena in nature.

Chinese medicine applies the laws of the five elements in characteristics, classification and promotion-restriction to summarize the functional attributes of the viscera and tissues, explain the inner relations among the five viscera system, and as such, to expound the human physiology, pathology, as well as the mutual relation between the human body and its environment, in order to guide treatment based on syndrome differentiation for the purpose of prevention and treatment of disease.

2.2.2 The Characters and the Categorization of the Five Elements

2.2.2.1 The Characters of the Five Elements

The characters of five elements are the theoretical meanings gradually developed by ancient people through extraction and sublimation of wood, fire, earth, metal and water, based on their simple reorganization. They are mainly used to analyze the attributes of various things in the five elements, and to study interrelations of things. The reorganization of the **characters of** five elements has exceeded the five things themselves, and what is more it is of extensive philosophic meaning.

(1) The characteristics of wood: "Wood bends and strengthens", which means the stem and branches can bend, strengthen, grow upward and outward. It is extended that anything that has the function or property of growing, developing and flourishing is attributed to wood.

(2) The characteristics of fire: "Fire burns and flares up", which means that the fire has the characters of warmth, heat, and ascending. It is extended that anything that has the function or property of warmth, heat, ascending is attributed to five.

(3) The characteristics of earth: "Earth provides for sowing and reaping", which means that the earth can be used for sowing and reaping. It is extended that anything that has the function or property of generating, holding and receiving is attributed to earth.

(4) The characteristics of metal: "Metal works for change", which means the metal can follow man's mind to change its shape. It is extended that anything that has the function or property of clearing, descending and astringing is attributed to metal.

(5) The characteristics of water: "Water moistens and flows downward", which means that the water has the characters of moistening and downward going. It is extended that anything that has the function or property of cold and coolness, moistening,

downward going is attributed to water.

2.2.2.2 Categorization of Things to the Five Elements

The basis for classifying the things and phenomena to the five elements is the characters of the five elements. The method includes direct categorization and indirect deduction.

(1) Direct categorization: This is to compare a part of properties of a thing or phenomenon with the characters of the five elements directly, so as to get the property of the thing or phenomenon in the five elements. That is, a thing similar to the wood in property pertains to wood; and a thing similar to the fire in property pertains to fire, etc. For instance, the east with more vital power where the sun rises, it is similar to growing, developing and flourishing of wood in property, so it pertains to wood. In the south it is hot, plants are flourishing, which is similar to burning and flaring of fire in property, so the south pertains to fire. The west with sign of decline where the sun sets, it is similar to purifying-killing and descending of metal in property, so it pertains to the metal. In the north it is cold, pets there are torpid; which is similar to cold and storage of water in property, so the north pertains to water. In the central region of China it is comfortable with distinct four seasons, every thing can grow there, and the four directions connect with the center, which is similar to generating and holding of earth in property, so the center pertains to earth.

(2) Indirect deduction: When a thing or phenomenon has been classified into one of the elements, some other things or phenomena that closely related with it can also be brought into the element. For example, in late summer it is humid, because of the close relationship of dampness with late summer, the dampness is also brought into earth following the categorization of late summer. In autumn it is dry, because of the close relationship of dryness with autumn; the dryness is also brought into metal following the categorization of autumn.

No matter by direct categorization or indirect deduction, among the things or phenomena that are classified into the same element the inner relationship of either one type or another must exist. The basement of this inner relation is the things or phenomena of one element all have some characters similar to the element.

The following table shows the attribution of things in nature and human to the five elements. (Table 2-1).

It may be seen from the table 2-1 that using the characters of the five elements to analyze, classify and deduct is to summarize the changeable things in nature into the system of the five elements of wood, fire, earth, metal and water. In terms of the human body it is to summarize the various tissues and functions of the body into the five physiological systems taking the five *Zang*-viscera as the center.

Table 2-1 The attribution of things to the five elements

		Jue	Zhi	Gong	Shang	Yu
	five notes	Jue	Zhi	Gong	Shang	Yu
	five times	early morning	noon	afternoon	evening	midnight
n	five flavors	sour	bitter	sweet	acrid	salty
a	five colors	green	red	yellow	white	black
t	five changes	germination	growth	transformation	reaping	storing
u	five climates	wind	summer-heat	dampness	dryness	cold
r	directions	east	south	center	west	north
e	seasons	spring	summer	late summer	autumn	winter
	five elements	wood	fire	earth	metal	water
h	five Zang-viscera	liver	heart	spleen	lung	kidney
u						
m	five Fu-viscera	gall-bladder	small intestine	stomach	large intestine	urinary bladder
a						
n	five constituents	tendon	vessel	muscle	skin	bone
	five brilliances	nail	face	lip	fine hair	hair
b	five emotions	anger	joy	thinking	sorrow	fear
o	five sense organs	eye	tongue	mouth	nose	ear
d	five secretions	tear	sweat	slobber	snivel	spittle
y	five voices	shouting	laughing	singing	crying	moaning
	five pulse	wiry	surging	moderate	superficial	deep

2.2.3 Essential Contents of Theory of the Five Elements

(1) Promotion and restriction among the five elements: ① Promotion means that one of the five elements promotes and helps another element in the five elements. The order of promotion among the five elements is: Wood promotes fire, fire promotes earth, earth promotes metal, metal promotes water and water promotes wood. In the relations among the five elements, each element has two sides of "being promoted" and "promoting". The one promoting me is called "mother" while the one being promoted by me is called "child". So the promotion relationship among the five examples is also named "mother-child relationship". Take wood as an example, the one that promotes fire is wood and the one that is promoted by wood is water. So wood is the mother of fire and wood is the child of water. ② Restriction means that one of the five elements restricts and checks another element in the five elements. The order of restriction is: Wood restricts earth, earth restricts water, water restricts fire, fire restricts metal and metal restricts wood. In the restriction relationships among the five elements, each element has two sides of "being restricted" and "restricting". The one being restricted by me is my "subordinate"; while the one restricting me is my "dominator". Take wood for example, the one that restricts wood is metal and the one that is restricted by wood is earth. Thus, metal is called the dominator of wood and earth is called the subordinate of wood.

Promotion and restriction among the five elements are two inseparable respects, which expresses concretely that "there is restriction within promotion" and "there is promotion within restriction". For example, wood promotes fire, also restricts earth; earth promotes metal, also restricts water. This relationships of restriction in the promotion and promotion in the restriction are both opposite and yet complementary to each other, with a balance between the promotion and restriction, so that the normal occurrence and development of things are maintained. (See Fig. 2-1)

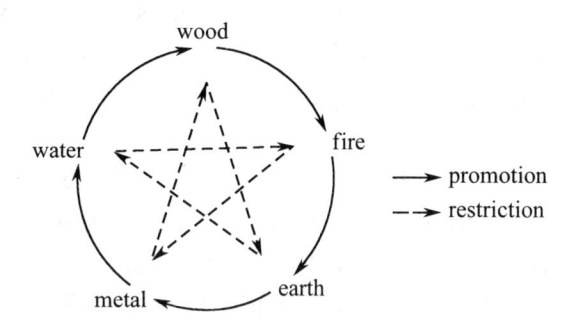

Fig. 2-1 The schematic diagram of the laws of promotion and restriction among the five elements

Promotion and restriction among the five elements reflect normal phenomena in nature. Every part of the system of the five elements is not isolated, but closely related. The change of each part will affect the states of others; at the same time, it is influenced and restrained by the structural whole of the five-element system.

(2) Abnormal promotion and restriction among the five elements

① The abnormal change of promotion: Since it happens between a mother and its child, it is called "mutual involvement of the mother and the child." It includes two conditions of the involvement of the mother by its child and the involvement of the child by its mother.

The involvement of the child by its mother means that a disorder of a mother-element involves or affects its child-element, leading to anomaly of both mother and child. Because a mother-element is weak, its child-element gets also deficient. For example, water is a mother and wood is its child. If water gets deficient, it fails to promote wood. As a result, both the mother and its child will be weak.

The involvement of the mother by its child means that a disorder of a child-element involves or affects its mother-element. It includes deficient and excessive types. One is that a child-element gets too excessive, it causes excess of its mother-element, and as a result both the child and its mother are hyperactive. For example, fire is a child and wood is its mother; hyperactivity of fire may affect wood, leading to superabundance of both wood and fire. Such a condition is called "Rchild's disorder affects its mother". The other is that deficiency of a child-element involves or affects its mother-element, leading to deficiency of the mother, thus both the mother and child are weak. For example, wood is a child and water is its mother. If deficiency of wood causes shortage of water, leading to deficit of both wood and water, this is called "Rchild's disorder steals its mother's qi".

② Abnormal restriction: the relations of abnormal restriction in the five elements are mainly reflected in two respects of subjugation and violation.

Subjugation: Subjugation refers to an abnormal condition in which one element of the five elements excessively restricts its restricting element. There are two causes for subjugation: One is that one element of the five elements becomes too powerful and in turn, excessively restrains the element that it normally restrains, leading to weakness of the element being restricted. For example, if wood is too powerful, it will excessively restrain earth, leading to deficient of earth; this is called "wood subjugates earth". The other is that one element of the five elements becomes too weak, and thus makes the element that restricts it relatively hyperactive, and it cannot stand the relatively stronger restriction from the element that originally restricts it, hence making it more deficient. For example, wood itself is normal and its restriction on earth is also normal. But if the earth itself gets weak, then the strength of restriction of earth by wood becomes relatively enhanced, it will make earth more deficient; this is called "wood subjugates earth with deficiency".

Violation: Violation refers to an abnormal condition in which one element of the five elements reversely restrains and bullies the element that restricts it. There are two causes responsible for violation: One is that one element of the five elements becomes very powerful, it is no longer restricted by the element that originally restricts it, but reversely restricts the element; so this is also called counter restriction. For example, wood is originally restricted by metal; however, under the condition of too much power of wood, it is not only restricted by the metal, but also reversely restricts metal; this is called "wood violates metal". The other is one of the five elements gets too weak, thus leading to relatively powerfulness of the element being originally restricted by it; as a result, this element is no longer restricted by it, but reversely restricts it.For example, when the metal gets too weak, it cannot restrict wood anymore, and will be reversely restricted by wood; this is called "wood violates metal".

Subjugation and violation are both phenomenon of abnormal restriction. The two are both different and relative. The difference is: Subjugation is an abnormal restriction going in the order of restriction among the five elements; while the violation is an abnormal restriction going in the opposite order of restriction among the five elements. The relation is: When a subjugation occurs, a violation will appear at the same time, and vice versa. For example, when wood gets too powerful, it may both subjugate earth and violate metal; if metal gets weak, it may both be violated by wood and subjugated by fire. The diagram taking wood as an example is shown in Fig. 2-2.

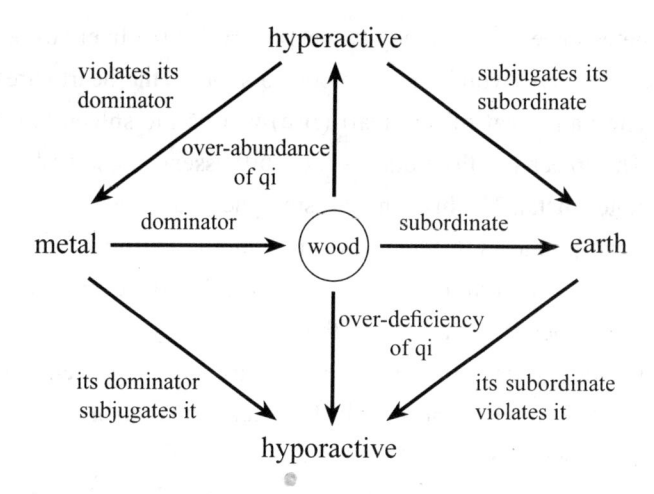

```
                    hyperactive
violates its           ↑           subjugates its
 dominator             |            subordinate
      ↘      over-abundance      ↗
              of qi
        dominator   ╱───╲  subordinate
metal  ─────────→ ( wood ) ──────────→ earth
                    ╲───╱
      ↗      over-deficiency    ↖
              of qi
its dominator          |           its subordinate
 subjugates it         ↓            violates it
                    hyporactive
```

Fig. 2-2 The diagram of the relationship between subjugation and violation among the five elements

2.2.4 Application of Theory of the Five Elements in Chinese Medicine

In Chinese medicine the application of the theory of the five elements is, by using the method of classification or attribution of things to the five elements and their change laws of promotion and restriction, to explain the physiological functions and pathological phenomena of the five *Zang*-viscera, and to guide clinical diagnosis and treatment.

2.2.4.1 To Explain Physiological Functions and Their Relationships

The theory of the five elements classifies the five *Zang*-viscera into the five elements so as to explain the characteristics of physiological functions of the five *Zang*-viscera according to the characters of the five elements. For example, wood is characterized by growing and flourishing, and the liver prefers free flow of qi; so the liver pertains to wood. Fire is hot and tends to flame up, and heart-yang has a warm action; so the heart pertains to fire. Earth is characterized by generating myriad of things, and the spleen is the source for production of qi and blood; so the spleen pertains to earth. Metal has the properties of purifying and astringing, and lung-qi is in charge of purification and descent; so the lung pertains to metal. Water has the properties of moistening and storage, and the kidney stores essence and governs water metabolism; so the kidney pertains to water. Through indirect deduction, those things that have relationships with the five *Zang*-viscera such as the five *Fu*-viscera, five constituents, five brilliances, five emotions, five orifices, and five secretions, are all attributed to the five elements along with the corresponding *Zang*-viscus.

The theory of the five elements can also be taken to explain the inner relations in physiological function among the viscera and tissues. For example, promotion among the five elements may be used to explain the generation relationships among the five

Zang-viscera. The essence in the kidney (water) nourishes the liver (wood), this is water promotes wood. The liver (wood) stores blood to support the heart (fire), this is wood promotes fire. The yang-heat of the heart (fire) warms the spleen (earth), this is fire promotes earth. The spleen (earth) produces foodstuff essence to nourish the lung (metal), this is earth promotes metal. The lung (metal) smoothes water passages to help the kidney (water), this is metal promotes water. The restriction relationships among the five Zang-viscera can be explained in term of restriction among the five elements. The purification and descent of lung (metal) qi can check the hyperactivity of the liver (wood), this is metal restricts wood. The free flow of liver (wood) qi may prevent the stagnation of spleen (earth) qi, this is wood restricts earth. The transformation and transportation by the spleen (earth) may prevent disorder of the kidney (water), this is earth restricts water. The kidney (water) yin goes up to prevent the hyperactivity of the heart (fire), this is water restricts water.

In addition, the relations between human being and its external environment such as four seasons, five climatic factors, and five flavors of the diet, may all be explained by the theory of the five elements. Therefore, application of the theory of the five elements in physiology consists in explanation of the unity among the viscera and tissues of the human body, as well as the unity between man and the environment.

2.2.4.2 To Explain Pathological Change and Their Inter-Influence

The theory of the five elements may be taken to explain the inter-influences in pathology among the viscera through the abnormal laws of promotion and restriction among the five elements. For example, if a liver disease affects the spleen, this is wood subjugates earth; if a spleen disease involves the liver, this is earth violates wood; If the liver and the spleen get disordered at the same time, and mutually influence, that is either wood stagnation leads to earth deficiency or earth stagnation leads to wood stagnation: A liver disease may also affect the heart, this is a child disease involves its mother; if it affects the lung, this is wood violates metal; if it affects the kidney, this is a child's disease involves its mother. Diseases of the other viscera can all be explained like this, by using the abnormal laws of promotion and restriction among the five elements.

2.2.4.3 To Guide Clinical Diagnosis

Abnormal changes in functional activities of the viscera and their relationships can all be reflected in the external appearances. The five Zang-viscera have a certain relations in the attribution to the five elements to the changes of five colors, five flavors and pulse condition. So, on diagnosing disease, according to its attribution to the five elements and the laws of promotion and restriction, one can judge the conditions of disease through comprehensively analyzing the data gained via the four diagnostic methods. For example, a patient whose complexion is greenish with a preference for sour food and a wiry pulse may be diagnosed as having a liver disease; a patient with a reddish complexion, bitter taste in the mouth, and a surging pulse may be diagnosed as having a heart disease. A patient with spleen deficiency accompanied with a greenish complexion implies that wood (liver) subjugates earth (spleen) with deficiency. A patient with heart disease with darkish complexion suggests that water (kidney) subjugates fire (heart) with deficiency.

2.2.4.4 To Guide Treatment of Disease

(1) Deciding therapeutic principles and methods:

1) The therapeutic principles and methods decided according to promotion law: The therapeutic principles decided according to promotion law include: "tonifying the mother and reducing the child".

Tonifying the mother: It is a therapeutic principle to treat a deficiency pattern in disorders of mother-child relationship. For example, if kidney yin gets deficient and fails to nourish the liver-wood, it may lead to deficiency of liver yin with hyperactivity of liver yang; this is called water fails to produce wood or water fails to nourish wood. The treatment for it is not only to deal with the liver, but also to nourish kidney yin. Since the kidney is the mother of the liver, kidney-water can promote liver-wood. Therefore by treating the kidney alone it can astringe liver-yang. Another example, when a deficiency of lung qi develops to a certain degree, it may affect the transformation and transportation, and thus leads to insufficiency of the spleen. The spleen-earth is the mother and the lung-metal is its child; earth can promote metal. So this case may be treated by the method of treating both the mother and its child in combination. This is the meaning of "tonifying the mother for a deficiency syndrome".

Reducing the child: It is a therapeutic principle to treat an excess pattern. For example, for a case that the liver fire gets too hyperactive with liver qi over ascending, showing as an excess syndrome of liver disorder, the treatment may be reducing heart fire as the subsidiary. The liver-wood is the mother and the heart-fire is its child. So reducing heart fire will help to reduce liver fire. This is the meaning of "reducing the child for an excess syndrome".

The therapeutic methods decided according to promotion relationship mainly include replenishing water to nourish wood, mutual promotion of metal and water, reinforcing earth to strengthen metal and assisting fire and strengthen earth.

The method of replenishing water to nourish wood: This method is also called replenishing the kidney to nourish the liver. It is a method to nourish the liver through supplementing the kidney so as to astringe liver yang. It is mainly suitable for deficiency of liver yin, even superiority of liver yang due to shortage of kidney yin. Its clinical manifestations may be dizziness and vertigo, dry and discomfort feeling of the eyes, tinnitus and flushed face, dry mouth, vexation with hot sensation of the five centers, soreness and weakness of the waist and knees, spermatorrhea in male, irregular menstruation in female, red tongue with little coating, wiry, thready and rapid pulse.

The method of mutual promotion of metal and water: It is also named "nourishing the lung and tonifying the kidney". This is a method to nourish deficient yin of both the lung and kidney. It is mainly suitable for a case that insufficient lung fails to distribute the fluid to nourish the kidney, or a case of yin deficiency of the lung and kidney because that kidney yin gets deficient, with failure of essence-qi to go up to nourish the lung. Clinically there may appear cough, dyspnea, dry cough or hemoptysis, hoarseness, bone steaming sensation with tidal fever, night sweating, spermatorrhea, soreness and weakness of the waist and knees, emaciation, dry mouth, red tongue with little coating, thready and rapid pulse.

The method of reinforcing earth to strengthen metal: It is also called "invigorating the spleen to benefit the lung". It is a method to replenish lung qi by replenishing spleen qi. It is mainly suitable for an insufficiency of both the spleen and lung because that the insufficiency of the spleen and stomach cannot nourish lung qi. Clinically there may appear chronic cough, copious sputum with thin quality, or a little sticky sputum, poor appetite, sloppy feces, lassitude, pale tongue, and weak pulse.

The method of assisting fire and strengthening earth: It is also named "warming the kidney and strengthening the spleen". It is a method to support spleen yang by warming and strengthening kidney yang. It is suitable for a syndrome of yang deficiency of both the spleen and kidney (or "fire fails to produce earth") due to great decline of kidney yang with resultant deficiency of spleen yang, or a part of patterns of spleen yang deficiency. Clinically there may occur cold pain in the lower abdomen, diarrhea at dawn, intolerance of cold with clod limbs, pale and enlarge tongue with white and glossy coating, deep and fast pulse.

It should be pointed out, in terms of promotion law among the five elements, the heart belongs to fire and spleen to earth. So fire promotes earth, that is, the heart promotes the spleen. That "fire fails to promote earth" should be understood to be failure of heart-fire to promote spleen-earth. However, since the time when the theory of life gate is established, there is a change for this concept. Clinically the fire specially means the kidney yang (or life gate fire), and seldom means the heart fire again. On treatment, the method of warming and strengthening kidney yang to help spleen yang really has a better effect. Nevertheless, the method of nourishing the heart to benefit the spleen also has its indications, and thus needs to be kept.

2) The therapeutic principles and methods decided according to restriction law: The therapeutic principles decided according to restriction law include checking the strong and strengthening the weak.

Checking the strong: This is a therapeutic principle to restrict the hyperactive viscus so as to benefit the recovery of the subjugated or violated viscus. For example, if the lever qi gets disordered and transversely affects the stomach or spleen, leading to disharmony of the liver and the stomach, or disharmony of the liver and spleen; this is a pattern of subjugation of earth by the hyperactivity of wood. On treatment, the method of soothing or pacifying the liver should be considered. If qi of the spleen and stomach gets stagnated, and thus it affects the liver, leading to failure of the liver to govern free flow of qi; this is a pattern of depressed wood due to stagnation of earth, being a case of violation (counter restriction). The treatment should be strengthening the spleen and normalizing the stomach. Restricting the strong one will make the functions of the subjugated ones naturally recovered.

Strengthening the weak: This is a therapeutic principle to support the functions of the subjugated or violated viscus so as to coordinate the strengths of both sides. This is mainly suitable for a case, in which the power for restriction gets lower, or subjugation or a violation due to insufficiency. For example, if the liver gets insufficient with qi depression, it affects the spleen and stomach, leading to disorders of receiving and transforming functions; this is called failure of wood to smooth earth. The treatment should be nourishing or harmonizing the liver, with strengthening the spleen and normalizing the stomach as the subsidiary. In a word, strengthening the weak will be conducive to reconcile the harmony of restriction relation.

The therapeutic methods decided according to restriction law include inhibiting wood to assist earth, banking up earth to treat water, assisting metal to subdue wood, reducing the south and tonifying the north.

Inhibiting wood to assist earth: It is also called smoothing the liver and strengthening the spleen. This is a method to treat the case of failure of the insufficient spleen in transformation and transportation due to hyperactivity of liver qi by soothing the liver and strengthening the spleen. It is mainly suitable for the pattern of depressed liver qi with insufficient spleen. The clinical manifestations are chest distress, hypochondriac distention, poor appetite, abdomen fullness with borborygmi, or sloppy feces, or gastric discomfort, fullness and pain, eructation, flatus, etc..

Banking up earth to treat water: It is also called strengthening the spleen, warming the kidney for diuresis. This is a method to treat a case of accumulation of water-dampness by warming and strengthening spleen yang, or strengthening the spleen and warming the kidney. It is mainly suitable for the pattern of flood of water-dampness due to failure of the insufficient spleen or yang deficiency of the spleen and kidney. The clinical manifestations are edema of lower limbs, abdominal fullness and distention, pale and enlarged tongue, wiry and slippery pulse.

Assisting metal to subdue wood: It is also called subduing the liver and clearing the lung. This is a method to inhibit the hyperactivity of liver fire by clearing and purifying lung qi. It is mainly suitable for a case of "torture of metal by wood-fire" due to failure of lung qi in purification resulting from reverse rise of liver fire to burn lung-metal. The clinical manifestations are hypochondriac pain, bitter taste in the mouth, cough with hemoptysis, or blood-tinged sputum, irritability, fidgets, wiry and rapid pulse.

Reducing the south and tonifying the north: It is also called reducing fire and replenishing water or nourishing yin and pursing fire. This method is to reduce heart-fire and nourish kidney-water, being manly suitable for a case of "non-coordination between the kidney and the heart" due to discordance of water and fire resulting from shortage of kidney yin and superiority of heart yang. The clinical manifestations are soreness and weakness of the lower back and knees, dysphor with insomnia, spermatorrhea, palpitation, amnesia, or tidal fever, and night sweating.

It should be pointed out that the kidney is a viscus with both water and fire in it. So a yin deficiency of the kidney can also lead to superiority or audacity of the ministerial fire, and thus resulting in symptoms of nocturnal emission, tinnitus, sore and dry throat. This belongs to the superiority or inferiority of the yin or yang of the kidney itself; and it is not the same as failure of water to check fire in the relations among the five *Zang*-viscera.

(2) To guide therapies for metal disease: The relationships in promotion and restriction among the five elements are of a certain guiding significance for therapies for mental diseases. The therapies are mainly suitable for disorders of emotions. The emotions originate from the five *Zang*-viscera, and among the latter there are relations of promotion and restriction, so among the emotions there are also these relations. Owing to there is inter-restriction in physiology among the emotional changes, and also the close relations in pathology among the viscera, clinically, these restriction relations among emotions may be taken to regulate the emotional disorders for the purpose of curing disease. This is named method of inter-check among the five emotions. For example:

Sorrow is the emotion of the lung, belonging to metal; and anger is the emotion of the liver, belonging to wood. Metal can restrict wood, so sorrow can check anger.

Fear is the emotion of the kidney, belonging to water; and joy is the emotion of the heart, belonging to fire. Water can restrict fire, so fear can check joy.

Anger is the emotion of the liver, belonging to the wood; and thinking is the emotion of the spleen, belonging to the earth. Wood can restrict earth, so anger can check thinking.

Joy is the emotion of the heart, belonging to fire; and worry is the emotion of the lung, belonging to metal. Fire can restrict metal, so joy can check worry.

Thinking is the emotion of the spleen, belonging to earth; and fear is the emotion of the kidney, belonging to water. Earth can restrict water, so thinking can check fear.

(3) To guide choice of acupoints in acumoxibustion: The theory of the five element may also be used to guide the choice of acupoint in acumoxibustion. In acumoxibustion therapy, when we match the "five *Shu*-points" of yin meridians of both hand and foot to the five elements, *Jing* (well) points belong to wood, *Ying* (spring) points to fire *Shu* (stream) points to earth, *Jing* (river) points to metal and *He* (sea) points to water. And when match the "five *Shu*-points" of yang meridians of both hand and foot to the five elements, *Jing* (well) points belong to metal, *Ying* (spring) points to water, *Shu* (stream)

points to wood, *Jing* (river) points to fire and *He* (sea) points to earth. On treatment by acumoxibustion, one may choose the points according to laws of promotion and restriction among the five elements for the disease patterns. For example, according to the principle of "reinforcing the mother for a deficiency", the *He* (sea) point (water-point) of the kidney meridian, Yingu (KI 10), or the *He* (sea) point (water-point) of the liver meridian, Ququan (LR 8), may be taken for treatment of a pattern of liver insufficiency. While according to the principle of "reducing the child for an excess", the *Ying* (spring) point of the heart meridian, Shaofu (HT 8), or the *Ying* (spring) point of the liver meridian, Xingjian (LR 2), may be chosen for treatment of a pattern of liver excess.

The laws of promotion and restriction among the five elements are of a certain significance to guide clinic. However this is not suitable for all cases, a flexible application according to the concrete conditions is needed.

To sum up the above mentioned, yin-yang and the five elements theories are of their own characters, and each has its stress. But they are related to each other. So only application of them in combination in the medical field, can one explain the physiological and pathological relations of the body more comprehensively. In the practical utilization, as applying yin-yang, one usually needs to involve the five elements, and vise versa. The association of yin-yang and five elements theories may not only explain the general relations of things, but also the concrete and complicated relations of things that are both inter-dependent and inter-restrictive. And as such, it is conducive to the complicated life phenomena and pathological process.

Review Questions

- Briefly describe the essential contents of yin-yang theory.
- What are the wane-wax and transformation of yin-yang? What is the relation of them?
- Try to explain tissue structure and physiological activities of the body by using yin-yang theory. How to use yin-yang theory to guide the diagnosis and treatment of disease?
- What are the five elements and the theory of the five elements? How to class the attribution of things to the five elements?
- What are contents of laws of promotion and restriction among the five elements?
- How to explain the physiological functions in the viscera and their relations by using the theory of the five elements?

3 VISCERAL PICTURE THEORY

The word of "visceral picture" comes from *Sù Wèn·Liu Jie Zang Xiang Lùn* (*Plain Question: On Visceral Picture of Six Periods in a Year*). Viscera means the internal organs hiding in the body; picture means the physiological and pathological signs reflected outside.

Visceral picture is a theory expounding the physiological functions and pathological changes of the internal organs of the body and the relationships among the organs through inspection of physiological and pathological signs outside. Chinese medicine holds that the human body is an organic whole; each viscus has its own outside signs, and is specially related with certain body constituents and orifices. Therefore the internal organs hide inside of the body, but their physiological functions and pathological changes have a certain signs externally. Thus through inspection of the corresponding external signs one can determine the functional status. For example, through inspection of the outside signs such as complexion, tongue color, pulse picture and sensation of the chest one can know whether the function of the internal organ or heart in governing the blood and vessels is normal.

The main contents studied in visceral picture are internal organs. According to the characteristics of the internal organs, they can be divided as *Zang*-viscera, *Fu*-viscera and extraordinary *Fu*-viscera. *Zang*-viscera are the heart, lung, spleen, liver and kidney, collectively called five *Zang*-viscera; their common functions are to produce and store essence-qi, and their characteristics are "they can be full of essence-qi instead of containing the foodstuff". *Fu*-viscera are gallbladder, stomach, small intestine, large intestine gladder and tri-Jiao, being collected called Six *Fu*-viscera; their common functions are to receive, digest and transmit the foodstuff, and their characteristics are "they can be full of foodstuff instead of storing essence-qi". And extraordinary *Fu*-viscera are brain, marrow, bone, vessel, gallbladder and uterus. The shapes of the extraordinary *Fu*-viscera are mostly hollow like the six *Fu*-viscera, but their physiological characteristics are to store the essence-qi like the five *Zang*-viscera; they are similar with *Zang*-viscera but not, and similar with *Fu*-viscera but also not, thus being called as "extraordinary *Fu*-viscera".

Visceral picture theory takes a given anatomic knowledge as its basis, but it is mainly guided under the ancient philosophical thinking in China. It seeks the activity of internal organs from the integral investigation, or "determining the viscera from their pictures" and "operating the external to surmise the internal". Therefore the viscera in the visceral picture, are not simply the organs in anatomy, what is more, they mean the physiological functions. The names of the viscera in Chinese medicine are generally the same as those of internal organs in Western medicine; however their connotations are quite different. The functions of a viscus in Chinese medicine visceral picture may include the functions of several internal organs in Western medicine; and the functions of an internal organ in Western medicine may also be decentralized among the functions of several viscera in Chinese medicine visceral picture.

3.1 Five *Zang*-Viscera

3.1.1 Heart

The heart is located in the thorax, its major functions are to govern blood and house spirit. The heart and small intestine form an internal-external relationship through mutual connection and affiliation of their meridians. The heart is associated with vessel in constituent, reflects its brilliance in the face, is associated with joy in emotion, with tongue in orifice, and with sweat in secretion. The heart plays a dominant role to the vital activity of the whole body, so it is called "monarch" and "the dominator of the five *Zang*-viscera and six *Fu*-viscera".

3.1.1.1 Major Functions of the Heart

(1) Governing blood: The function of governing blood by the heart includes two respects of circulating and producing blood. ① The heart circulates blood: This means the heart-qi is of action to drive and regulate circulation of blood within the vessels. Continuous flow of blood in the vessels depends upon the action of heart-qi. The heart-qi maintains blood flow free and the vessels smooth through propelling blood circulation and regulating dilation and contraction of the vessels. Therefore if the heart-qi is sufficient, and the function of the heart in governing blood is normal, then the complexion will be rosy and lustrous, the thorax be comfort, and pulse be even, moderate and forceful. On the contrary, if the heart-qi is insufficient, and the function of the heart in governing blood is disordered, then the blood flow will get unsmooth, the pulse be forceless; or even there occur stagnation of qi-blood and obstruction of the vessels, then there will occur dark and gray complexion, cyanoses of the lips and tongue, precordial oppression, stuffiness and stabbing pain, as well as knot, intermittent and hasty pulse. ② The heart produces blood: Blood is mainly composed of nutritive qi and body fluid, but the action of hear-yang is necessary for nutritive qi and body fluid to compose blood, or changing them into red to become blood.

The heart can both circulate and produce blood so as to guarantee sufficient nourishment of blood for all tissues of the whole body.

(2) Housing spirit: The function of housing spirit of the heart means the heart has the function of dominating the mental activities such as in psychology and emotion, and life activities of the whole body. Man's psychological and emotional activities are closely related with the five *Zang*-viscera, performed by coordination of the five *Zang*-viscera, however dominated by the heart. The heart houses spirit which can control qi. The heart-spirit controls and coordinates the movement of the visceral qi so as to drive and regulate the function of the viscera. When the function of the heart in housing spirit is normal, there will be high spirit, clear consciousness, quick thinking and acute response, then the functions of the viscera are coordinative and the whole body is healthy. On the contrary, if the function of the heart in housing spirit is abnormal, there will appear clinical manifestations of insomnia, dreamfulness, restlessness, delirium and madness; or tardy response, amnesia, listlessness, and even coma; it may also affect the functions of other viscera, or so called in Chinese medicine "dysfunction of the heart would cause the disorders of the five *Zang*-and six *Fu*-viscera", even endanger the life.

The function of housing spirit and the function of governing blood of the heart are closely related. The function of housing spirit of the heart can regulate the heart qi in its driving blood to circulate within the vessels, being helpful to the heart in its governing blood. While the heart by governing blood can supply material basis for mental activities, being beneficial to the heart in its housing spirit, for blood is the major material basis for mental activities. Therefore the dysfunction of the heart in governing blood will inevitably lead to disorder of the heart-spirit; contrarily, the dysfunction of the hear in housing spirit may also result in anomaly of blood flow..

3.1.1.2 Relations of the Heart with Constituent, Emotion, Orifice and Secretion

(1) The heart is associated with vessel in constituent, and reflects its brilliance in the face: Vessel means blood vessel, being the passageway of qi-blood circulation. What the heart is associated with vessel in constituent signifies that the blood vessels of the whole body are dominated by the heart. The heart directly connects with the vessels; the dilation and constriction of the vessels are regulated by the heart-qi. When the heart qi is sufficient, the pulsation will be moderate and forceful with an even rhyme; if the heart-qi is insufficient, the pulsation will be thready and forceless. Its reflection of brilliance in the face means the state of the physiological function of the heart may be reflected as the changes of color and luster in the face. The heart is associated with the vessels, and the face is rich in distribution of vessels. Therefore when the heart-qi is sufficient and blood vessels are full of blood, the face will be red and lustrous; if the heart-qi is insufficient, the face will get pale or dark and gloomy; if the heart-blood is deficient, the face will become illustrious; and if the heart-blood gets stagnated, the face will get cyanotic.

(2) The heart is associated with joy in emotion: The function of the heart is closely related with "joy" of emotion. An appropriate joy is a reaction of the body to an optimal stimulation, and it is good to the physiological functions of the heart such as governing blood. However, over-joy may make the heart-spirit lax, leading to clinical manifestations such as endless joy and mental disorder. Besides, the heart houses spirit, so not only over joy injures the heart, but also the extreme of the five emotions can all disturb the heart-spirit.

(3) The heart is associated with tongue in orifice: The heart connects with the tongue through the meridians, "the divergence of the hand Shaoyin meridian... along with its meridian enters into the heart and connects with the root of tongue." The conditions of the functions of the heart influence and are reflected in the tongue, so the heart is associated with tongue. When the functions of the heart in governing blood and sousing spirit are normal, the tongue will be red and moist, soft and flexible, with acute sense of test and fluent speech. If the function of the heart gets disordered in governing blood and the blood is deficient, the tongue will become pale; if the heart-yang gets short, the tongue will be pale and enlarged; if the heart-blood gets stagnated, the tongue will become dark and purplish or with ecchymoses. If the function of the heart in housing spirit gets abnormal, there may be symptoms of curled tongue, stiff tongue with dysphasia or aphasia.

(4) The heart is associated with sweat in secretion: This means that sweat is closely related with the heart-blood and heart-spirit. Sweat is transformed from body fluid, and the body fluid shares the same source with blood, and the two transform themselves into each other. The body fluid, as it permeates into the vessels, will become blood; while blood, as it permeates out of the vessels, will become body fluid. Furthermore blood is governed by the heart. So when the heart-blood is abundant, body fluid will be ample, thus sweat will have its source for production. In addition, the heart houses spirit, and the production and secretion of sweat are regulated by the heart-spirit. Mental stress may cause perspiration; hence the saying sweat is the secretion of the heart.

Appendix: Brain

Brain, called also sea of marrow, is located in the cranial cavity.

The major functions of the brain are to dominate life activity, mentality and consciousness and sense movements. When the brain functions normally, the human body will be full of vitality with clear consciousness, acute senses and agile movements. On the contrary, if the brain functions abnormally, the body will be disordered in vital activity with listlessness, unconsciousness, dull senses and slow movements.

3.1.2 Lung

The lung is of two lobes, each being situated in one side of the thorax. The major functions of it are governing respiratory qi and qi of the whole body, smoothing water passage and connecting with vessels. The lung and large intestine form an exterior-interior relationship through connection and affiliation of their meridians. The lung is associated with the skin in constituent, reflects its brilliance in the fine hair, and is associated with sorrow (worry) in emotion, with nose in orifice, and with snivel in secretion. The lung is located at the highest position among the viscera and covers the others; it is thus called the "canopy". Because its lobes are delicate and communicates with outside environment, it is subject to invasion of pathogens, hence the name of "fragile organ".

The movements of the lung-qi are of two models of diffusion and descent. Diffusion includes diffusing and dispersing. Diffusing and dispersing of lung-qi means the lung-qi can diffuse upwards and disperse outwards. The physiological function of the lung-qi in diffusion mainly embodies three respects. Firstly, exhaling turbid gases in the body; next, transporting the foodstuff essence and fluid transported by the spleen upward to the head and face, outward to the surface of the body; and last, diffusing defensive qi to the body surface to warm the muscle and skin, to regulate opening-closing of the striae so as to control the excretion of sweat. Therefore as the lung-qi fails in diffusion, there will occur cough, aversion to cold, anhidrosis, etc.. Descent includes purifying and descending. Purifying and descending of the lung-qi means the lung-qi can go downward and keep the respiratory tract pure and clear. The physiological function of the lung-qi also embodies three respects. Firstly, inhaling the clear air of nature; next, distributing the foodstuff essence and fluid transported by the spleen downward and inward to other viscera and tissues; and last, eliminating clearly the foreign body in the lung and respiratory tract so as to keep the respiratory clear. Therefore if the lung-qi fails in descent, there will appear expiratory dyspnea, wheezing and panting.

Diffusion and descent of the lung-qi are two aspects both opposite and complementary to each other. Under the physiological conditions, they depend upon each other and restrict each other; under the pathological conditions, they often impact each other. When the lung-qi diffuses and descends normally, the respiration will be even and freely, and water spreads out normally. If the coordination of two aspects gets disturbed, there will appear disorders of "failure of lung-qi in diffusion" and "failure of lung-qi in purification and descent", manifesting as chest distress, cough, panting, expectoration, etc..

3.1.2.1 Major Functions of the Lung

(1) The lung governs respiratory qi: This function means the lung possesses the actions to inhale the clear air of nature and exhale the turbid gases in the body so as to achieve gas exchange between the interior and exterior of the body. Government of respiratory qi by the lung is actually the embodiment of diffusion and purification-descent

of the lung-qi in the process of gas exchange between the interior and exterior of the body. Diffusion of lung-qi exhales turbid gases; and descent of lung-qi inhales clear air, so that it guarantees normality of the lung in governing respiratory qi. If the lung-qi fails in diffusion, or descent, it will definitely influence the respiratory movement of the lung, thus abnormally manifesting as chest distress, cough, panting, etc..

(2) The lung governs qi of the whole body: This function means the lung has the actions to govern the production and circulation of the whole body's qi. It first embodies the production of qi of the whole body. The whole body's qi is mainly composed of pectoral qi and primordial qi. The pectoral qi is mainly produced by combination of the clear air inhaled by the lung and the essential qi of foodstuffs transformed and transported by the spleen and stomach. The pectoral qi forms in the thorax and accumulates in the thorax. The lung governs respiratory qi, which influences the production of pectoral qi; in turn it influences the production of the whole body's qi. Next, the government of whole body's qi by the lung again embodies regulation of qi dynamic of the whole body. The process of the lung's respiratory movement is the motion of qi in ascending, descending, exiting and entering. The inhalation and exhalation by the lung in rhyme plays an important role for the motion of qi of the whole body in ascending, descending, exiting and entering.

The two functions of the lung in governing respiratory qi and the whole body's qi are closely related and inseparable, and depend upon the respiratory function of the lung. The lung governs respiratory qi through exhaling the turbid and inhaling the clear, promoting production and regulating the motion of qi in ascending, descending, exiting and entering, thus it guarantees the normal process of metabolism of the body. When the lung functions normally in governing the whole body's qi, the production and circulation of the whole body's qi will be normal. On the contrary, the lung functions abnormally in governing the whole body's qi, there will appear symptoms of qi deficiency such as low voice, breathlessness and lassitude; and disturbance of qi in motion of ascending, descending, exiting and entering.

(3) Smoothing water passage: Smoothing here means dredging and regulating. Water passageway signifies the passage for circulation and excretion of water. This function connotes the lung possesses the actions to dredge and regulate distribution, circulation and excretion of water in the body. The function of the lung in smoothing water passageway is actually the complete expression of the diffusing and descending motion of lung-qi in water metabolism. Diffusion of the lung-qi not only diffuses the fluid upward to the head and face and disperses the fluid outward to the body surface; but also can diffuse the defensive qi to control the opening-closing of the striea, regulating excretion of sweat. Purification and descent of the lung-qi not only transports the fluid downward to the other viscera and tissues, but also can transport the turbid liquid produced by metabolism of the viscera into the kidney as the source of urine formation. Only the lung

functions normally in smoothing water passageway, can the water metabolism be normal. Contrarily if the lung's function of smoothing water passageway gets weak, it will lead to accumulation of water, manifesting as disorders of water, dampness, phlegm and stagnant fluid.

(4) Connecting with vessels: This function of the lung means blood of the whole body converges in the lung through the vessels, carries out gas exchange through the lung's function of inhaling the clear and exhaling the turbid, then, by the diffusing and descending motion of lung-qi, the blood richly containing clear qi goes through the vessels again to the whole body.

The circulation of blood is propelled by the heart-qi, but the lung possesses the action of assisting the heart in circulating blood. The circulation of blood depends upon the driving action of qi, and the production and flow of qi of the whole body is governed by the lung. So when the lung-qi is sufficient, the production and flow of qi will be normal, being conducive to smooth blood circulation. Conversely, if the lung qi gets declined and fails to assist the heart in circulating blood, the blood will flow unsmoothly, thus there will appear the signs of qi deficiency and blood stasis such as chest distress, palpitation, cyanotic lips and purplish tongue.

3.1.2.2 Relations of the Lung with Constituent, Emotion, Orifice and Secretion

(1) The ling is associated with the skin, and reflects its brilliance in the fine hair: The skin and fine hair are the exterior of the body. The lung possesses the physiological function of diffusing the defensive qi and transporting the essence onto the skin and fine hair, so it guarantees the skin and hair to get the warning and nourishing and moistening of the defensive qi and foodstuff essence. Therefore the lung is closely related with the skin and fine hair. When the lung-qi is sufficient, the function of the lung in diffusing defensive qi and transporting essence onto the skin and hair will be normal, then the skin will be compact and the fine hair be lustrous; on the contrary, if the lung-qi gets declined and fails to diffuse the defensive qi and essence onto the skin and hair, there will occur polyhidrosis, being subject to catch cold, or haggard skin and hair.

(2) The lung is associated with sorrow (worry) in emotion: Sorrow and worry are the emotional changes to an pessimistic stimulation. The major influence of them is constant consumption of qi, or so called "grief makes qi consumed". The lung governs qi, so sorrow and worry are apt to consume the lung. Over sorrow and worry may cause deficiency of lung qi manifesting as shortage of breathing. Contrarily, if the lung qi gets deficient, the tolerance of pessimistic stimulation by human body will decrease, and thus it is likely to lead to the changes of sorrow and worry. The lung and sorrow-worry interact on each other; therefore, the lung is associated with sorrow (worry) in emotion.

(3) The lung is associated with nose in orifice: The nose is the passageway for entrance and exit of breathing qi. It communicates with the lung, so the lung is associated

with the nose in orifice. The normality of the nose in ventilation and smelling depends upon the action of the lung qi. When lung qi diffuses smoothly, the nose will be free from obstruction with keen swelling. On the contrary, if the lung qi fails in diffusion, it will lead to nasal obstruction and hyposmia. Since the lung opens into the nose, exogenous pathogens often invade the body through the nose.

(4) The lung is associated with snivel in secretion: Snivel is the nasal discharge, and the nose is the orifice of the lung, therefore the lung is associated with snivel in secretion. When the essential qi in the lung is sufficient, the snivel moistens the nasal cavity and does not flow outward. If the lung is invaded by cold pathogen, it will cause clear nasal discharge; if the lung is invaded by heat pathogen, it will cause yellow and tick nasal discharge; if the lung is invaded by dryness pathogen, it will cause dry nose.

3.1.3 Spleen

The spleen is located under the diaphragm. Its main functions are to govern transformation and transportation, send up the clear and control blood. The spleen and stomach form an exterior-interior relationship through mutual affiliation and connection of their meridians. The spleen is associated with the muscles in constituent, dominates the four limbs, reflects its brilliance in the lips, is associated with thinking in emotion, with mouth in orifice and with slobber in secretion. The spleen transforms the foodstuff into essence, thus provides substantial basis for postnatal life activity and production of qi-blood, it is thus called "the root of acquirement" and "the origin for qi-blood production".

3.1.3.1 Major Functions of the Spleen

(1) The spleen governs transformation and transportation: This function of the spleen means the actions of the spleen in transforming the foodstuff into essence, and absorbing and transporting it to the whole body. This function can be divided into two aspects of transforming and transporting foodstuff and transforming and transporting water.

Transforming and transporting foodstuff: The spleen is in charge of transforming and transporting foodstuff signifies that the spleen qi has the actions to promote the digestion of food taken in and the absorption of the foodstuff essence and further to distribute the essence. The digestion of the food takes place in the gastrointestinal tract, but it must depend on the transformation of the spleen to make the food transform into the essence; and the essence again must depend upon the transportation by the spleen to be absorbed and sent up to the lung and spread to the whole body. When the spleen filctions soundly, the body's digestion, absorption and transportation will be sufficient, then it provides sufficient nutriment for production of essence, qi, blood and fluid so that the viscera, meridians and collaterals, four limbs and skeleton, as well as tendons, muscles, skin and fine hairs can get enough nutritious materials and thus perform their normal physiological activities. Contrarily, if the spleen's function in transforming and transporting foodstuff decreases, the body's digestion, absorption transportation will get disordered, then there may appear failure of the spleen in sound transformation and transportation, manifesting as flatulence, diarrhea and poor appetite; or under-production of qi-blood presenting with lassitude and emaciation.

Transforming and transporting water: The spleen is in charge of transforming and transporting water connotes that the spleen possesses the action to absorb and transport body fluid so as to regulate water metabolism. The spleen qi can make the water taken in by the body absorbed, and transport it onto the whole body so that the water plays its moistening and nourishing roles. It can also timely transport the surplus water in the body into the lung and kidney where the surplus water, through the qi transformation of the lung and kidney, is transformed into sweat and urine which are discharged out of the body. Therefore when the spleen factions soundly in transforming and transporting water, it will guarantee the moistening of the whole body's tissues by the fluid; on the other hand, it can also prevent the abnormal stagnation of the water in the body. If the function of the spleen in transforming and transporting water decreases, it will inevitably lead to stagnation of water in the body, and thus the pathological products such as water-dampness and phlegm-stagnant-fluid will develop.

The two aspects of the spleen's actions of transforming and transporting foodstuff and water are inseparable; they are related with each other and influenced mutually. The spleen's function in transformation and transportation provides the material basis for production of qi and blood, and it is very important to maintenance of the body's vital activity. Therefore, one should protect the spleen carefully to make the spleen qi sound in transformation and transportation, so that qi and blood are sufficient and the body free from invasion of pathogens.

(2) The spleen is in charge of sending up the clear: This denotes that the spleen qi goes upward and thus transports the nourishment of foodstuff essence by its transformation up to the heart, lung, head and eye; and further the foodstuff essence is transformed into qi-blood by the functions of the heart and lung so as to nourish the whole body. The sending up the clear by the spleen is mentioned just to compare with the sending down the turbid by the stomach. "The spleen will function soundly as its qi goes up normally, and the stomach will function soundly as its qi goes down normally," Only when the ascent of spleen qi and descent of stomach qi coordinate, can the function of the body in digestion and absorption keep normal. Besides, it is owing to the ascent of the spleen qi that the positions of the internal organs are kept relatively fixed, and the ptoses of them avoided. If the spleen qi fails to send up the clear, the foodstuff essence cannot be transported up to the heart and lung, generation of qi-blood is short of source, and the head and eyes lose their nourishment, then there may appear symptoms of listlessness, dizziness and vertigo; if the spleen qi loses its power to lift or conversely sinks down, there may appear symptoms of chronic diarrhea with proctoptosis, or ptopses of some

other viscera.

(3) The spleen controls blood: This function of the spleen signifies that the spleen possesses the action of keeping blood circulating within the vessels and preventing it from extravasation. The reason for the spleen to control blood lies in its function of transformation and transportation, being the source for production of qi-blood. When the spleen qi is sound in transformation and transportation, the generation of qi-blood will have the source, and qi-blood will be abundant; as qi is sufficient so that its power in controlling blood is powerful, then blood cannot escape from the vessels and cause bleeding. On the contrary, if the spleen gets insufficient and fails to transform and transport, qi and blood will be deficient because generation of qi-blood is short of source; as qi is deficient, its function of controlling blood will decline, thus it will lead to extravasation of blood, with resultant bleeding. Since the spleen qi is in charge of ascending and the spleen is associated with the muscle in constituent, so the failure of spleen in controlling blood is often presented as the bleeding in the lower part of the body such as hemafecia, hematuria, metrorrhagia and metrostaxis, as well as perpura.

3.1.3.2 Relations of the Spleen with Constituent, Emotion, Orifice and Secretion

(1) The spleen is associated with the muscles in constituent, dominates the four limbs, and reflects its brilliance on the lips: The muscles of the whole body and four limbs all depend upon the nutrition of foodstuff essence transformed and transported by the spleen. So the spleen is associated with the muscles and dominates the four limbs. When the spleen functions normally in transformation and transportation, the muscles and four limbs can get the nourishment of the foodstuff essence, then the muscles are well developed, thick and strong, the four limbs are nimble and forceful. If the spleen's function in transformation and transportation gets disordered, the muscles and four limbs will lose their nourishment of foodstuff essence, thus it definitely cause severely-thinning of the muscles and flaccidity and weakness of the four limbs, even atrophy with motor impairment. The color of the lips is related with the abundance of qi-blood of the whole body; and the spleen is the source for production of qi-blood, therefore the color and luster of lips can reflect the strength of the spleen's function, or the spleen reflects its brilliance in the lips. When the spleen functions normally in transformation and transportation, qi-blood will be abundant, then the lips will be ruddy and moist with luster; contrarily, if the spleen's function of transformation and transportation gets disordered, qi-blood will be deficient, then there will be abnormal manifestation of pale lips with no luster.

(2) The spleen is associated with thinking in emotion: Over thinking may influence the normal activity of qi, leading to qi stagnation, especially in the meddle, thus it will influence the functions of the spleen in transformation and transportation, and sending up the clear, then there may appear symptoms of poor appetite, distending and stuffiness of

the epigastrium, dizziness and vertigo. Therefore it is said the spleen is associated with thinking in emotion.

(3) The spleen is associated with the mouth in the orifice: The spleen is in charge of transformation and transportation. When the spleen qi is sufficient in transformation and transportation, the taste and appetite will be normal, namely "the spleen qi communicates with the mouth, as the spleen functions normally the mouth can taste the five flavors." If the spleen fails in normal transformation and transportation, there will appear poor appetite, and some abnormal sensations of tastelessness, or sweet, greasy and bitter tastes of the mouth. The appetite and taste are closely related with the spleen's function of transformation and transportation, so the spleen is associated with the mouth in orifice.

(4) The spleen is associated with slobber in secretion: Slobber is the liquid in the mouth, and the mouth is the orifice of the spleen, so the spleen is associated with lobber in secretion. When the spleen functions normally in transformation-transportation and sending up the clear, the body fluid will go up to the mouth, becoming slobber to help swallowing and digestion of the food taken in. If the spleen and stomach function abnormally, it will lead to disorder of slobber production.

3.1.4 Liver

The liver is situated in the upper part of the abdominal cavity and at the inside of the right hypochodrium. Its major functions are to govern free flow of qi and store blood. The liver and gallbladder form an exterior-interior relationship through affiliation and connection of their meridians. The liver is associated with tendons in constituent, reflects its brilliance in the nails, and is associated with anger in emotion, with the eye in orifice, and with tear in secretion. The liver is characterized by ascent and motion of its qi, and its qi tends to be flourishing and free from obstruction, therefore the liver has its name of "resolute organ".

3.1.4.1 Major Functions of the Liver

(1) The liver governs free flow of qi: This function connotes that the liver possesses the action to smooth the qi dynamic of the whole body. Qi dynamic means the motion of qi. The function of the liver in governing free flow of qi plays an important regulatory role of ascending, descending, exiting and entering of qi in every viscus and tissue so as to guarantee the freedom of the whole body's qi dynamic, and in turn to promote the circulation and distribution of essence, blood and body fluid, transformation and transportation by the spleen and stomach, secretion and excretion of bile, smoothness of sentiment, ejaculation in men and menstruation in women, influencing the body extensively. The major effects of the governing free flow of qi by the liver are as follows.

Smoothing qi dynamic: The liver is physiologically characterized by ascent and motion of its qi. The government of free flow of qi by the liver can both make qi dynamic free from obstruction and avoid qi stagnation. So when the liver functions normally in government of free flow of qi, the qi dynamic will be smooth, with harmony of qi and blood, smoothness of meridians and collaterals and normal activities of the viscera. If the liver gets abnormal in government of free flow of qi, it may present with hypofunction in government of qi flow, then the ascent of qi will be insufficient, the qi dynamic will be obstructed, with resultant pathological changes of un-freedom and stagnation of qi dynamic manifesting as distending pain and discomfort of the chest, hypochondria, two breasts, or lateral parts of the lower abdomen; on the other hand it also may present with hyperfunction, then the ascent of qi will be hyperactive, with resultant pathological changes of adverse rising of liver qi manifesting as distending pain of the head and eyes, red face and eyes, irritability, or even adverse rising of blood following qi with hematemesis and hemoptysis.

Promoting circulation of blood and body fluid: Blood and body fluid belong to yin and are characterized by stillness; their distribution depends upon the propelling action of qi. When the liver functions normally in government of qi flow, the ascending, descending, exiting and entering motion of qi will be free, then the circulation of blood and distribution of body fluid will be smooth along with it. On the contrary, if liver qi gets stagnated, it will lead to disturbance of blood circulation with formation of blood stasis; if liver qi rises adversely, it will force blood to go upward and lead to bleeding like hematemesis and hemoptysis. Besides, the abnormality of the liver's governing free flow of qi may also lead to disturbance of body fluid metabolism, causing pathological changes of water, dampness, phlegm and fluid retention.

Promoting transformation and transportation of the spleen and stomach: Spleen qi ascends and stomach qi descends in property, the spleen is in charge of sending up the clear and the stomach is in charge of sending down the turbid. Only ascent and descent coordinate with each other, can the function of the spleen and stomach in transformation and transportation be normal. The normality of the liver's governing free flow of qi serves as an important condition for normal ascent and descent of qi of the spleen and stomach. When the liver functions normally, qi flows freely and smoothly, the spleen qi can ascend, and stomach qi can descend, then the function of the spleen and stomach in transformation and transportation will be normal. As the liver functions abnormally in governing free flow of qi, it will not only affect the spleen in sending up the clear manifesting as dizziness and vertigo in the upper and diarrhea in the lower, but also affect the stomach in sending down the turbid manifesting as hiccup and eructation in the upper, epigastric distention and fullness in the meddle, and constipation in the lower.

Helping secretion and excretion of bile: The bile is produced by the surplus qi of the liver, so its secretion and excretion are controlled by the liver's function of governing free flow of qi. When the liver functions normally in transformation and transportation with smooth flow of qi dynamic, then the bile will be normally secreted and excreted, thus it is conducive to spleen's transformation and transportation and stomach's decomposition. If the liver qi gets depressed, it will affect the secretion and excretion of bile, resulting in pathological changes of distension, fullness and pain in the hypochondria, bitter test in the mouth, indigestion, and even jaundice.

Smoothing emotion: Normal activity of emotion is mainly dependent upon the normal circulation of qi-blood. The government of qi flow by the liver is conducive to smoothness of qi dynamic; sooth flow of qi will make blood circulate smoothly because qi can circulate blood. Normal circulation of qi-blood provides material basis for emotional activity, then the mood will be happy. On the contrary, if the liver functions insufficiently in governing free flow of qi, the liver qi will be stagnated, then the mood will be easily depressed, and a little stimulation may cause refractory melancholy; if the liver hyper-functions in governing free flow of qi with hyperactive rise of qi, then the mood is liable to be irritable, and a little stimulation will easily cause rage.

Being conducive to ejaculation in men and menstruation in women: Ejaculation in men and menstruation in women are closely related with the function of the liver in governing free flow of qi. When the liver functions normally in government of qi flow, the qi dynamic will be free and smooth, then the ejaculation in men will be smooth and proper, and the menstrual cycle in women will be regular with smooth menstruation. Contrarily, if the liver's function in governing free flow of qi gets abnormal, the qi dynamic will get disordered, then the ejaculation in men will become un-smooth, and the menstrual cycle in women will become disturbed with obstructed menstruation..

(2) The liver stores blood: This function signifies that the liver has the action to store blood, regulates blood volume and prevents bleeding. The liver's function of storing blood firstly means the liver can store a certain amount of blood so as to check the yang qi of liver to prevent its over-rise, and thus to maintain the normal process of the liver's function of governing free flow of qi. Next, the liver stores a certain amount of blood, which, assisted by the governing free flow o f qi, can effectively regulate the amount of blood demanded by every tissue according to the physiological conditions of the body. As a person is in movement his blood will circulate throughout all the meridians and collaterals, and as he is in rest, his blood will return to the liver. In addition, storage of blood by the liver is also conducive to holding blood within the vessels to prevent its loss unduly. Therefore there is a saying "the liver is the origin for blood coagulation". So, if the liver fails to store blood, it will not only lead to shortage of liver blood and over rise of yang qi, but also may result in various kinds of bleeding.

The liver is in charge of storing blood, its body proper belongs to yin; and it governs free flow of qi, its function belongs to yang. So there is saying "the liver pertains to yin in substance and yang in function". The two functions of the liver of storing blood and governing free flow of qi are dependent upon each other. As the liver governs free flow of qi, qi dynamic will be unimpeded, then blood can normally return into the liver for storage and regulation. Blood is stored by the liver, it can nourish liver qi to check over rise of yang qi, then the liver can normally govern free flow of qi.

3.1.4.2 Relations of the liver with Constituent, Emotion, Orifice and Secretion

(1) The liver is associated with the tendons in constituent, reflects its brilliance in the nails: the tendons of the body depend upon the nourishment of liver blood. As the liver blood is sufficient, the tendons can be nourished, and then their movement is flexible and powerful. If the liver blood gets deficient, the tendons will lose their nourishment, then the power of tendons will be weak and the motion be impaired, or there appear tremors of hand and foot, numbness of the limbs with impaired flexion and extension, or even spasm and convulsion. Nails are the extension of the tendons. They need the nourishment of liver blood all the same. The abundance of liver blood may influence the soundness of the nails, so it is said the liver reflects its brilliance in the nails. When the liver blood is abundant, the nails will be tough and tensile, ruddy and lustrous. If the liver blood gets deficient, the nails will become soft, thin and withered with no luster, or even deformed, fragile with cracks.

(2) The liver is associated with anger in emotion: Anger is a emotional change as a person gets excited in mind or feelings. Over-anger may make qi-blood rise adversely, yang qi goes upward and outward. Since the liver governs free flow of qi, rise of yang qi represents the function of the liver; therefore the liver is associated with anger in emotion. Anger is apt to injure the liver. Over anger may cause liver's yang qi to rise too much to make blood ascend adversely along with rise of qi, resulting in hematemesis, or even sudden coma. On the contrary, if the liver yin gets deficient, the liver yang can not be checked, whenever there is a little unease of mood, it will cause anger.

(3) The liver is associated with the eyes in orifice: The liver meridian of foot Jueyin ascends to link with the eye, the qi-blood of the liver goes up into the eye through the meridian of the liver to maintain the version of the eye. When the liver blood is abundant and the liver qi is harmonious, the eye will be able to see things and differentiate colors. Contrarily, if the liver blood gets deficient, the eyes will be dry and discomfortable feelings, blurred vision or color blindness; invasion of the liver meridian by the wind-heat will cause red eye with itching pain; flaming of liver fire will cause red eye with nebula; hyperactivity of liver yang will cause dizziness and vertigo; and stirring up of liver wind will cause deviated eye or upward-stared eye.

(4) The liver is associated with tear in secretion: Tear is secreted by the eye, and the liver opens into the eyes; so the liver is associated with tear in secretion. When the qi-blood of the liver is harmonious, the tear can moisten the eye and does not flow out. If the liver blood gets deficient, there may appear dry and discomfortable feelings in the eye; and in case of red eye with invasion of wind and fire, or dampness-heat in the liver meridian, there may appear too much caked secretion in the eye and epiphora induced by

irritation of wind.

3.1.5 Kidney

The kidneys are located in the lumbar region; there is one at both right and left side. The major functions of the kidney are storing essence, governing water and governing reception of qi. The kidney and bladder form an exterior-interior relationship through mutual connection and affiliation of their meridians. The kidney is associated with the bone in constituent, reflects its brilliance in the hair, is associated with fear in emotion, with ear and two yin organs in orifice, and with spittle in secretion. The kidney stores the innate essence, is the origin of life, so it is called "the root of innateness".

3.1.5.1 Major Functions of the Kidney

(1) The kidney stores essence: This function means that the kidney possesses the action to store essence-qi. The kidney is the root for storage, being in charge of storing essence. The essence stored in the kidney includes "innate essence" and "acquired essence". The innate essence originates from the reproductive essence of the parents, it comes from the birth, and is stored in the kidney. The acquired essence originates from the foodstuff essence transformed and transported by the spleen and stomach. After birth, the foodstuff essence produced by the spleen and stomach, through the transportation by the spleen qi, is conveyed to the viscera to become visceral essence. After supporting the functions of every viscus, the residual part of the visceral essence is transported into the kidney to supplement and nourish the innate. The innate essence and the acquired essence combine with each other to form the kidney essence. The kidney essence is the material basis for generation of kidney qi.

That the kidney stores essence is mainly to avoid undue loss of essence-qi in the kidney, and thus provide a good condition for the essence-qi to play its necessary physiological effects in the body.

The physiological effects of the essence-qi in the kidney are firstly to promote the growth, development and reproduction. There is a life law of birth, growth, prime, aging and death in human body, and the whole process of life is influenced by the kidney-essence-qi. After birth, a person's essence-qi in the body begins to grow gradually, in the childhood; there appear phenomena of dental transition and growth of hair. In the young and prime period, the kidney-essence-qi further develops and flourishes, then there occur phenomena of growth of wisdom tooth, strong and firm tendons and bones, strong and healthy physique. Up to the elderly period, the kidney-essence-qi gradually declines, there appear phenomena of withered look, hoar hair, odontoptosis, and weak physique. It can thus be seen that the kidney-essence-qi determines the process of human growth and development. The development of human's reproduction organs and its reproductive power are also influenced by the abundance of the kidney-essence-qi. As a person grows to his adolescence stage, following his kidney-essence-qi gets abundant to a certain degree, within his body a kind of essential substance is produced, which possesses the actions of promoting development and maturity of sexual organs and maintaining the reproductive power, being called *Tiangui* (sex promoters). Thus in men there may appear ejaculation, and in women, menstruation; or one then possesses the genitality. Hereafter, the kidney-essence-qi gets more and more flourishing within the body and the sex promoters are continuously produced to maintain the genital function. As a person gets his senile stage, his kidney-essence-qi becomes declined, thus the sex promoters decrease and exhaust, the genitality also declines and disappear. Therefore the root factor for determining the reproduction function lies in the abundance of the kidney-essence-qi, and there is a saying "the kidney dominates reproduction". When the kidney-essence-qi is sufficient, the growth and development will be normal, and the reproduction be sound. Contrarily, if the kidney-essence-qi gets deficient, there will appear maldevelopment in children, early senility in adult, and there may appear hypo-genetality. So importance should be ever attached to replenishing the kidney-essence-qi for betterment of birth and breeding, health care, and protecting from senility.

Next, the kidney-essence-qi performs propelling and regulating actions to physiological activities of all human's viscera. The kidney essence can transform into kidney qi, and the kidney qi can present with physiological effects of two respects of kidney yin and kidney yang. The kidney yin plays moistening, calming and inhibiting Toles; while the kidney yang plays warming, propelling and exciting roles. The kidney stores the innate essence, being the origin of life; and the kidney yin and yang are the root of yin and yang for every viscus. The yin of the five *Zang*-viscera and the sex *Fu*-viscera depends upon the nourishment of kidney yin; and the yang of the viscera depends upon the reinforcement of kidney yang. The kidney yin and the kidney yang restrict each other and depend on each other so as to maintain the balance of yin and yang of every viscus, guaranteeing the normality of metabolism and physiological activity of the body. In case of development of kidney yin deficiency because of some reasons, there may appear internal heat, dizziness, tinnitus, sore and weak feeling in the waist and knees, nocturnal spermatorrhea, red tongue with little liquid; and in case of development of kidney yang deficiency, there may occur listlessness and lassitude, cold appearance with cold limbs, clod pain and weakness of the waist and knees, clear urine of increased volume, or dysuria, or enuresis, or incontinence of urine, pale tongue; as well as sexual hypofunction and edema. The kidney yin and yang are very important to human life, so the kidney yin is also called "genuine yin" and "original yin", and the kidney yang is also called "genuine yang" and "original yang".

(2) The kidney governs water: The function signifies that the kidney has the actions to control and regulate the distribution and excretion of water in the body so as to keep water metabolism balance. The procedure of water metabolism is: Through reception by

the stomach, transformation and transportation by the spleen, diffusion and descending by the lung, steaming and qi transformation by the kidney, and taking the tri-Jiao as the passageways, water is transported throughout the whole body; the water after being metabolized can be transformed into sweat and urine to be discharged out of the body. The whole process of water metabolism is concerned with a series of physiological activities of several viscera, however the kidney-essence-qi plays controlling and regulating role. The kidney yin and yang transformed from the essence-qi in the kidney are the root of yin and yang of every viscus of the body, they maintain the balance for yin and yang of every viscus so as to guarantee normal participation of every viscus in water metabolism. In addition, in the water metabolite process, the turbid fluid produced by viscera, body constituents and orifices is transported into the kidney through the tri-Jiao. The turbid is, under the qi transformation of the kidney, divided as two parts of clear and turbid fluid again. The clear part is re-absorbed and transported by the spleen qi up to the lung to be used further; and the turbid part, through the qi transformation of the kidney, is transformed into urine and pored into the urinary bladder to be further discharged out of the body under the qi transformation of the kidney and urinary bladder. It can thus be seen that the production and discharge of urine are directly related to the steaming and qi transformation of the kidney, which is important to maintain the balance of water metabolism of the body. If the steaming and transformation of essence-qi in the kidney get disordered, it will lead to disorders of production and discharge of urine, resulting in pathological phenomena of oliguria and edema.

(3) The kidney governs reception of qi: This function means the kidney possesses the action of receiving the fresh air inhaled by the lung so as to keep the depth of inspiration. The respiratory function of the body is governed by the lung, but it must be through the reception and storage by the kidney qi to keep a certain depth. Performance of normal respiratory movement depends upon the coordination of the lung and kidney, so there is saying "the lung is the ruler of qi and the kidney is the root of qi. The lung governs exhalation of qi and the kidney governs reception of qi." When the essence-qi in the kidney is sufficient and with ability to receive qi, the respiration will be even and harmonious. On the contrary, if the essence-qi in the kidney gets deficient and with little power to receive qi, then there will appear pathological phenomena of tachypnea, gasp induced by a little exertion, or dyspnea with prolonged expiration. The function of the kidney in governing reception of qi is actually the complete embodiment of storing action of the kidney in respiratory movement.

3.1.5.2 Relations of the Kidney with Constituent, Emotion, Orifice and Secretion

(1) The kidney is associated with the bone in constituent, generates marrow, and reflects its brilliance in the hair: The bone, or skeleton, is of the function to support the body, protect the internal organs and perform movement. The kidney stores essence that

generates morrow, which is within the bone to nourish it, so the kidney is associated with the bone in constituent. When the kidney essence is sufficient, the bone will be strong and firm. If the kidney essence gets deficient, the bone marrow will be short, and the bone will lose its nourishment, then there may appear delayed closure of the fontanel and weak bone in children, and fragile and weak bone subjected to fracture in adults.

"The tooth is the extension of the bone", the tooth depends upon the nourishment of the kidney essence too. When the kidney is sufficient, the tooth will be firm. Contrarily, in case of kidney essence deficiency there will occur slow growth of tooth in children, and looseness and falling off of the tooth in adults.

The hair is dependent upon the nourishment by essence and blood. The kidney stores essence, which can generate blood. When essence-blood is abundant, the hair will glow and is moist and lustrous. Contrarily, as the essence-blood gets deficient, the hair will lose its nourishment, leading to withering and falling off of the hair. So the kidney reflects its brilliance in the hair.

The bone, tooth and hair are all closely related with essence-qi in the kidney. The growth state of the bone, tooth and hair reflect the ups and downs of the kidney-essence-qi, therefore they are the objective marks for determining the growth and developing conditions and the senile degree of the human body.

(2) The kidney is associated with fear in emotion: Fear is a kind of emotional activity of timidity or cowardic. The close relation of the kidney with fear is from the long observation by ancient people. The kidney is located in the lower-Jiao, the kidney essence transforms into kidney qi. The kidney qi must ascend through the middle- and upper-Jiao to spread onto the whole body. "Great fear (terror) makes qi sinking". If a person is in a state of great fear, the kidney qi will fail to go up and conversely go downward, thus the kidney qi cannot normally spread, so the kidney is associated with fear in emotion.

(3) The kidney is associated with the ear and two yin organs in orifice: That the kidney is associated with the ear signifies the sharpness of hearing is closely related to the abundance of the kidney-essence-qi. "The kidney qi is communicated with the ear, as the kidney qi is sufficient the ear can differentiate the five notes of voices". The kidney essence can generate marrow, and "the brain is the sea of marrow". When the essence-qi in the kidney is sufficient, the marrow sea will get its nourishment, and then the hearing will be sharp. On the contrary, if the essence-qi in the kidney gets deficient, the marrow sea will lose its nourishment, and then it may lead to blunt hearing, tinnitus, or even deafness.

The two yin organs are anterior and posterior yin organs. The anterior yin organ is an urino-sexual organ, and the posterior is the passage for defecation. The reproduction function of human body depends upon the abundance of the kidney-essence-qi. The discharge of urine and feces are closely related to the qi transformation and regulation of the kidney. Therefore there is saying "the kidney is associated with the two yin organs".

(4) The kidney is associated with spittle in secretion: The spittle is transformed from the kidney essence; it has the action to moisten the mouth and tongue. The kidney essence goes up to Jinjin (EX-HN 12) and Yuye (EX-HN 13) points beneath the lower surface of the tongue through the kidney meridian of foot Shaoyin to excrete out as the spittle. So the kidney is associated with the spittle in secretion. Since the spittle originates from the kidney, swallowing down of it can in return nurture the essence-qi in the kidney. And too much or prolonged excretion of the spittle will be apt to consume the kidney essence.

Appendix: Womb

Womb, also called uterus, is located in the lower abdomen. Its lower opening is communicated with the vagina.

The major function of the womb is to control menstruation, and form and culture the fetus. The production of menstruation and formation and cultivation of the fetus are the outcome that the viscera, sex promoters, meridians and qi-blood act on the womb. So whether the womb functions normally or not directly influence the production of menstruation and formation and cultivation of the fetus. When the womb functions normally, the menstruation and the development of the fetus will be normal. On the contrary, if the womb functions abnormally, there will appear disturbance of menstruation, and anomaly of the pregnancy and development of the fetus.

The physiological functions of the womb are related to the viscera and meridians; of which the more closely related are the heart, liver, spleen and kidney; as well as the Chong and Ren meridians.

3.2 Six *Fu*-Viscera

3.2.1 Gallbladder

The gallbladder is located under the right hypochondrium, attaching to between the short lobes of the liver. The major function of the gallbladder is to store and excrete the bile.

The gallbladder connects with the liver; the surplus of the liver qi generates the bile that flows into the gallbladder to be stored. The bile is pure and clear; so it is called "refined juice", and the gallbladder is also named "the *Fu*-viscus containing refined juice". The bile stored in the gallbladder, under the control and regulation by the function of the liver in governing free flow of qi, is excreted into the intestine to help to digest and absorb the foodstuff. When the liver's governing free flow of qi functions normally, the excretion of bile is free, and then the digestion and absorption of the foodstuff will be normal. Contrarily, if the liver functions abnormally in governing free flow of qi, the excretion of bile is obstructed, thus it will affect the digestion and absorption of the foodstuff, there may appear distending pain in the hypochondrium, poor appetite and abdominal distention; if the bile goes adversely upward, there may occur bitter taste in the mouth, or vomiting with bitter liquid yellowish and green in color; if the bile spreads out from the bile tract, there may appear jaundice.

In addition, the gallbladder also has the function to govern decision, can judge things and make decision.

In morphology the gallbladder is an organ hollow inside and with a cavity, just similar to the other *Fu*-viscera; so it belongs to six *Fu*-viscera. In function it stores the bile, being similar to "storing essence-qi" of the five *Zang*-viscera; so it is also called extra ordinary *Fu*-viscus.

3.2.2 Stomach

The stomach is located in the upper abdomen; it connects superiorly with esophagus and inferiorly with the small intestine. The major functions of the stomach are to receive and decompose the foodstuff.

Receiving the foodstuff means the stomach possesses the actions to accept and contain the food and drink taken in. The foodstuff taken in through the mouth is contained in the stomach under the action of stomach qi. So the stomach is called "granary" and "the sea of foodstuff".

Decomposing the foodstuff indicates the stomach has the action to primarily digest the foodstuff to make it become the chyme. When the stomach functions normally in receiving and decomposing the foodstuff, the appetite will be normal. If the stomach's functions of receiving and decomposing the foodstuff get disordered, there will appear poor appetite, eructation with fetid odor, etc..

Reception of foodstuff is the basis for decomposing it. The foodstuff entering the stomach transforms into chyme through the decomposition by the stomach, and then the chyme must smoothly go down into the small intestine so as to be further digested and absorbed; at the same time this also creates the condition for the stomach to receive further. So the stomach dominates dredging and descending, taking descent as its normality. If the stomach fails in dredging and descending, and stomach qi gets stagnated, there will appear symptoms of poor appetite, epigastric distention, stuffiness and pain, constipation, etc.. If the stomach qi fails to descend, and further it develops into adverse rise of stomach qi, there will appear belching, nausea, vomiting, hiccup, etc..

3.2.3 Small Intestine

The small intestine is situated in the abdomen. Its upper end connects with the stomach, and its lower end connects with the large intestine. The major physiological functions of the small intestine are to dominate reception and digest the chyme, and to separate the clear from the turbid.

Reception and digestion of the chyme means that the small intestine accepts the chyme sent down by the stomach and holds it for a longer time so as to facilitate further digest on of it into the essence. If the small intestine functions abnormally in reception and digestion of the chyme, it will result in abdominal distention, diarrhea or sloppy stool.

Separation of the clear from the turbid signifies that the small intestine separates its digested foodstuff into two parts of foodstuff essence and waste, and absorbs the essence and sends the waste down into the large intestine. At the same time of absorbing foodstuff, the small intestine also absorbs a great amount of water, so there is a saying "the small intestine dominates thick fluid". If the small intestine functions abnormally in separation of the clear from the turbid, it may lead to mix-up of the clear and the turbid, manifesting as sloppy stool or diarrhea, etc..

The functions of the small intestine in reception of the chyme and separation of the clear from the turbid are very important in the process of transformation of the foodstuff into the essence. However the functions of the small intestine must coordinate with the transformation and transportation of the spleen qi so that the work can be smoothly accomplished.

3.2.4 Large Intestine

The large intestine is located in the abdomen. It connects superiorly with the small intestine and inferiorly with the anus. The major function of the large intestine is to transform and convey the waste. The large intestine accepts the foodstuff residue from the small intestine by its separation, and reabsorbs the redundant water in the waste so as to make the waste become stool; then conveys the stool down and discharges it via the anus out of the body. The conveyance and transformation of waste by the large intestine is the continuance of the separation of the clear from the turbid; it is related with the dredge and descent by the stomach qi, the purification and descent by the lung qi and qi transformation of the kidney qi. If the large intestine functions abnormally in conveyance and transformation of waste, it will cause abnormality in quality and quantity of stool and frequency of defecation. Since the large intestine reabsorbs the redundant water in the foodstuff residue, there is saying "the large intestine dominates thin fluid".

3.2.5 Urinary Bladder

The urinary bladder is located in the lower abdomen. Its upper outlets communicate with the kidneys through the ureters; and its lower outlet connects with the urethra. The major function of the urinary bladder is to store and discharge urine. The urine is produced from the water under the qi transformation of the kidney, then poured into the bladder for storage. When the urine in the bladder gets to a certain amount, it will be discharged out of the body. The storage and discharge of urine by the bladder is regulated by the kidney. When kidney qi is sufficient, the bladder will close and open orderly, thus the function of storing and discharging urine will be normal. If the kidney qi fails in control, there will appear enuresis, or even incontinence of urine. If the qi transformation of the kidney gets disordered, there will appear dysuria, or even anuria.

3.2.6 Tri-Jiao

The tri-Jiao is a collective term for the upper-, middle- and lower-Jiao. The meaning of the tri-Jiao is of two: One is one of the six *Fu*-viscera, which are the passageways formed by the mutual communication of the spaces among the viscera and within the interior of the viscera. The other is a concept of simple regions, or the part above the diaphragm as the upper-Jiao, the part from below the diaphragm to the umbilicus as the diddle-Jiao, and the part below the umbilicus as the lower-Jiao.

The major functions of the tri-Jiao as one of the six *Fu*-viscera are to pass primordial qi and transmit water. The primordial qi originates from the kidney; it flows into the five *Zang*- and six *Fu*-viscera and spreads through the whole body via the tri-Jiao to play its physiological effect. The water metabolism of the whole body is accomplished by the coordination among the viscera such as the lung, spleen, stomach, kidney and urinary bladder; however, it must take the tri-Jiao as its passages to ascend, descend, exit and enter normally. If the water passageways of the tri-Jiao get obstructed, the lung, spleen and kidney will hardly perform their physiological effects in distributing and regulating water metabolism.

As viewing the simple regions as meanings of the tri-Jiao, the physiological functions of the upper Jiao (including the heart, lung and head and face) are to dominate the diffusion and dispersion. *Lín Shū* (*Miraculous Pivot*) summarizes this as "the upper-Jiao works like a sprayer". The physiological functions of the middle-Jiao (including the spleen, stomach, liver and gallbladder) are to digest foodstuff, absorb and distribute foodstuff essence to produce qi and blood. *Lín Shū* summarizes this as "the meddle-Jiao works like a fermentation tun". The physiological functions of the lower-Jiao (including the small intestine, large intestine, kidney and urinary bladder) are to dominate discharge of the waste and urine. *Lín Shū* summarizes this as "the lower-Jiao works like a drain".

3.3 Relationships among the Viscera

Human body is an organic whole. There are among the viscera close relationships of mutual promotion, restriction, dependence and coordination.

3.3.1 Relationships among the Five *Zang*-Viscera

3.3.1.1 Heart and Lung

The relationship between heart and lung is mainly marked in two respects of blood circulation and respiratory movement.

Blood circulation is dependent upon the propelling of heart qi, and also upon the assistance of lung qi. The lung connects with vessels to assist the heart in circulating blood, thus keeping normal blood circulation. If the lung qi gets insufficient or the lung is invaded by cold, and thus the lung fails in assisting the heart to circulate blood, it will lead to stasis of heart blood with obstructed circulation of blood.

The lung controls respiration, inhaling the clear and exhaling the turbid, so as to maintain the normal respiratory movement; while the heart governs circulation of blood, only when blood circulates normally, and the lung gets its nourishment of blood, can the lung's function of controlling respiration keep normal. If the heart qi gets weak and fails to circulate blood, blood circulation will be unsmooth, then it may affect the lung in controlling respiration, resulting in chest distress, cough, panting, etc..

Pectoral qi is produced through combination of the fresh air inhaled by the lung and foodstuff essence-qi transformed and transported by the spleen and stomach. The pectoral qi can both go along the gas tract to promote respiration, and permeate through the heart vessels to circulate qi-blood; thus it strengthens the mutual relation between the blood circulation and respiratory movement.

3.3.1.2 Heart and Spleen

The relationship between heart and spleen is mainly marked by the two respects of generation and circulation of blood.

The heart governs blood circulation to provide nourishment of blood for the spleen to maintain its normal function of transformation and transportation. The spleen governs transformation and transportation, being the source for generation of qi and blood. When the spleen qi is sound in transformation and transportation, generation of blood will possess its source, the blood will be kept abundant. If the heart blood gets deficient, it may affect the spleen in governing transformation and transportation. On the contrary, if the spleen qi gets weak with deficient source for blood generation, then the heart will lose what it governs due to blood deficiency.

The heart governs blood circulation; heart qi drives blood to circulate in the vessels. The spleen controls blood; spleen qi holds blood to keep it circulate within the vessels without extravasations. The two are opposite and yet complementary to each other and thus guarantee normal circulation of blood. If the heart qi gets too weak to circulate blood, it may lead to some disorders of qi deficiency with blood stasis. If the spleen qi gets too deficient to control blood, it may lead to some disorders of qi deficiency with bleeding.

3.3.1.3 Heart and Liver

The relationship between heart and liver is mainly shown as mutual coordination in blood circulation and interaction in mental activity.

The heart governs blood circulation. When blood circulates normally, the liver will have what it stores. The liver stores blood to keep in storage of blood, regulate blood volume and prevent bleeding. As the storage and regulation are coordinative, the heart will have what it governs. The two viscera cooperate with each other and commonly maintain normal blood circulation. In pathology, heart blood and liver blood often affect each other; as a result, there appear disorders of blood deficiency of both the heart and liver, or blood stasis of both the heart and liver.

The heart governs mental activity; it dominates human's psychological and emotional activities. The liver governs free flow of qi; it smoothes qi dynamic, makes qi and blood harmonious and mind ease. The two functions supplement each other to commonly maintain normal psychological and emotional activities. If the functions of the heart in governing mental activity and the liver in governing free flow of qi get disordered, there will appear abnormal psychological and emotional activities, manifesting as being in a trance, depressed emotion, or vexation, insomnia, irritability, being easy to get angry, etc..

3.3.1.4 Heart and Kidney

The relationship between heart and kidney is mainly manifested as "mutual assistance between the water and the fire" and "independence of essence and spirit".

The heart is located in the thorax, belongs to fire in the five elements; and so it pertains to yang. The kidney is situated in the lumbar region, belongs to water in the five elements; and so it pertains to yin. According to the theory of ascent-descent of yin-yang or water-fire, what is located superiorly should descend, and what is situated inferiorly should ascend. So the heart fire should go down to warm the kidney water, and the kidney-yin should go up to assist heart yin for restricting heart yang. If the heart fire fails to go down for warming the kidney or the kidney water fails to go up to assist the heart, there will appear pathological changes of "discordance between heart and kidney".

The heart houses spirit, which can control essence. The kidney stores essence, which can generate spirit. The spirit and the essence depend upon each other. The essence is the material basis of spirit; and the spirit is the external expression of the essence. If the kidney essence gets deficient, and the generation of spirit is short of source; there may appear symptoms of listlessness, slowness in thinking, etc.. Contrarily, if the spirit fails in control, it will easily lead to failure in storage of essence, manifesting as nocturnal spermatorrhea, dreamy sexual action, etc..

3.3.1.5 Lung and Spleen

The relationship between lung and spleen is mainly reflected in the two respects of generation of qi and water metabolism.

The fresh air inhaled by the lung and the foodstuff essential qi are the main material basis for generation of qi; the combination of the two generates pectoral qi. The pectoral qi is the cardinal component part of whole body's qi. So the function of the lung in governing respiration and the function of the spleen in governing transformation and transportation are of important role to generation of qi. Pathologically, the lung qi deficiency and the spleen qi deficiency usually affect each other, thus to develop into a syndrome of dual deficiency of the lung and spleen.

The lung regulates water passage, freeing and regulating the distribution, flow and excretion of water. The spleen transforms and transports water to guarantee generation, and distribution of water. The distribution of water by the spleen is the prerequisite for the lung to regulate water passage. The coordination and cooperation of the spleen and lung maintain normal metabolism of water. If the spleen functions abnormally in governing transformation and transportation of water, water-dampness may be produced internally, which can often affect the lung to result in failure of the lung in diffusion and descent, and thus there appear symptoms of phlegm, fluid retention, cough and panting.

3.3.1.6 Lung and Liver

The relationship between lung and liver is essentially marked by mutual coordination between ascent and descent of qi dynamic.

The liver is characterized by ascending of its qi; and the lung by descending of its qi. The liver qi ascends and disperses, and the lung qi purifies and descends. The coordination between ascent and descent is of important regulatory role to freedom of the whole body's qi dynamic. Pathologically, the disorders of the liver and lung often affect each other. Adverse rising of liver qi, or up-flaming of liver fire consumes lung yin, which may lead to failure of lung qi to purify and descend. Contrarily, if the lung fails to purify, dry-heat will get hyperactive internally; as it involves liver yin and then yin fails to restrict yang, it may further result in hyperactivity of liver yang.

3.3.1.7 Lung and Kidney

The relationship between lung and kidney is mainly manifested in mutual dependence in respiratory movement and water metabolism.

The lung controls respiration, inhales the fresh air and exhales the turbid gas, so as to perform the exchange of gas between the interior and exterior of the body. The kidney governs reception of qi, the lung's function of controlling respiration needs assistance by the kidney's function of reception of qi; and thus the body can keep the depth of inspiration and prevent hypopnea, guaranteeing the evenness and harmony of respiratory movement. In pathology, protracted deficiency of lung qi with disturbance of purification and descent often results in the failure of the kidney in receiving qi with deficiency of kidney qi; and vise versa.

The lung governs water passage; the function of the lung in freeing and regulating distribution and excretion of water depends upon the kidney in qi transformation. The kidney governs water; the function the kidney in sending up and down the water by qi transformation is also dependant upon the descending action of lung qi to make the water go down into the kidney. The lung and kidney act on each other to maintain the normal process of water metabolism. If the lung's or kidney's function gets disordered, it will cause disturbance of water metabolism, and then there will appear symptoms like edema.

In addition, yin qi of the lung and kidney promote each other. When lung yin is sufficient, it will go down into the kidney and make the kidney yin abundant. As kidney yin is sufficient, it will go up into the lung and make the lung yin full enough. Pathologically, lung yin deficiency and kidney yin shortage usually are of causality to get disordered commonly.

3.3.1.8 Liver and Spleen

The relationship between liver and spleen is mainly manifested as two aspects of foodstuff transformation and transportation and blood circulation.

The spleen governs transformation and transportation, possessing the functions to transform the foodstuff into essence, and absorb and transport it onto the whole body. The liver governs free flow of qi to smooth qi dynamic for coordinating the ascending of the spleen qi and descending of the stomach qi and, to smooth the bile, for helping the spleen in transformation and transportation. If the liver fails in governing free flow of qi, the qi dynamic will get obstructed, and then it will lead to failure of the spleen in transformation and transportation, there will appear syndrome of disharmony between liver and spleen.

The spleen controls blood; spleen qi holds blood to prevent its escape from the vessels. the liver stores blood. When liver blood is sufficient, the liver proper will get its nourishment, then the liver's function in governing free flow of qi will be normal, qi dynamic be smooth, and thus blood flow will be free from obstruction. The liver and spleen cooperate with each other to guarantee both smooth blood flow and non-escape of blood from the vessels. If the liver and spleen get injured, the control and storage of blood will become disordered, then it may lead to abnormal blood flow, with manifestation of bleeding.

3.3.1.9 Liver and Kidney

The relationship between liver and kidney is mainly marked by mutual transformation between essence and blood, and interdependence of storage and discharge.

The liver stores blood, and the kidney stores essence. The kidney essence is one of the essential materials for generation of blood; the generation of blood depends upon the sufficiency of essence qi in the kidney. And the sufficiency of the essence-qi is also dependent upon the nourishment of the liver blood. The liver blood and the kidney essence are physiologically supplementary to each other, and they also mutually affect each other pathologically. Shortage of liver blood may result in deficiency of kidney essence, and vise versa, thus there appear dual deficiency of kidney essence and liver blood, manifesting as dizziness, vertigo, tinnitus, deafness, soreness and weakness of the waist and knee.

The liver governs free flow (discharge) of qi, and the kidney dominates storage; both are opposite and yet complementary to each other. The discharge of liver qi is conducive to reasonable opening-closing of the kidney qi. Contrarily, the storage of kidney qi can prevent over-discharge of the liver qi. The two respects support each other to coordinate the functions of menstruation in women and ejaculation in men. If the discharge of the liver and storage of the kidney get disharmonious, then there may appear disorder of menstruation in women; impotence, spermatorrhea or priapism with spermatemphraxis.

In addition, the liver and kidney are closely related in yin-yang. The kidney yin can nourish the liver yin so as to restrict liver yang to keep balance of yin-yang. If the kidney yin gets deficient and fails to nourish liver yin, it may lead to yin deficiency of both liver and kidney with resultant hyperactivity of liver yang, and thus there appear disorders of dizziness and apoplexy.

3.3.1.10 Spleen and Kidney

The relationship between spleen and kidney is essentially reflected by mutual promotion of innateness and acquirement, and mutual cooperation in water metabolism.

The kidney is the root of innateness, and the spleen is the root of acquirement. Sound transformation and transportation through spleen qi to produce foodstuff essence depends upon the help and promotion by kidney qi. And the abundance of essence-qi in the kidney is also dependent upon the culture and nourishment of foodstuff essence. Pathologically, the spleen insufficiency and the kidney asthenia often affect each other, leading to both weakness of the spleen and kidney. If qi of the spleen and kidney gets deficient, there may appear symptoms of abdominal distention, sloppy stool, sourness and coldness of the waist and knees, diarrhea at dawn, or diarrhea with undigested foodstuff.

The spleen governs transformation and transportation to distribute water so as to prevent effusion of water-dampness. The kidney governs water to manage and regulate distribution and excretion of water. The spleen and kidney cooperate with each other to maintain equilibrium of water metabolism. If there appears insufficiency of both spleen and kidney, and water-dampness stagnates internally, there may appear symptoms of oliguria, edema, abdominal distention, sloppy stool, sourness and weakness of the waist and knees.

3.3.2 Relationships among the Six *Fu*-viscera

The relationships among the six *Fu*-viscera are mainly manifested as association and cooperation in the process of digestion, absorption and transportation of foodstuff, and excretion of the waste as well.

The foodstuff entering the stomach is, through the decomposition by the stomach, sent down into the small intestine. After reception and digestion of the chyme, and separation of the clear and turbid by the small intestine, the clear is transported throughout the whole body under the function of the spleen; and the turbid is transported down into the large intestine, which, through dryness and conveyance by the large intestine, becomes stool to be discharged out of the body. The water permeating into the urinary bladder is, through qi transformation, turned into urine to be discharged out of the body. The above process of digestion and absorption of foodstuff and excretion of the waste is also dependent upon the gallbladder to excrete the bile to help digestion, and the tri-Jiao to sooth water passageways to circulate water. The six *Fu*-viscera constantly receive, digest and transport the foodstuff, and yet excrete the waste, which is a process that demands for no stagnation but freedom. Therefore there is a saying "the six *Fu*-viscera are to dredge functionally".

The six *Fu*-viscera coordinate functionally and affect pathologically one another. For example, rampancy of gallbladder fire may often invade the stomach to make it fail in normal descent of stomach qi, thus there appear symptoms like vomiting with bitter liquid. If stomach heat consumes the liquid, it will lead to constipation with obstructed conveyance of the large intestine.

3.3.3 Relationships between *Zang*- and *Fu*-Viscera

3.3.3.1 Heart and Small Intestine

The heart meridian of hand Shaoyin affiliates to the heart and connects with the small intestine, and the small intestine meridian of hand Taiyang affiliates to the small intestine and connects with the heart, thus the heart and the small intestine form an exterior-interior relation through their meridians' connection and affiliation.

Heart yang goes down to the small intestine to warm it so that it benefits the small intestine in its reception and digestion of the chyme, and separation of the clear from the turbid. The small intestine absorbs foodstuff essence and sends it up to the heart; and then the heart reddens the essence to make it become blood so as to nourish the heart-vessels. The heart and small intestine functionally serve each other and pathologically affect each other. If heart fire gets hyperactive, the heat may be transported into the small intestine, then there appear symptoms of dysphoria, red tongue with sore, scanty urine that is hot and red, dysuria.

3.3.3.2 Lung and Large Intestine

The lung meridian of hand Taiyin affiliates to the lung and connects with the large intestine, and the large intestine meridian of hand Yangming affiliates to the large intestine and connects with the lung, thus the lung and the large intestine form an exterior-interior relation through their meridians' connection and affiliation.

The purification and descent of lung qi is conducive to the large intestine in conveyance of the waste. The smooth conveyance by the large intestine is also beneficial to lung qi's purification and descent. If the lung qi fails in purification and descent, and the fluid cannot be sent down, then the liquid in the large intestine will be short, there will appear constipation due to intestinal dryness. If the large intestine fails in smooth conveyance, and the intestine qi gets obstructed, it may also affect the diffusion and descent of lung qi to cause the symptoms of chest fullness, cough and panting.

3.3.3.3 Spleen and Stomach

The spleen meridian of foot Taiyin affiliates to the spleen and connects with the stomach, and the stomach meridian of foot Yangming affiliates to the stomach and connects with the spleen, thus the spleen and the stomach form an exterior-interior relation through their meridians' connection and affiliation

The stomach dominates reception, and the spleen governs transformation and transportation; reception and transformation depend on each other. The reception and decomposition of the foodstuff by the stomach is the prerequisite for the transformation and transportation by the spleen. The spleen governs transformation and transportation, conveying the essence to the body, which provides the condition for further reception of foodstuff by the stomach.

Spleen qi is characterized by ascent and stomach qi by descent; the two condition each other by coordination of ascent and descent, commonly accomplishing the distribution of essence and conveyance of waste.

The spleen is a *Zang*-viscus, it belongs to yin, and likes dryness and hates dampness. The stomach is a *Fu*-viscus, it belongs to yang, and likes moisture and hates dryness. Only when dryness and dampness supplement each other, and yin and yang are harmonious, can reception and transportation and, ascent and descent coordinate normally.

The spleen and stomach serve each other functionally, and influence each other pathologically. If the spleen is encumbered by dampness, spleen qi fails to ascend, and the spleen gets insufficient in transportation, it will affect reception and descending of the stomach; then there may appear symptoms of abdominal distention and diarrhea.

3.3.3.4 Liver and Gallbladder

The liver meridian of foot Jueyin affiliates to the liver and connects with the gallbladder, and the gallbladder meridian of foot Shaoming affiliates to the gallbladder and connects with the liver, thus the liver and the gallbladder form an exterior-interior relation through their meridians' connection and affiliation.

The bile originates from the surplus qi of the liver. The secretion and excretion of the bile are regulated and controlled by the liver's function in governing free flow of qi. When the function of the liver performs normally, the secretion and excretion of the bile will be normal. Contrarily, the smooth excretion of the bile is also beneficial to the liver's function in governing free flow of qi. If the liver qi gets stagnant, the secretion and excretion of the bile will become disturbed. If the gallbladder is invaded by dampness-heat, and the excretion of bile gets obstructed, it will affect the free flow of liver qi, thus there will appear the syndromes such as qi stagnation of the liver and gallbladder, dampness-heat in the liver and gallbladder, and blazing of liver and gallbladder fire. In addition, the liver is in charge of making strategy, but to make decision depends upon the gallbladder. The two organs cooperate closely.

3.3.3.5 Kidney and Urinary Bladder

The kidney meridian of foot Shaoyin affiliates to the kidney and connects with the urinary bladder, and the urinary bladder meridian of foot Taiyang affiliates to the urinary bladder and connects with the kidney, thus the kidney and the urinary bladder form an exterior-interior relation through their meridians' connection and affiliation.

The bladder is a yang *Fu*-viscus. Its major function is to store and discharge urine. However, the urine storing function depends upon the controlling action of kidney qi, and urine discharging function also upon the qi transformation of the kidney. If the kidney fails in qi transformation or controlling, there will appear disturbance for the bladder to store and discharge urine, with manifestations of scanty urine, anuria, or incontinence of urine. The kidney is a "water-viscus". The function of the kidney in governing water is also influenced by the bladder's function in storing and discharging urine. If the bladder functions abnormally in storing and discharging urine, it may affect the kidney's function in qi transformation and controlling, manifesting as the changes of urine in color, quality, and quantity.

In relationships between *Zang*- and *Fu*-viscera, besides the close relations between the exterior-interiorly related *Zang*- and *Fu*-viscera, a *Zang*-viscus also has relations with other non-exterior-interiorly related *Fu*-viscera. For example, that the liver governs free flow of qi influences the dredging and descending of stomach qi. When the liver qi keeps free flow, the stomach qi can normally descend. If the liver qi loses its free flow, then the stomach will fail to descend normally, and there may appear disorder of disharmony between liver and stomach, manifesting as distending pain in chest, hypochondrium and epigastrium, hiccup, belching, acid regurgitation, epigastric upset, etc..

Review Questions

- What are the visceral picture and visceral picture theory?
- What are the differences among the five *Zang*-, six *Fu*-and extra *Fu*-viscera?
- Please recount major functions of the fve *Zang*-viscera.
- Please describe major functions of the five *Fu*-viscera.
- Please expound the relations among the *Zang*-viscera, and those between *Zang*- and *Fu*-viscera.

4 ESSENCE, QI, BLOOD AND BODY FLUID

The essence, qi, blood, body fluid are the basic substances which constitute the human body and maintain its life activity. They are produced by the functional activities of the viscera, meridians, tissue and organs. Therefore, they are closely related to the viscera, meridians, tissues and organs in physiology and pathology.

4.1 Essence

4.1.1 Concept of Essence

The essence is a type of refined nutritious substances in the body. It usually has two meanings. In a broader sense, it refers to the refined nutritious substances transformed by qi and constituting the human body and maintaining its life activity, including qi, blood, body fluid, marrow, foodstuff essence, etc.; in a narrow sense, it means the reproductive essence having the function of producing offspring and stored in the kidney, being the basic substance promoting growth, development and reproductive function of the human body.

4.1.2 Production of Essence

The essence of human body is endowed by the parents and is constantly replenished and nourished after birth. Viewing from the origin of production, there are the innate and acquired essences.

4.1.2.1 Innate Essence

The innate essence is inherited from the parents, and the original substance constituting the embryo. The life material endowed by the parents is an essence coming from birth, being called the innate essence. Through the observation and experience of the multiplying process of the mankind, the ancients recognized that the combination of reproductive essence of parents can produce a new individual life. However from the embryo's formation to the fetus' maturity, the breeding of it all depends on the nutrition of the qi-blood in uterus. Therefore, the innate essence is an original substance of life, mainly stored in the kidney.

4.1.2.2 Acquired Essence

The acquired essence comes from foodstuffs, and is called "foodstuff essence". After birth, a man depends on the spleen-stomach to digest and absorb the foodstuff, converting it into the foodstuff essence so as to nourish every viscus, thus maintaining its normal life activity. Because this part comes from the acquirement, it is called the acquired essence.

Although the innate essence different from the acquired essence, they depend on each other and promote mutually. The innate essence must be constantly replenished by the acquired essence so as to maintain its normal physiological function, and in turn the production of the acquired essence must depend on the vitality of the innate essence to subsidize. Therefore the deficiency of either the innate or the acquired essence can all produce the pathological changes of essence deficiency.

4.1.3 Functions of Essence

The essence has functions of producing offspring, promoting growth and development, transforming itself into marrow and blood, producing qi and spirit.

4.1.3.1 Producing Offspring

The reproductive essence is the congenital material of life origin. Combining the reproductive essences of the couple can produce a new life individual. The reproductive essence has the function of reproduction. It comes from combination of the innate and acquired essence and stores in the kidney, constituting essence-qi of the kidney. With its abundance that is marked by full development of the body, to the period of youth, in the body "*Tiankui*"(sex promoters) is generated, thus the person possesses function of producing offspring. Therefore, essence-qi of the kidney can not only contain the reproductive essence but also transform into kidney qi to promote reproduction. This genetic substance that gives life to the offspring is "the innate essence" of the new life. If the kidney essence is ample, the reproductive function is normal; if it is short, it will affect the reproductive power. So supplementing the kidney essence is an important method to treat sterility in men and women clinically.

4.1.3.2 Promoting Growth and Development

The essence-qi of the kidney has the function of promoting growth and development. After birth, the body constantly grows and develops till matures as the essence-qi of the kidney gradually becomes abundant; then the body gradually gets senile along with continual decline of the essence-qi of the kidney. As a result, with the changes of the essence-qi from abundance to decline, the human body presents with a life regularity of birth, growth, prime, senility and death. If the kidney essence is abundant, the growth and development of the body will be normal; if the kidney essence gets deficient, it will result in pathological changes marked by hypoevolutism, five kinds of flaccidity and retardation.

4.1.3.3 Transforming Itself into Marrow and Blood

The kidney stores essence which can transform itself into the marrow including brain marrow and bone marrow. The brain marrow can nourish the brain. So as it is sufficient, there will be alert mind, agile thinking and clear speech. The bone depends upon nourishment of marrow. As the kidney essence is sufficient, the bone marrow will be abundant, and then the skeleton will be firm and powerful with a flexible movement. The teeth are the extension of the bones which are nourished by the marrow transformed from the kidney essence. As the kidney essence is abundant, the teeth are firm and lustrous. If kidney essence is deficient, it will affect the production of the marrow, and then the skeleton loses its nourishment, leading to looseness, even loss of teeth. If the brain marrow is deficient, it will result in symptoms such as dizziness, vertigo, mental weakness, amnesia and retarded intelligence.

The essence produces marrow which is one of the sources for blood production. Sufficient essence in the kidney provides necessary nourishment for the liver, and then blood will be replenished. Essence and blood promote each other, so there is a saying "essence and blood have the same origin". In clinical, medicinals derived from the animals, such as Lujiaojiao (*Corne Cervi*) and guijia (*Caraoax Trionycis*), which have the functions of supplementing both blood and essence, are used in treating syndrome of blood deficiency.

4.1.3.4 Moistening and Nourishing the Viscera

The essence can moisten and nourish the viscera, tissues, sense organs and orifices. As the essence is sufficient, the human body can get necessary nourishment to perform its normal physical function. If the kidney essence is deficient due to inadequate natural endowment or disturbed production of the acquired essence, the essence of five *Zang*-viscera will decline, and the viscera, tissues, sense organs and orifices fail to get the nourishment and supplement, then their physical functions will be insufficient or even fail. If the kidney essence gets deficient, there will appear hypoevolutism or senility in adults. If lung essence gets short, it will cause hypopnea, dry and illustrious skin. If the liver essence is short, the liver blood will be deficient, then the tendons cannot get enough nourishment, there will come convulsion, tremor and spasms.

4.1.3.5 Producing Qi and Spirit

The innate essence can generate the innate qi (primordial qi). The foodstuff qi which is transformed from the foodstuff essence combines with the fresh air inhaled by the lung to form the acquired qi. Qi constantly drives and regulates the metabolism of human body, maintaining the life activity. The essence can produce both qi and spirit. It is the substantial basis for mental activity. Only the essence is enough, can the spirit be sound, which is the basic assurance for life existence. On the contrary, the shortage of the essence will lead to weariness of spirit, and depletion of the essence will cause loss of spirit. A sound spirit gives a healthy physiques; a lowered spirit causes disease of the body.

4.2 Qi

The theory concerning "qi" in Chinese medicine comes from "monoism of qi" in ancient philosophy, which is originally a kind of abstract understanding to the nature and its material origin. The monosism of qi holds that qi is the most basic material of world and the constant movement of qi produces all the things in the universe. When this viewpoint infiltrates through medical science realm, it urged medical specialist to combine together with medical knowledge, constructing theory of qi in Chinese medicine.

4.2.1 Concept of Qi

Qi in the body is a kind of very active and refined substance that is in constant movement, which constitutes the human body and maintains its life activity.

Qi is the basic material constituting the human body. The constant movement of qi produces all the things in the universe. So there is no exception for man. The man's body takes qi as basic material, so there is a saying "the gathering of qi produces life while the dispersion of qi puts an end to life".

Qi is the basic material maintaining life activity. All the life activities of human body are produced by qi transformation. So, qi is the most important for life activity, also being seen as the root of life.

Qi is a kind of very active and essential substance which constantly circulates inside the body. The vitality of qi mainly expresses in the aspects of invigorating and promoting functions of the viscera, as well as circulation of essence, blood and body fluid. Therefore, the motion and changes of qi is used to explain the life activity of human body in Chinese medicine.

4.2.2 Production of Qi

The origin of production of qi is divided into two aspects: the innate qi and the acquired qi. The essential qi inherited from the parents before birth is called "the innate qi"; after birth, the essential qi acquired from the nature (such as nutrients from the food and fresh air from nature) is known as "the acquired qi".

The production of qi mainly depends on integral action of physiological functions of the viscera such as the lung, spleen-stomach and kidney, combining the innate essence with the acquired essence. Among them, the innate essence-qi is stored in the kidney, the fresh air is inhaled by the lung, and the foodstuff essence-qi is transformed by the spleen. Whether the physiological functions of the lung, spleen-stomach, and kidney are normal and their inter-relations are harmonious or not, usually influence the formation of qi. Among them the spleen-stomach is a key.

4.2.3 Movement of Qi

Qi, as an essential substance that is the most active and constantly moving, flows every parts of the body, constantly drives and maintains various physiological activities of human body. Therefore, the movement of qi determines the states of life activity.

The motion of qi is also called "qi dynamic". The moving style of qi can usually be classified into four kinds, namely ascending, descending, exiting and entering. Ascending is a sort of motion of qi from the lower to the upper, descending is a sort of motion of qi from the upper to the lower, exiting is a sort of motion of qi from the interior to the exterior; entering is a sort of motion of qi from the exterior to the interior. With regard to human body, the movement of qi universally exists without intermission. For example, in the respiration of the lung, the process of exhaling the turbid, in which the lung breathes out the turbid qi through throat, nose, skin and fine hair, contains the movement of exiting and ascending; while the process of inhaling the clear, in which the lung breathes the fresh air through nose and throat, contains the movement of entering and descending.

It should be pointed out, each *Zang* or *Fu*-viscus may differ from others in its moving style of qi. Among the five *Zang*-viscera, the moving style of liver qi and spleen qi is ascending, the moving style of heart qi and lung qi is descending; the qi of six *Fu*-viscera are to descend normally with an exception of the gallbladder. Viewing from the whole, the ascending, descending, exiting and entering are in a coordinative balance. For example, the liver qi is in charge of ascending and the lung qi is in charge of descending; the spleen qi governs the elevation of the clear while the stomach qi controls the lowering of the turbid, the lung governs the discharge of qi while the kidney governs the reception of qi; heart fire descends while kidney water ascends.

The ascending, descending, exiting and entering of qi are very important to life. The movement of qi can regulate the physiological function so as to attain the relative equilibrium. The concrete performance consists in two aspects: On the one hand, the viscera, meridians, body, sense organs and orifices are harmonious and sequential in physiological function through the movement of qi. For example, the kidney essence, foodstuff essence, fresh air spread over the whole body to exert various physiological effects must take the tri-Jiao as the passage and through the ascending, descending, exiting and entering of qi. The essence, blood and body fluid have to depend upon the movement of qi to constantly circulate, so as to nourish and moisten the viscera, tissues, body constituents, sense organs and orifices. On the other hand, the exchange of qi between outside and inside of the body, or absorbing essence-qi from the nature and expelling the turbid qi and terminal metabolic products, makes human qi renew and supply continuously so as to maintain life activity and regulate the physiological balance. If the movement of qi is broken down, it will result in pathological changes due to imbalance among the viscera, tissues, body, sense organs and orifices.

The state of coordinative balance without obstruction among ascending, descending, exiting and entering of qi is known as "free flow of qi". On the contrary, if the motion of qi in ascending, descending, exiting and entering gets obstructed, or it fails to be harmonious, this state will be called "disorder of qi dynamic".

There are five kinds of forms of "disorder of qi dynamic", namely: ① qi stagnancy, refers to unsmooth flow of qi or obstructed flow of qi, also called "inhibited qi dynamic" or "qi depression"; ② regurgitation of qi, refers to hyper-ascending of qi or hypo-descending of qi and/or transversely adverse movement; ③ qi sinking, refers to hypo-ascending of qi or hyper-descending of qi; ④ qi blockage, refers to failure of qi to exit and accumulation of qi in the interior; ⑤ qi exhaustion, refers to outside escape of qi due to its failure in holding itself inside.

4.2.4 Functions of Qi

Qi of human body is the source maintaining the life activity, and power of physiological functions of the viscera, meridians, tissues and other organs. Generally, the function of qi exerting in the life activity can be summarized as six aspects.

4.2.4.1 Propelling Function

Qi is the refined substance with very strong activity. Qi, with its vitality and motion, can invigorate and propel the growth and development of human body, the physiological functions of the viscera, meridians, tissues and other organs, and promote the formation and circulation of liquid substances such as blood and body fluid. When qi within body is abundant, the physiological functions are sound and normal, life is full of vitality. If qi is deficient, it may result in the hypofunction of the viscera as well as metabolite disorders of essence, blood, body fluid, even retarded growth and development, marked by various pathological states with hypofunction.

4.2.4.2 Warming Function

The warming function of qi means qi can produce thermal energy and make the body warm and remove the cold. The concrete performance is in three aspects: ① to maintain the body temperature relatively constant; ② to ensure the physiological functions of the viscera, meridians, body, sense organs and orifices; ③ to propel normal circulation of the essence, blood, body fluid without coagulation and stagnation, so as to promote metabolism of human body. If qi, because of deficiency, fails to warm, it will give rise to non-warm limbs, intolerance of cold, hypofunction and sluggish circulation of essence, blood and body fluid.

4.2.4.3 Defending Function

The defending function of qi means qi can guard the body surface and resist the invasion of exogenous pathogens or drive the pathogens out. When human body is invaded by exogenous pathogens, qi has the function of fighting against the pathogens and expelling them out. When exogenous pathogens invade into a part of the body, qi will gather in the affected place and exert its defending function to fight against the pathogens. When the defending function of qi is normal, the human body will be hardly invaded by pathogens; or one is invaded by pathogens, he is hardly diseased; even though when one is suffering, he will be cured easily. If the defending function of qi gets weakened, the resistant ability will fall down gradually, and exogenous pathogens will take advantage of the insufficiency to invade and make the body contracted.

4.2.4.4 Controlling Function

The controlling function of qi means qi has the action to control the liquid materials, such as blood, body fluid and sperm so as to prevent them from losing unduly. The concrete performance is in three aspects: ① to control blood, making the blood circulate inside the vessels and preventing it from extravasation; ② to control sweat, saliva, urine, adjusting their secretive and excretive volumes to make them discharge normally, in order to prevent the body fluid from excessive loss; ③ to control sperm, preventing its undue emission. If the controlling function of qi is weakened, it will lead to loss of liquid materials inside the body in great quantities. For example, failure of qi to control blood may cause bleeding; failure of qi to control body fluid may lead to polyhidrosis, polyguria or urinary incontinence, slobbering or salivation; failure of qi to control sperm may result in emission or spermatorrhea. In addition, such conditions as diarrhea, prolapse of the rectum, leukorrhagia and threatened abortion are mostly related with failure of qi in controlling.

4.2.4.5 Nourishing Function

The nourishing function of qi mainly manifests in three aspects: ① to nourish the body surface through the defensive qi flowing the muscular striae. ② to transport nutrients so as to moisten and nourish the tissues and organs through the meridian qi; ③ to nourish the whole body through the nutritive qi transforming into blood.

4.2.4.6 Qi Transforming Function

The qi transforming function means qi can produce and promote changes of various materials and energy through the motion of qi. Inter-transformation among the essential substances, various functions transformed by substance metabolism, and excretion of the wastes within the body are all dependent on the qi transformation. This is the most basic characteristic of life activity. If qi transformation is out of order, it will influence digestion and absorption of foodstuffs, the normal conversions of essence, qi, blood and body fluid, and the discharge of sweat, urine and stool, leading to various pathological changes of metabolic disturbance.

4.2.5 Classification of Qi

Qi of the human body, according to its production, distribution and functional characteristics, is classified into different kinds, i.e. the primordial qi, pectoral qi, nutritive qi and defensive qi.

4.2.5.1 Primordial Qi

The primordial qi refers to the most fundamental and important qi of the human body and is the motivating power of life activity. So, the primordial qi is also called "the innate qi", or "genuine qi".

(1) Production and distribution of the primordial qi: The primordial qi comes mainly from the innate essence stored in the kidney, being continuously supplemented and nourished by the acquired essence produced by the spleen-stomach. Therefore, the rise and fall of the primordial qi has direct relation with natural endowment. In addition, the food condition, physical exercises and the metal adjustment can influence the primordial qi. Insufficient primordial qi due to inadequate natural endowment can usually become sound through the cultivation after birth. The primordial qi is stored in the kidney and distributed to all parts of the body through tri-Jiao. It goes everywhere inward to the five *Zang*-viscera and the six *Fu*-viscera and outward to the body constituents, sense organs and orifices.

(2) Functions of the primordial qi: The physiological functions of the primordial qi mainly manifest two aspects: ① to boost and regulate growth, development and reproduction of the body. ② to activate, promote and regulate the physiological activities of the viscera, meridians, tissues and organs. Among them, the primordial yang can foster the yang of the whole body; the primordial yin can nourish the yin of the whole body. Sufficient primordial qi keeps normal growth, development and reproduction, normal viscera function, and strong vital qi. If there appears inadequate natural endowment, or inappropriate adjustment after birth, or prolonged disease, thus essence-qi in the kidney gradually declines, it will lead to shortage of source for producing the primordial qi; or the primordial qi is consumed too much. Both cases can cause various pathological changes due to decline of the primordial qi.

4.2.5.2 Pectoral Qi

The pectoral qi is the qi accumulated in the thorax and it is an acquired essential qi.

Because the thorax is the part where the pectoral qi gathers, it is called "the sea of qi".

(1) The formation and distribution of the pectoral qi: The pectoral qi is a combination of the natural fresh air inhaled by the lung and the foodstuff essence-qi transformed by the spleen-stomach. Accumulating in the thorax, the pectoral qi goes up along the upper respiratory tract, permeates the heart and the lung, and distributes to the whole body by continuously going downward through the tri-Jiao. On the one hand, the pectoral qi goes up out of the lung and flows along the respiratory tract to the throat to promote respiration. On the other hand, it permeates the heart and the vessels to propel blood circulation. tri-Jiao is the passage for all qi to circulate. Through the tri-Jiao the pectoral qi continues to go downward and to be stored in the elixir field so as to supply the primordial qi, and permeates the foot Yangming meridian via the point Qijie (ST 30).

(2) Function of the pectoral qi: The pectoral qi mainly has three functions: ① It flows through the respiratory tract to promote the respiratory movement of the lung. The condition of its sufficiency concerns the intensity of speech, voice and respiration. ② It permeates the heart and vessels to promote circulation of blood and qi. The strength of the pectoral qi is closely related to the rhythm and strength of throbbing of the heart, circulation of qi-blood, body temperature, and movement of the limbs, as well as the vision and hearing. ③ It accumulates in the elixir field to subsidize the innate endowment. The pectoral qi has important subsidiary function to the primordial qi. Taking tri-Jiao as its passages, the pectoral qi goes from the upper to the lower, storing in the elixir field to support the innate endowment. If the pectoral qi gets insufficient, it will lead to feeble breath, weak and low voice, arrhythmia, retarded blood circulation, cold limbs, lassitude, etc.

4.2.5.3 Nutritive Qi

The nutritive qi refers to a kind of qi circulating within the vessels and having nutritive action. It is the important component of the blood. It can be different but cannot be separated from blood, hence the name of "nutritive-blood". Compared with the defensive qi, the nutritive qi pertains to yin, so it is also called "nutritive-yin".

(1) Production and distribution of the nutritive qi: The nutritive qi comes from the most refined and nutritive part of foodstuff essence. The nutritive qi flows inside the vessels to circulate throughout the body, interiorly into the viscera and exteriorly onto the limbs and joints, repeatedly in cycle without an end.

(2) Functions of the nutritive qi: The physiological functions of the nutritive qi shows two aspects: ① to produce blood: Containing rich nutrient, as the nutritive qi flows into the vessels it will become the important part of blood. Therefore, it is the main material basis of the generation of blood. ② to nourish the whole body: The nutritive qi comes from the pure and most essential part of foodstuff essence. It follows inside the vessels, provides essential nutritive materials for the physiological activities of all the

viscera, meridians, tissues and organs.

The functions of producing blood and nourishing the whole body of the nutritive qi are closely related. Insufficiency of the nutritive qi will cause blood deficiency, and then all the viscera, meridians, tissues and organs cannot get enough nourishment, the physiological functions will decline gradually.

4.2.5.4 Defensive Qi

The defensive qi means the qi circulating outside the vessels and having protective function to the body. Compared with the nutritive qi, it belongs to yang, so there is name of "defensive-yang".

(1) Production and distribution of the defensive qi: The defensive qi comes from the fierce and swift part of the foodstuff essence. Because of quick activity and strong vitality, the defensive qi does not be limited by the vessels and goes outward over the skin and muscular striae, inward onto the thorax and abdomen, spreading the whole body.

(2) Functions of the defensive qi: The physiological functions of the defensive qi can be generalized as three aspects: ① to guard the surface of the body: The defensive qi distributes over the superficial to resist the invasion of the exogenous pathogens, embodying the defensive function of qi concretely. ② to warm the body: The defensive qi spreads all over the body, going to viscera inside, reaching the skin outside, exerting the warming function to the viscera, muscles, skin and fine hair. It both contributes to the physiological activities of the viscera, and makes the muscle strong and the skin lustrous. ③ to regulate the opening and closing of the striae: The defensive qi spreads to the body surface and regulates the opening and closing of the striae according to the need of the physiological activity, keeping a relatively constant body temperature by adjusting the excretion of sweat.

Although the nutritive qi and the defensive qi all come from the foodstuff essence, they have difference in the property, distribution and the physiological function. The nutritive qi comes from "the most essential part" of foodstuff essence, flowing inside the vessels and having the function to produce blood and nourish the whole body, so it belongs to yin. The defensive qi comes from "the most active and powerful part" of foodstuff essence, flowing outside the vessels and having the function to defend the body surface and warm the body, so it belongs to yang. Only when the nutritive qi and the defensive qi coordinate with each other, can they exert their own physiological function respectively.

Besides the above mentioned qi, there are also "visceral qi", "meridian qi", they all derive from the primordial qi which is distributed to a viscus or meridian and combined with foodstuff essence or fresh air so as to become qi of a viscus or meridian. In clinical, according to the functional conditions of them, the rise and fall of visceral qi and meridian qi can be determined.

4.3 Blood

4.3.1 Concept of Blood

The blood is a red liquid material circulating within the vessels and possessing the stronger nourishing and moistening functions.

Under normal conditions, blood circulates along the relatively closed vessels without extravasation. Blood of the whole body circulates within the vessel, so the vessel is called "the house of blood". If some reasons make the blood extravasate, it is called "bleeding"; and the blood escaping out of the vessels is called "extravasated blood".

4.3.2 Production of Blood

Generally speaking, the blood is composed of the nutritive qi and body fluid. In addition, essence can also be converted into blood.

4.3.2.1 Transformation of Foodstuff Essence into Blood

The foodstuffs are converted into foodstuff essence through the decomposition by the stomach and transformation and transportation by the spleen, the pure and refined part of which is transformed into the nutritive qi. The nutritive qi permeates the vessels and combines with body fluid to become blood. The nutritive qi comes from the most pure and refined part of the foodstuffs. It insures that the blood has extremely abundant nourishing composition. The body fluid is also the important part of the blood, and has the functions of maintaining and regulating blood volume, diluting blood and lubricating the vessels, thus guaranteeing ample blood and its enduring circulation. The nutritive qi and body fluid are the main material basis of blood production. The balanced diet and robust spleen-stomach function are important assurance for the blood production, so there is a saying "the spleen and stomach are the source for production of qi and blood".

4.3.2.2 Transformation of Essence into Blood

Essence can be transformed into blood because essence is the source of life. The essence and blood are the same kind, being of inter-promotion and inter-transformation. Essence is the beginning of life, and blood belongs to a kind of essence. Essence stores in the kidney. Sufficient kidney essence can provide necessary nourishment for the liver. The liver stores blood, as the essence enters the liver it will change into blood. The mutual supporting and conversion of essence and blood outstandingly reflect the close relationship of the liver and the kidney in the physiological function, so there are the saying "the liver and the kidney share the same source" and "essence and blood have the same origin". If the function of the liver or the kidney is weakened, particularly deficiency of kidney essence or kidney yin, it will affect the formation of blood, resulting in syndrome of blood deficiency.

Generally, the formation of blood mainly depends upon transformation and transportation by the spleen-stomach, and blood can be sufficient under the coordination of physiological function of the heart, liver, kidney.

4.3.3 Circulation of Blood

The blood circulates endlessly within the vessels, like a circle without an end, thus to nourish the whole body to satisfy the need of the life activity of human body.

4.3.3.1 Conditions for Maintaining Normal Blood Circulation

(1) The propelling and controlling function of qi: The circulating blood within the vessels must depend on propelling function of qi. Only qi is abundant, can blood circulation acquires enough power. At the same time, blood circulation also depends on controlling function of qi. Only when qi is abundant, can blood not escape out of the vessels. Therefore, coordinative balance between the propelling and controlling functions of qi is the important guarantee for maintaining the normal blood circulation.

(2) The integrity and smoothness of vessels: The vessel is the house of blood. The integrity, lubrication and smoothness of the vessels are important factors for blood circulation. Injuries from falls, or contusions and strains often damages vessels, hence bleeding; improper diet and phlegm retention often obstruct the vessels, leading to obstruction of the vessel passages, with an unsmooth or even obstructed blood circulation.

(3) Quality and temperature of blood: Quality and quantity of blood usually influence blood circulation directly. The viscosity and volume of blood will change blood circulation. Deficient body fluid results in stagnated blood circulation due to high viscosity of blood, insufficient blood volume results in unsmooth circulation. The blood is a kind of flowing liquid substance. It coagulates as it is exposed to cold, flows as exposed to warmth, rampantly circulates as exposed to heat. So temperature is also one of the common factors for influencing the blood circulation.

4.3.3.2 Relation of Blood Circulation to the Heart, Lung, Spleen and Liver

The heart, lung, spleen and liver play important roles in maintenance of normal blood circulation.

(1) The heart governs blood circulation: The heart qi is the main motive power of blood circulation. The normal circulation of blood along a certain direction within the vessels mainly depends on the propelling function of the heart qi.

(2) The lung connects with many large vessels: The lung governs qi of the whole body, particularly determines the rise or fall of the pectoral qi. The pectoral qi permeates the heart and vessels to propel the flowing of qi-blood. The vessels of the whole body converge in the lung, where blood is through a process of getting rid of the stale and

taking in the fresh, and then transported to the whole body's vessels by the heart. The lung participates in blood circulation directly, becoming another basic motive power of assisting the heart to propel blood circulation.

(3) The spleen controls blood: The normal blood circulation with no escape mainly depends on the controlling function of spleen qi. Prosperous spleen qi not only ensures the source for the formation of blood, but also controls blood to prevent it from extravasation.

(4) The liver stores blood: The liver can keep effective volume of circulating blood constant by storing blood and regulating its volume, so as to prevent it from flowing out of the vessels. Moreover, the liver governs free flow of qi and adjusts qi dynamic; this is one of the important factors for normal blood circulation.

Briefly, the normal blood circulation mainly depends on coordinating function of the viscera, such as the heart, lung, spleen and liver. Concretely, the heart drives blood circulation, the lung and the liver promote blood circulation and keep smoothness of the vessels, the liver and the spleen store blood and control its circulation, preventing blood from bleeding. In addition, the heart yang and the kidney yang keep blood vessels warm and relaxing.

4.3.4 Functions of Blood

The blood is the life material with abundant nourishment and yin-liquid. Its function mainly embodies two aspects:

4.3.4.1 Nourishing and Moistening Function

The blood, constantly circulating through the vessels to every part of the body, performs nourishing and moistening function to the whole body so as to meet the need of life activity. When the blood is sufficient, the viscera can get enough nourishment, marked by ruddy and shining complexion, strong muscle, lustrous hair and skin, sharp senses, and free movement. If blood is deficient, its function will decline, presented by pale complexion, dizziness, vertigo, withered hair or even loss of hair, rough skin, numbness or impaired movement of limbs, scanty menstruation, delayed menstruation, or even amenorrhea in women, etc..

4.3.4.2 Material Basis for Mental Activities

The blood is the main material basis for mental activities, which have to get nourishment from blood. When blood is sufficient, people will be full of vitality, acute in thinking, alert in consciousness, keen in response, and free in movement. If blood is deficient, and the blood cannot flow smoothly, there will appear a series of mental disorders which are presented by insomnia with dreaminess, fidgety, amnesia, absent mindedness, dispiritedness, even delirium, menia, unconscious, etc..

In addition, the blood is the material basis for generation of the sperm, menstrual blood, and milk.

4.4 Body Fluid

4.4.1 Concept of Body Fluid

Body fluid is a general term for all normal liquids in the body. It mainly exists in the viscera, tissues and organs. In addition, before being discharged out of the body, some normal secretions such as the gastric juice, intestinal juice, snivel, and saliva also belong to the category of body fluid. The body fluid spreads over the whole body, becoming a component of blood when it flows inside the vessels, being interstitial fluid permeating the viscera, organs and tissues when it flows outside of the vessels.

Body fluid can be subdivided into two parts of *Jin* (thin fluid) and *Ye* (thick fluid). Although they all come from foodstuffs, and are transformed by the spleen-stomach and distributed inside and outside the vessels, they are different in the characteristic, distribution and function. Generally speaking, the lucid and thin type with more fluidity, mainly spreading onto the skin, muscles and orifices, and seeping into the vessels as a component part of blood to play the moistening and nourishing function, is called *Jin* (thin fluid); the dense and thick type with less fluidity, mainly pouring into the skeleton, joints, viscera, brain-marrow and skin to play the nourishing and lubricating function, is called *Ye* (thick liquid).

The *Jin* and the *Ye* are of no difference in nature, and can mutually supply and convert during the process of metabolism, so they are often collectively termed as "body fluid". In pathology, it is necessary to differentiate "consumption of thin fluid" from "exhaustion of thick fluid".

4.4.2 Metabolism of Body Fluid

The metabolism of body fluid includes production, distribution and excretion.

4.4.2.1 Production of Body Fluid

Body fluid mainly comes from foodstuffs, including daily drinking and a certain amount of moisture contained in food. The production of body fluid involves physiological activities of several viscera. Speaking concretely, it is mainly produced by digesting-absorbing moisture and nourishing component of foodstuffs through the stomach, spleen, liver, small intestine and large intestine. It comes into being through a series of physiological activities: preliminary digestion by the stomach, transformation and transportation by the spleen, governing free flow of qi by the liver, separating the clear from the turbid by the small intestine, and dominating thin fluid by the large intestine; among them, the function of the spleen-stomach is predominant.

On the whole, the production of body fluid is determined by two aspects: One is the sufficient origin as the material basis for producing the body fluid; the other is normal function in absorbing and digesting, so that water and nourishment taken in are transformed into body fluid. If water intake is short, or the functions of such viscera as the spleen-stomach get weakened, it may all cause the deficiency of body fluid.

4.4.2.2 Distribution of Body Fluid

After the production of body fluid, under the function of transformation and transportation by the spleen, a part of body fluid is directly spread to the body, while a great deal of body fluid is sent up to the lung. By diffusing action, the lung further disseminates body fluid upward and outward; by descending action, it further sends body fluid inward and downward. After metabolism, body fluid is transported to the kidney. The kidney governs water. Through the steaming action and qi transformation by the kidney yang, the kidney steams the clear and secretes the turbid: the clear part of the fluid is steamed and sent up to the lung and the spleen to be used again; and the turbid part of the fluid is transformed into urine to be sent down into the urinary bladder. In addition, smoothness of water passage of tri-*Jiao* and free flow of the liver qi can also help the distribution of body fluid.

4.4.2.3 Excretion of Body Fluid

After body fluid is utilized by human body, its surplus and the metabolized wastes should be discharged outside of the body timely. Its excretion ways are mainly of four: ① excretion of sweat through skin: the lung disseminates body fluid to the surface of the body through its diffusing action, and through steaming action of yang qi the fluid is transformed into sweat and to be excreted outside of the body via the pores; ② excretion of urine through the urinary bladder: The urine is the terminal metabolic product of body fluid stored in the urine bladder and discharged outside of the body through the qi transformation of the kidney and the urinary bladder. This is the most important excretive pathway of waste fluid inside the body; ③ parts of water carried out through feces: The feces discharged by the large intestine also contain parts of water; ④ moisture carried out with exhalation: The lung controls respiration and also continuously disperses a certain amount of moisture in the process of breathing.

Generally, the metabolism of body fluid is coordinated by many viscera, among which the lung, spleen and kidney are the most important. If the function of these three viscera is disordered, it will influence the metabolic process of body fluid, thus producing phlegm, stagnant fluid, retention of urine, dropsy, etc..

4.4.3 Functions of Body Fluid

4.4.3.1 Moistening and Nourishing Function

Body fluid is extensively distributed in the viscera, sense organs, orifices, body constituents and limbs. Body fluid contains not only a great deal of moisture, but also various nourishing substance, with moistening and nourishing function to the whole body. For example, it is distributed onto the body surface to moist the skin, and luster the hair; it flows into orifices to make the sensory organs smooth and acute; it spreads into the joint to make the movement free and flexible; it permeates into the marrow to strengthen the skeleton; it permeates into blood vessels to increase blood volume and lubricate the vessels; and it gets into the viscera to nourish them.

4.4.3.2 Transforming and Regulating Function

Body fluid is one of the important components of blood. The body fluid, which combines with the nutritive qi to transform into the blood under the function of heart yang, circulates thought the whole body, exerting its moistening and nourishing function. Moreover, body fluid also has the function of regulating blood concentration. As blood concentration is higher, body fluid seeps into the vessels to dilute blood and complement blood volume. When the body is short of fluid, the fluid in blood will seep out of the vessels to supplement the body fluid and rectify dehydration. Through permeation of the fluid into and out of the vessels, human body can regulate blood concentration according to the physiological or pathological changes, thus maintaining normal effective blood volume, and ensuring integrity and smoothness of the vessels so as to contribute to blood circulation.

4.4.3.3 Regulating and Neutralizing Function

Body fluid pertains to yin, also called "yin liquid", have the function of regulating yin-yang, moderating the cold and hot, and keeping equilibrium of body temperature. Yin can inhibit yang. If the body fluid is abundant, deficiency-fire is difficult to rise. The deficiency of body fluid may result in excess heat and dryness. As it is cold, body fluid cannot excrete as sweat through the pores, but flows down into the urinary bladder, making the urine increase; as it is hot, body fluid spreads outward through the widely opened pores so as to help discharge heat, thus the fluid flows down less and the urine decreases. When the body loses moisture, it can be corrected by drinking beverage or taking in the medicinals that can produce fluid to quench thirst.

Body fluid belongs to liquid material, so it has neutralizing action. It can moderate and dilute the toxin or partiality in flavors and natures so as to reduce stimuli and damages, and accelerate excretion. The neutralization of body fluid is very important for the maintenance of physiological function.

4.4.3.4 Function of Excreting the Wastes

Through the metabolic process, the body excretes metabolic products outside of the body in time through the ways of urine, sweat and feces. etc., thus the normal physiological activity can be kept. If this function is out of order, causing retention of metabolic products in the body, this can produce various pathological changes.

4.5 Relationships among Essence, Qi, Blood and Body Fluid

The essence, qi, blood and body fluid are of their own different characters in the property, production, distribution and function; however, they are all the basic substances for constituting human body and maintaining its life activity. Therefore, they depend on, promote and coordinate with each other in physiology, as well as influence and affect each other in pathology.

4.5.1 Relationship between Essence and Qi

Compared with essence, qi is active and pertains to yang; essence is quiet and pertains to yin. There is a close relationship between the two. This is concretely manifested in three aspects: Essence can generate qi, qi can produce essence and qi can control essence.

4.5.1.1 Essence Generates Qi

Essence of human body can transform itself into qi under invigorating and promoting function of qi. The essence of five *Zang*-viscera turns into qi of the five *Zang*-viscera, but the innate essence stored in the kidney transforms into the primordial qi, the foodstuff essence into foodstuff qi. Essence is the origin of production for qi. Sufficient essence makes qi abundant, so as the essence spreads onto the viscera and meridians, the visceral qi and meridian qi are also ample. When the essence of five *Zang*-viscera is sufficient, qi of the five *Zang*-viscera will be produced abundantly, and thus can propel and control physiological activity of the whole body. Therefore abundant essence makes qi prosperous, and insufficient essence results in decline of qi. In clinic, the patient with essence deficiency and loss of essence usually presents the sign of qi deficiency.

4.5.1.2 Qi Produces Essence

Prosperous function of qi transformation can promote the production of essence. The essence stored in the kidney takes the innate essence as foundation, and can get prosperous through the continuous nourishment of the acquired essence. Only visceral qi of the whole body is sufficient and their function is normal, can the foodstuff essence be transported and transformed, making the essence of the viscera abundant, and flowing into the kidney to be stored. As a result, the production of essence depends on prosperous qi.

4.5.1.3 Qi Controls Essence

Qi can both promote the production of essence and control essence, making the essence abundant without losing unduly. This is the embodiment of controlling function of qi. If qi in deficiency fails to produce essence, it will lead to essence deficiency. If qi in deficiency fails to control essence, it will cause loss of essence. In clinical, the remedies of invigorating qi to produce or control essence are usually used in treating this kind of disorders.

4.5.2 Relationship between Essence and Blood

Essence and blood all belong to liquid life substances. Because they have the relationship of mutual supplement and transformation, there is a saying "essence and blood are of the same origin".

4.5.2.1 Essence Produces Blood

Essence is one of the basic materials to produce blood. When the essence of five *Zang*-viscera permeates and blends with blood flow, it will become blood. Under qi transformation of the kidney, the essence in the kidney that enters the liver can turn into blood. Under qi transformation of the spleen, the refined part of the foodstuff essence can turn into the nutritive qi, and the clear and lucid part of it into body fluid. As the nutritive qi and body fluid go into the vessels and are reddened under the function of heart yang, they can change into blood. Therefore in treating liver blood deficiency syndrome, the method of invigorating kidney and supplementing essence can often gain satisfactory effect.

The kidney stores essence, so it is particularly important for the kidney essence to transform into blood. The kidney essence can transform into blood to nourish the hair, so there is a saying "the kidney reflects its brilliance in the hair", and "the hair is the extension of blood". Therefore, in deficiency of kidney essence there may appear the manifestation of blood deficiency, such as dry lusterless hair and loss of hair.

4.5.2.2 Blood Generates Essence

Blood takes the foodstuff essence as main source for production. The essence in the kidney also depends on continuous nourishment of the foodstuff essence. Therefore, the blood can also transform itself into essence so as to continuously enrich and nourish the kidney essence, making it prosperous. Sufficient blood gives rise to abundance of essence, and insufficient blood causes shortage of the essence.

4.5.3 Relationship between Qi and Blood

Qi belongs to yang, being invisible and active. It is in charge of propelling and warming. Blood belongs to yin, being visible and quite. It has the function of nourishing and moistening. They are opposite to and dependent on each other; they inter-generate and cannot be separated from each other for a while. The relation of qi and blood can usually be generalized as "qi is the commander of blood and blood is the mother of qi." The former refers to the action of qi on blood, including three aspects: Qi can produce blood, circulate blood and control blood. The latter refers to the action of blood on qi, including two aspects: Blood can nourish qi and carry qi.

4.5.3.1 Qi Produces Blood

This means qi participates in and promotes the formation of blood. It concretely embodies two aspects: ① The nutritive qi is the main part constituting the blood: The nutritive qi circulates in the vessels. It is not only the basic material promoting the formation of blood, but also the motive power in combining with body fluid infused into the vessels; ② Visceral qi produces blood: Under the function of qi of the spleen-stomach, the small intestine, the heart, the lung. etc., foodstuff essence originated from the food and drink further transforms itself into the nutritive qi and body fluid which are reddened to become blood. The kidney essence can also be transformed into blood. Each link cannot do without qi transformation. Because prosperous qi makes the blood sufficient, deficient qi may lead to shortage of blood. So qi deficiency may further cause blood deficiency, resulting in manifestations of deficiency of both qi and blood, such as dizziness and giddiness, shortness of breath, disinclination to speak, lassitude, spontaneous sweating, pale complexion, palpitation, unbearable throbbing, insomnia, forgetfulness, pale and tender tongue, feeble and thready pulse.

4.5.3.2 Qi Circulates Blood

This means that the driving action of qi is the motive force to propel blood circulation. The blood pertains to yin and is characterized by quiet. Its flowing depends on the driving action of qi. Concretely speaking, the heart controls the flow of blood; the heart qi is the basic motive power to propel the blood circulation. The lung governs qi and connects with many large vessels; the lung qi is main assistant strength for the heart in governing blood. The liver governs free flow of qi and adjusts qi dynamic; the liver qi is the important link keeping normal blood circulation. The coordination among the functions of the three Zang-viscera makes the blood circulation smooth and free.

If qi gets deficient and fails in propelling or qi gets depressed, it will cause retarded, stagnated blood circulation and lead to formation of stagnant blood. The disorder of qi dynamic can also cause disturbance of blood circulation, such as bleeding superiorly caused by adverse rise of qi, or bleeding inferiorly due to qi sinking.

4.5.3.3 Qi Controls Blood

This means that qi has the function to keep blood circulating within the vessels and prevents it from extravasation. This is the specific embodiment of controlling function of qi, mainly related with the controlling function of spleen qi on blood. If deficiency of the spleen qi fails to control blood within the vessels, it will cause various kinds of hemorrhage, such as hematochezia, subcutaneous hemorrhage, metrorrhagia and metrastaxis in women. In clinical, this phenomenon is called "failure of qi to control blood" or "failure of the spleen to control blood".

4.5.3.4 Blood Nourishes Qi

Blood contains abundant nourishment. It can provide material foundation for generation and functional activity of qi so as to make qi replenished timely and appropriately. The abundant blood provides qi with nourishment. If blood gets deficient and fails to nourish qi, it may cause qi deficiency.

4.5.3.5 Blood Carries Qi

Qi is invisible and active, so it must attach to blood that is visible and quiet to perform its physiological effect that it should has. When blood is sufficient, it can carry qi. If blood loses in a great quantity, it will cause collapse of qi following blood.

4.5.4 Relationship between Qi and Body Fluid

Qi is invisible and active, belonging to yang. Body fluid is visible and quiet, belonging to yin. Their relationship can be generalized as "qi dominates body fluid and body fluid carries qi". Among them, qi as the dominator of body fluid refers to the function of qi on body fluid, including three aspects, i.e. qi generates fluid, circulates fluid and controls fluid.

4.5.4.1 Qi Generates Fluid

This means that qi has the effect of promoting the production of body fluid, which is produced by the absorption and digestion of foodstuffs by spleen-stomach qi. If the spleen-stomach qi is sufficient with a sound digestive and absorptive function, the production of body fluid will be prosperous. Contrarily, if the spleen-stomach qi gets insufficient, and the function in digesting and absorbing decreases, the generation of body fluid will be short. So there is a saying "prosperous qi makes body fluid sufficient" and "weak qi makes body fluid deficient".

4.5.4.2 Qi Circulates Fluid

This means that qi has the effect of propelling the distribution and excretion of body fluid. Through propelling function of qi, body fluid can spread over the whole body. By qi transformation, terminal metabolic products of body fluid can be discharged out of the body timely. The distribution and excretion of body fluid depend on qi transformation and coordination of the viscera such as the lung, spleen, kidney, and tri-Jiao. If qi of the above mentioned viscera gets deficient or qi dynamic gets disordered, it may cause obstacle in distribution and excretion, producing the pathological products such as water, dampness, phlegm, and stagnant fluid. This is called "failure of qi to circulate water".

4.5.4.3 Qi Controls Fluid

This means that qi has the effect to astringe body fluid and prevent it from losing unduly. This is the specific embodiment of controlling function of qi, mainly related to the regulating and controlling actions of the defensive qi on sweat and the kidney qi on urine. If qi of the lung and kidney get deficient and fail in controlling, it will cause abnormal loss of body fluid, showing polyhidrosis and polyuria.

4.5.4.4 Fluid Conveys Qi

This means that body fluid has the function of carrying qi. Qi has to attach to body fluid so as to exist inside the body and spread to the whole body, so there is a saying "fluid conveys qi". It concretely embodies two aspects: One refers that fluid inside the vessels as the constituting part of blood can carry the nutritive qi; the other refers that fluid outside the vessels can carry the defensive qi. Because fluid can carry qi, when body fluid loses in a great quantity, such as polyhidrosis, polyuria, severe vomit and diarrhea, qi will immediately escape out of the body, resulting in "collapse of qi following fluid", which is marked by shortness of breath, feeble breath, lassitude, faint and thready pulse. Since body fluid is the carrier of qi, there also is also the condition of qi stagnation due to obstruction of body fluid pathologically, namely, retention of body fluid hinders the movement of qi.

4.5.5 Relationship between Blood and Body Fluid

Blood and body fluid are all liquid substance, belonging to yin. They all come from foodstuff essence and have the moistening and nourishing functions. Because blood and body fluid promote and transform into each other, their relation can be generalized as that "body fluid and blood have the same origin".

4.5.5.1 Blood Generates Body Fluid

Blood usually circulates inside the vessels. When the fluid as the composition of blood leaks out of the vessels, separating from the nutritive qi, it can be integrated into body fluid outside of the vessels. If blood gets consumed, particularly in excessive loss of blood, which cause blood in the vessels reduced, then body fluid outside the vessels will permeate into the vessels in great quantity so as to complement the reduced blood volume. As a result it will cause relative shortage of body fluid outside the vessels, showing thirsty, dry throat, oliguria, dry skin, etc. Therefore the patient with loss of blood should not be treated with diaphoresis in order to prevent the malignant result of exhaustion of body fluid and blood.

4.5.5.2 Body Fluid Produces Blood

Body fluid circulating outside the vessels seeps into the vessels and combines with the nutritive qi under the function of heart yang, becoming the constituting part of blood. Under the conditions such as intake shortage of water, hypofunction of the spleen and stomach, or profuse sweat, severe vomit, server purgation, or serious burns and scalds, the body fluid outside the vessel gets short, then the fluid inside the vessels will leak out in great quantity, resulting in the sudden decrease of blood volume. This can make blood viscosity higher and cause pathologic changes of "fluid exhaustion with blood dryness" or "fluid consumption with blood stasis". Therefore for the patient with loss of fluid, the therapeutic methods such as breaking blood and bloodletting should not be taken.

Review Questions

- What is the concept of essence? What origins for production does the essence have?
- What viscera are closely related to the formation of qi?
- What is the qi dynamic? How many basic styles are there?
- What physiological functions does qi have?
- What viscera are closely related to the circulation of blood?
- What viscera are closely related to the distribution of body fluid?

5　MERIDIAN THEORY

Meridian theory is a basic theory studying the concept, composition, running course, physiological function, pathological change of the meridian system and its relationships with the viscera, constituent, sense organ, orifice, qi, blood, essence and mind. It is an important component part of theoretical system of Chinese medicine. The meridian theory and the visceral theory together make up the core of theoretical system of Chinese medicine.

The meridian theory runs through every aspect of human physiology, pathology, and the diagnosis, prevention and treatment of disease. It is mutually complementary with those theories of yin-yang, the five elements, visceral picture, and essence, qi, blood and body fluid. It deeply expounds the human body's physiological activity and pathological changes, playing very efficacious guiding role for acupuncture and moxibustion, massage, qigong, etc..

5.1　Concept of the Meridian and Its Composition

5.1.1　Concept of the Meridian

The meridian is a system of passages consisting of meridians, collaterals and its affiliated portions. It transports qi-blood of the whole body, communicates with the viscera and other tissues and organs so as to make the five *Zang*-viscera, six-*Fu* viscera, four limbs, skeleton, five sense organs, nine orifices, skin, muscles, tendons, vessels, etc. link up to be an organic whole. It is an important component part of the human tissue structure. The meridian is not only a passage system for internal communication of the body, but also a bridge for correspondence of the body with nature so as to maintain the coordination and unity of the body's internal and external environments. The viscera and tissues of the body are constantly carrying the exchanges of material, energy and information with nature so as to guarantee normal process of vital activity of the body.

Meridians here mean tracks; and collaterals mean network. Meridians are the major trunk, and collaterals are the branches. The physicians of later ages mostly hold that meridians run generally through the deeper parts of the body or among the muscles; while the collaterals run through the more superficial parts, and some even appear in the body surface. Meridians mainly run vertically, and have a certain running courses; while the collaterals criss-cross to network the whole body. However, meridians mostly "run deeper among the muscles", actually some of them may also appear in the body surface; and there are some of collaterals "running superficially and appearing in the body surface", but most of the collaterals actually distribute among the viscera and tissues. Further more, there are meridian such as Dai meridian running transversely; and collaterals criss-cross in a network, but there are definitely collaterals running vertically.

The meridians and collaterals are the major body of the meridian system, undertaking the role to circulate qi-blood and communicate so as to connect all the viscera, organs, orifices, skin, muscles tendons, bones, etc. to form an integral organic whole.

5.1.2 Composition of the Meridian System

The meridian system connects internally with the viscera and externally with the tendons, muscles and skin.

Meridians include three large groups of regular meridians, extra meridians and meridian divergences. The regular meridians are of twelve, including three yin meridians of hand, three yang meridians of hand, three yin meridians of foot and three yang meridians of foot, which are collectively called "twelve meridians" or "twelve regular meridians", and the major tracks for qi-blood circulation. The twelve meridians have their own starting and terminating points, running regions; connecting orders; certain regularities in distribution and course in the limbs and trunk. They have direct relationships of connection and affiliation with viscera within the body, and external-internal relationships among themselves. The twelve meridians are the necessary passages for qi-blood circulation.

Extra meridians are of eight, namely Ren, Du, Chong, Dai, Yinwei, Yangwei, Yinqiao and Yangqiao meridians, collectively called eight extra meridians. They have the actions to govern, communicate and regulate qi-blood within the twelve meridians. The eight extra meridians are different from the twelve meridians, having no direct relationships of connection and affiliation with viscera, and also no external-internal relationship among themselves, hence the name of "extra meridians".

The twelve meridian divergences are the meridians branching out from the twelve meridians. They originate respectively from the four limbs and run through the deeper parts of the body cavity and reach up the superficial parts of the neck. The meridian divergences of yang meridians branch out from their meridians-proper and still return to the meridians-proper after running through the body internally; while the meridian divergences of yin meridians branch out from their meridians-proper, after running through the interior of the body, however, they join their external-internally related yang meridians respectively. The functions of the twelve meridian divergences are mainly to strengthen the communication between the two external-internally related

```
                                              ┌─ The lung meridian of hand Taiyin
                                    ┌─ Three Yin ─┤  The heart meridian of hand Shaoyin
                                    │             └─ The pericardium meridian of hand Jueyin
                           ┌─ Hand ─┤
                           │        │             ┌─ The large intestine meridian of hand Yangming     ┐
                           │        └─ Three Yang ┤  The tri-Jiao meridian of hand Shaoyang            │
                           │                      └─ The small intestine meridian of hand Taiyang      │  the major passages
          ┌─ The twelve ───┤                                                                            │  of qi-blood; being of
          │  regular       │                      ┌─ The spleen meridian of foot Taiyin                │  directly relationships
          │  meridians     │        ┌─ Three Yin ─┤  The liver meridian of foot Jueyin                 │  of connection and
          │                │        │             └─ The kidney meridian of foot Shaoyin               │  affiliation with
          │                └─ Foot ─┤                                                                   │  internal viscera
          │                         │             ┌─ The stomach meridian of foot Yangming             │
          │                         └─ Three Yang ┤  The gallbladder meridian of foot Shaoyang         │
          │                                       └─ The bladder meridian of foot Taiyang              ┘
┌─ The ───┤
│ meridian│                         ┌─ The Du meridian
│         │                         │  The Ren meridian        ┐
│         │                         │  The Chong meridian      │
│         │                         │  The Dai meridian        │  being of the actions
│         └─ The eight     ─────────┤  The Yinqiao meridian    ├─ to command,
│            extra                  │  The Yangqiao meridian   │  communicate and
│            meridians               │  The Yinwei meridian     │  regulate the twelve
│                                   └─ The Yangwei meridian    ┘  meridians
│
│         ┌─ The twelve meridian ─┬─ branching out from the twelve meridians, functioning to strengthen the communication
│         │  divergences          └─ between the two external-internally related meridians in the twelve meridians
│         │
│─ The ───┤  The fifteen      ┌─ each of the twelve, Ren and Du meridians has one plus the other large collateral of the
│  collaterals  divergent    ─┤  spleen meridian, functioning to strengthen the communication in the exterior of the body
│         │  collaterals       └─ between the two external-internally related meridians and to ooze qi-blood
│         │
│         │  The minute collaterals──tiny and small collaterals
│         └─ The superficial collaterals──collaterals superficially appearing in the body surface
│
│         ┌─ The twelve       ┌─ the system of tendons-muscles where the twelve meridian qi concentrate,
│         │  meridian         ─┤  accumulate, distribute and connect, with the actions of linking up
└─ The ───┤  musculatures     └─ the four limbs and bones, and dominate the motion of
   affiliated
   portion  └─ The twelve skin areas──the sites in the body surface reflecting the functions of the twelve meridians
```

Fig. 5-1 The Meridian System

MERIDIAN THEORY

211

meridians in the twelve meridians; they can also severe as the supplement for regular meridians by reaching some organs and components where the regular meridians do not reach.

In addition, there are many types of collateral distributing all of the body. Collaterals are the branches of the meridians. They are divided as divergent collaterals, superficial collaterals and minute collaterals. The divergent collaterals are the larger and major collaterals; each of the twelve meridians, Ren and Du meridians has one plus the other large collateral of the spleen meridian, they collectively known as "fifteen divergent collaterals". The major functions of the divergent collaterals are to strengthen the communication in the exterior of the body between the two external-internally related meridians, to serve as the supplement for the regular meridians by reaching some parts where the regular meridians do not reach, and also to command all the yin and yang collaterals of the whole body. The superficial collaterals are those collaterals running superficially and often appear in the surface. They distribute widely and are without fixed region, playing roles of communication among the meridians and transporting qi-blood onto the body surface. The minute collaterals are the tiniest and smallest collaterals, belonging to the sub-branches of the collaterals, distributing the whole body and being numerous.

The meridian musculatures and skin areas are the affiliated portions in tendons-muscles and skin of the twelve meridians. The meridian musculatures of the body are the systems of tendons-muscles and joints where the qi of the twelve meridians "concentrate, accumulate, distribute and connect". They are the affiliated portions of the twelve meridians, with the actions of linking up the four limbs and bones, and dominating the motion of the joints. The skin of the whole body is the superficial regions reflecting the functional activities of the twelve meridians, and also the sites where the meridian qi distributes. Therefore the skin of the whole body is divided into twelve parts respectively belonging to the twelve meridians and being called "twelve skin areas".

The above mentioned twelve meridians, eight extra meridians, twelve meridian divergences, divergent collaterals, minute collaterals and superficial collaterals, as well as the meridian musculatures and skin areas connected and affiliated by the meridian together compose the meridian system (See Fig. 5-1), becoming an inseparable integrity.

5.2 Twelve Meridians

The twelve meridians are the core part of the meridian system. The twelve meridian divergences and collaterals in the meridian system all branch out from the twelve meridians, and they communicate with and coordinate each other to play the roles synergetically.

5.2.1 Nomenclature of the Twelve Meridians

The twelve meridians are the general name for three yin meridians of hand (the lung, pericardium and heart), three yang meridians of hand (the large intestine, tri-Jiao and small intestine), three yang meridians of foot (the stomach, gallbladder and bladder) and three yin meridians of foot (the spleen, liver and kidney). They are the main trunk of the meridian system, so they are also called "regular meridians". The twelve meridians symmetrically distribute on the right and left sides of the body, respectively running along the medial or lateral side of the upper or lower limbs; and each of them respectively belongs to a Zang-viscus or a Fu-viscus. Therefore, the twelve meridians are of different names. Nomenclature of a meridian in the twelve is based on the viscus, hand or foot, yin or yang. They respectively affiliate to the twelve viscera, so each of them is named with its affiliated viscus; combining with its distribution portion of hand or foot, medial or lateral, and anterior or posterior side; they are further divided into three yin or yang according to the theory of yin-yang and the principle of yin-yang evolution. Thus the twelve meridians such as the lung meridian of hand Taiyin and the large intestine meridian of hand Yangming are named.

Concretely speaking, the meridian that starts or terminates at the hand is called hand meridian; and the one that starts or terminates at the foot is called foot meridian. The meridians that run in the medial sides belong to yin and those in the lateral sides belong to yang, yin meridians are affiliated to the Zang-viscera and yang meridians are affiliated to the Fu-viscera. According to the principle of yin-yang evolution, yin is further divided into Taiyin, Jueyin and Shaoyin and yang into Yangming, Shaoyang and Taiyang. Among the three *Zang* viscera in the thorax the lung pertains to Taiyin, the pericardium to Jueyin and the heart to Shaoyin; their meridians run mainly in the upper limbs, thus the lung meridian is called hand Taiyin, the pericardium meridian called hand Jueyuin and the heart meridian called hand Shaoyin; they orderly run along the anterior, middle and posterior lines of the medial side of the upper limb. The large intestine, tri-Jiao and small intestine that are exterior-interiorly related with the three *Zang* viscera respectively belong to Yangming, Shaoyang and Taiyang; their meridians are respectively called hand Yangming, hand Shaoyang and hand Taiyang, which run orderly along the anterior, middle and posterior lines of the lateral side of the upper limbs. Among the three *Zang* viscera in the abdomen, the spleen pertains to Taiyin, the liver to Jueyin and the kidney to Shaoyin; their meridians mainly run in the lower limbs, thus respectively called foot Taiyin meridian, foot Jueyin meridian and foot Shaoyin meridian; they orderly run along the anterior, middle and posterior lines (in the regions below the site 8 *cun* above the medial malleolus Jueyin meridian runs along the anterior line and Taiyin meridian along the middle line) of the medial side of the lower limb. The stomach, gallbladder and bladder that are exterior-interiorly related with these three *Zang* viscera respectively belong to Yangming, Shaoyang and Taiyang; their meridians respectively called foot

Yangming, foot Shaoyang and foot Taiyang, which orderly run along the anterior, middle and posterior lines of the lateral side of the lower limb (see Table 5-1).

Table 5-1 Nomenclature and classification of the twelve meridians

	Yin meridian (affiliates to *Zang*-viscus)	Yang meridian (affiliates to *Fu*-viscus)		Running rout (Yin meridian in the medial side, Yang meridian in the lateral side)
hand	Lung meridian of Taiyin	Large litestine of Yangming	upper limb	Anterior line
	Pericardium meridian of Jueyin	Tri-Jiao meridian of Shaoyang		Middle line
	Heart meridian of Shaoyin	Small intestine meridian of Taiyang		Posterior line
foot	Spleen meridian of Taiyin*	Stamoch meridian of Yangming	lower limb	Anterior line
	Liver meridian of Jueyin*	Gallbladder meridian of Shaoyang		Middle line
	Kidney meridian of Shaoyin	Baldder meridian of Taiyang		Posterior line

*In the lower part of the leg and dorsum of the foot, the liver meridian runs along the anterior-line, while the spleen meridian along the mid-line. At the site 8 cun above the medial malleolus the two meridians cross each other, then the spleen meridian runs in front of the liver meridian.

5.2.2 Running Course, Interconnection, Distribution, Exterior–Interior Relationship and Flow Order

5.2.2.1 Regularity in Course and Connection

The three yin meridians of hand in the twelve meridians run from the internal viscera of the thoracic cavity to the ends of fingers, and connect the three yang meridians of hand there; the three yang meridians of hand run from the ends of fingers to the head and face, and connect the three yang meridians of foot there; the three yang meridians of foot run from the head and face to the ends of toes, and connect three yin meridians of foot there; the three yin meridians of foot run from the ends of toes to the abdomen and thorax, and connect the three yin meridians of hand in the viscera of the thoracic cavity. In this way, the hand meridians connect at the hand and the foot meridians connect at the foot, yang meridians connect at the head, and yin meridians connect at the viscera in the thoracic cavity. Thus the twelve meridians form "a circulatory cycle in which yin meridians and yang meridians communicate with each other" (see Fig. 5-2).

There are three models of connection in the twelve meridians:

Firstly, the exterior-interiorly related yin and yang meridians connect with each other at the ends of limbs. There altogether 6 pairs of exterior-interiorly related yin and yang meridians. Among them, the exterior-interiorly related three yin of hand and three yang of hand meridians connect at the ends of upper limbs (fingers), and the exterior-interiorly related three yin of foot and three yang of foot meridians connect at the ends of lower limbs (toes). Specifically, the lung meridian of hand Taiyin and the large intestine meridian of hand Yangming connect at the end of index finger; the heart meridian of hand Shaoyin and the small intestine meridian of hand Taiyang connect at the end of little finger; the pericardium meridian of hand Jueyin and the tri-Jiao meridian of hand Shaoyang connect at the end of ring finger. The stomach meridian of foot Yangming and the spleen meridian of foot Taiyin connect at the end of big toe; the bladder meridian of foot Taiyang and the kidney meridian of foot Shaoyin connect at the end of little toe; the gallbladder meridian of foot Shaoyang and the liver meridian of foot Jueyin connect at the posterior region of big toe nail.

Secondly, the yang meridian of hand and foot with the same name connect in the head and face. There are 3 pairs of yang meridian of hand and foot with the same name. Specifically, the large intestine meridian of hand Yangming and the stomach meridian of foot Yangming connect at the side of nose wing; the small intestine meridian of hand Taiyang and bladder meridian of foot Yangming connect at the inner canthus; and the tri-Jiao meridian of hand Shaoyang and gallbladder meridian of foot Shaoyang connect at the outer canthus.

Thirdly, yin meridians of foot and hand connect in the thorax. The yin meridians of foot and hand are also called "different named meridians". There are 3 pairs of them. They connect in the viscera of the thoracic cavity. Specifically, the spleen meridian of foot Taiyin and the heart meridian of hand Shaoyin connect in the heart; the kidney meridian of foot Shaoyin and the pericardium meridian of hand Jueyin connect in the chest; and the liver meridian of foot Jueyin and the lung meridian of hand Taiyin connect in the lung.

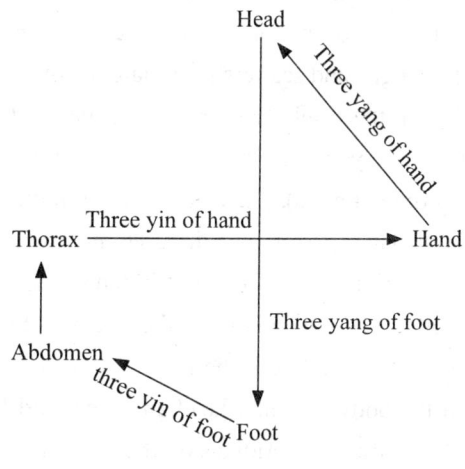

Fig. 5-2 Regularity in Course and Connection of the Twelve Meridians

5.2.2.2 Distribution and Exterior-Interior Relationship

The running courses of the twelve meridians in the body are circuitous and criss-crossing, however they basically run vertically. Yin meridians all run in the medial sides of the limbs and chest-abdominal aspect of the trunk, and yang meridians all run in the lateral sides of the limbs and dorsal aspect of the trunk, with an exception of the stomach meridian. The hand meridians run in the upper limbs, and foot meridians run in the lower limbs. The characteristics of the twelve meridians in distribution of different regions are as follows:

In the four limbs, yin meridians distribute in the medial sides, and yang meridians in the lateral sides. There are three yin meridians in the medial side, so are yang meridians in the lateral side. In the medial side of upper limb, Taiyin meridian runs in the anterior aspect,

Jueyin meridian in the middle, and Shaoyin in the posterior aspect. In the lateral side of upper limb, Yangming runs in the anterior aspect, Shaoyang meridian in the middle, and Taiyang meridian in the posterior aspect. In the medial side of lower limb, at the region 8 *cun* below the medial malleolus, Jueyin meridian runs in the anterior aspect, Taiyin meridian in the middle, and Shaoyin meridian in the posterior aspect; in the region 8 *cun* above the medial malleolus, Taiyin meridian in the anterior aspect, Jueyin meridian in the middle and Shaoyin meridian in the posterior aspect. In the lateral side of lower limb, Yangming meridian run in the anterior aspect, Shaoyang meridian in the middle and Taiyang meridian in the posterior aspect.

In the head and face, hand Yangming meridian runs in the face and foot Yangming meridian in the forehead; Taiyang meridians run in the zygomatic regions, vertex and posterior side of the head; Shaoyang meridians run in the two lateral sides of the head. All yin meridians arrive not at the neck. But some of them run in the deeper parts of the head and face or the vertex. Among them, the heart meridian of hand Shaoyin and the liver meridian of foot Jueyin go up into the eye connector; the liver meridian of foot Jueyin meets the Du meridian at the vertex; the kidney meridian of foot Shaoyin ascends to the root of the tongue, and the spleen meridian of foot Taiyin connects with the root of the tongue and scatters its collaterals over the lower surface of the tongue.

In the trunk, the three yang meridians of hand run in the scapular regions. Among the three yang meridians of foot, Yangming meridian runs in the ventral part (chest and abdominal parts), Taiyang meridian in the dorsal part (back side), and Shaoyang meridian in the lateral sides. The three yin meridians of hand all run out from the axillae. The three yin meridians of foot all run in the ventral part. Thus the order of meridians running in the ventral from the medial to the lateral is Shaoyin, Yangming, Taiyin and Jueyin meridians of foot. In addition, the twelve meridians run symmetrically on the left and right sides of the body in trunk, head and face, and limbs, in each side there are twelve meridians. Generally, the meridians on the left and right sides not go to the opposite side, except for the special case such as the large meridian of hand Yangming running to the opposite side in the face. The yin and yang meridians exterior-interiorly related respectively affiliate and connect the exterior-interiorly related viscera.

The twelve meridians form six pairs of exterior-interior relationships through communication of their meridian divergences and collaterals, namely, the small intestine meridian of hand Taiyang and the heart meridian of hand Shaoyin exterior-interiorly relate with each other, so do the tri-Jiao meridian of hand Shaoyang and the pericardium meridian of hand Jueyin, the large intestine meridian of hand Yangming and the lung meridian of hand Taiyin, the bladder meridian of foot Taiyang and the kidney meridian of foot Shaoyin, the gallbladder meridian of foot Shaoyang and the liver meridian of foot Jueyin, the stomach meridian of foot Yangming and the spleen meridian of foot Taiyin. Each pair of meridians with exterior-interior relationship run respectively in the opposite regions in the two medial and lateral sides of the limb (the liver meridian of foot Jueyin and the spleen meridian of foot

Taiyin, after crossing each other at the site 8 *cun* above the medial malleolus, change their place, or the foot Taiyin runs in the anterior aspect and foot Jueyin in the middle line), and they respectively connect and affiliate the exterior-interiorly related viscera.

The exterior-interior relationships in the twelve meridians not only enhance the communication between the two exterior-interiorly related meridians, but also make the exterior-interiorly related viscera coordinate physiologically, and influence pathologically. For example, invasion of the lung meridian by a pathogen may influence the smooth movement of qi in the large intestine, leading to constipation. If heart fire gets exuberant, it may descend through the meridians to the small intestine, resulting in stranguria and red urine. In treatment, based on the principle that the meridian qi of the exterior-interiorly related meridians communicate with each other, the points of the two exterior-interiorly related meridians may be used crossly. For example, the points of the lung meridian may be taken to treat the diseases of the large intestine or its meridian.

5.2.2.3 Flow Order

The twelve meridians are the main passageways for circulation of qi-blood; they communicate with each other from the head to the tail, orderly connecting. So the flow of qi-blood within them is also in a definite order. Since qi-blood of the whole body are produced from foodstuff essence through transformation and transportation by the spleen and stomach, the flow of qi-blood within the twelve meridians starts from the lung meridian of hand Taiyin that origins from the middle-Jiao, in turn it pours into the liver meridian of foot Jueyin, then it runs back into and starts again from the lung meridian of hand Taiyin. It is thus communicated from the head to the tail, and endless like a cycle. The following table shows its flow order (see Fig. 5-3).

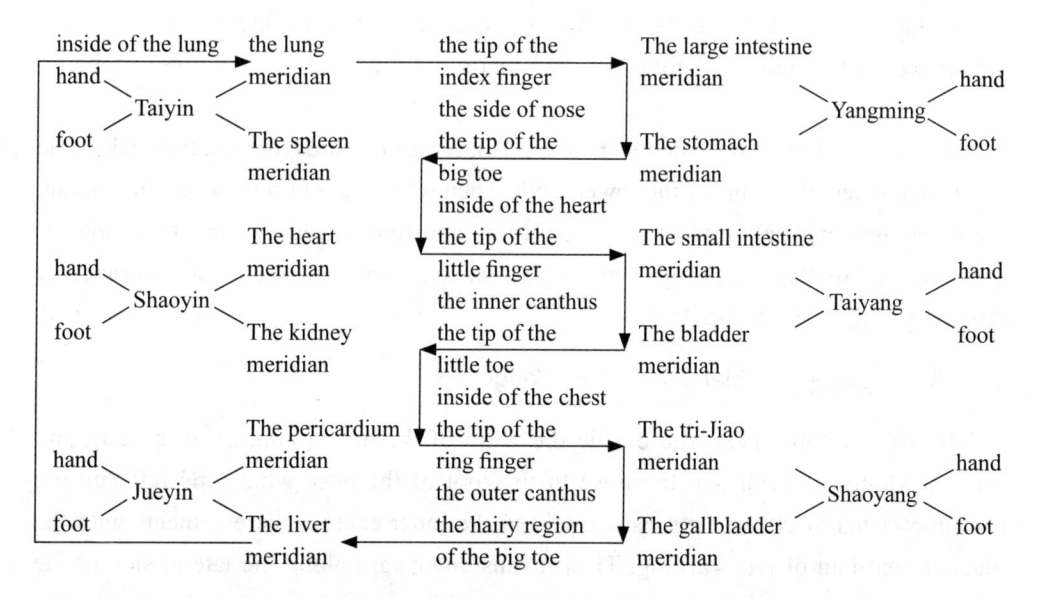

Fig. 5-3 The Order of Flow of Qi and Blood in the Twelve Meridians

5.2.3 Running Routes of the Twelve Meridians

5.2.3.1 The Lung Meridian of Hand Taiyin

It originates from the middle-Jiao, running downward to connect with the large intestine; winding back, it runs along the openings of the stomach (the lower opening is pylorus and the upper one is cardia), passes through the diaphragm, and enters the lung, its belonging viscus. It then ascends to the throat, and transversely runs to the superolateral aspect of the chest (Zhongfu, LU 1), it comes out from the axilla, and descends along the anterior border in the flexor aspect of the upper limb, passing through the cubital fossa, and entering *cunkou* (the radial artery at the wrist for pulse feeling); then it arrives at the thenar eminence and reaches the radial side of the tip of the thumb (Shaoshang, LU 11).

The branch: Emerging from the proximal part of the wrist (Lieque, LU 7), it runs along the dorsal aspect of the palm to the radial side of the tip of the index finger (Shangyang, LI. 1) where it links the large intestine meridian of hand Yangming (See Fig. 5-4 p58).

5.2.3.2 The Large Intestine Meridian of Hand Yangming

It originates from the radial side of the tip of the index finger (Shangyang, LI. 1). Passing through the dorsum of the hand, it runs upward along the anterior border in the extensor aspect of the upper limb and arrives at the anterior aspect of the shoulder joint. Then it runs backward to the site beneath the spinous process of the 7th cervical vertebra (Dazhui, GV 14), and runs forward and downward to the supiaclavicular fossa (Quepen, ST 12), there it enters the thoracic cavity to connect with the lung, and further passes through the diaphragm, terminating at the large intestine, its belonging viscus.

The branch: Emerging from Quepen (ST 12), it runs upwards through the neck to the cheek, and enters the gums of the lower teeth. Then returning and running by the mouth, it crosses the opposite meridian at the philtrum, and runs further to the site beside the opposite wing of the nose (Yingxiang, LI 20), where it connects the stomach meridian of foot Yangming (See Fig. 5-5 p59).

5.2.3.3 The Stomach Meridian of Foot Yangming

It originates from the site beside the wing of the nose (Yingxiang, LI 20), and ascends along the bridge of the nose to the root of the nose where the left and the right meridians meet, then it runs laterally to the inner cantus where it meets with the bladder meridian of foot Taiyang. Then it runs downward along the lateral side of the bridge of the nose, and enters the upper gums of the teeth. Returning, running by the mouth, and curving around the lips, it meets the opposite meridian at the mentolabial groove (Chengjiang, GV 24). Turning back, it runs along the posterior-inferior border of the mandible to the site anterior to the angle of the mandible (Daying, ST 5); then it ascends in front of the ear, passing through Shangguan point (GB 3), it runs along the anterior hairline and reaches the forehead.

Branch 1: Emerging in front of Daying point, it runs downward to Renying point (ST 9). Along the throat it runs backward and downward to Dazhui (GV 14). Turning back it runs forward to Quepen (ST 12); then it runs deep into the cavity of the body, descends through the diaphragm, enters the stomach, its belonging viscus, and connects with the spleen.

The straight portion: Starting from Quepen (ST 12), it runs downward along the midclavicular line and by the umbilicus to Qijie (ST 30) superior to the inguinal groove.

Branch 2: Coming out from the lower opening of the stomach (pylorus) it descends along the inside of the abdomen to Qijie (ST 30), where it joins the straight portion. Then it runs downward along the anterior aspect of the thigh to the knee. Descending along the anterior border of the lateral aspect of the tibia it arrives at the dorsum of the foot, then enters the lateral side of the tip of the 2nd toe (Lidui ST 45).

Branch 3: Emerging from the site 3 *cun* below the knee (Zusanli, ST 36), it descends and enters the lateral side of the tip of the middle toe.

Branch 4: Arising from Chongyang (ST 42) it runs forward to the medial side of the tip of the big toe (Yinbai, SP 1), where it links the spleen meridian of foot Taiyin (See Fig. 5-6 p60).

5.2.3.4 The Spleen Meridian of Foot Taiyin

It originates from the medial side of the tip of the big toe (Yinbai, SP 1). It runs along the junction of the red and the white skin in the medial aspect of the foot, then ascends by the anterior border of the medial malleolus and along the mid-line of the medial aspect of the leg to the site 8 *cun* above the medial malleolus, where it crosses over and further runs in front of the liver meridian of foot Jueyin. It ascends along the anterior border of the medial aspect of the thigh, enters the abdomen, arrives at the spleen, its belonging viscus, and connects with the stomach. Running upward through the diaphragm, it runs alongside the esophagus, reaches the root of the tongue, and scatters its collaterals over the lower surface of the tongue.

The branch: Arising from the stomach, it ascends through the diaphragm and enters the heart, linking the heart meridian of hand Shaoyin (See Fig. 5-7 p61).

5.2.3.5 The Heart Meridian of Hand Shaoyin

It originates from the heart, then enters the heart connector, runs downward through the diaphragm and connects with the small intestine.

The branch: Coming out from the heart connector, it runs upward alongside the esophagus to connect the eye connectors.

The straight portion: Emerging from the heart connector, it runs through the lung. Then it descends and runs superficially from the axilla, (Jiquan, HT 1). Along the posterior border of the medial aspect of the upper limb, it runs and passes through the cubital fossa; by the styloid process of the ulna proximal to the palm, it enters the palm. Then it runs along the radial side of the little finger to its tip (Shaochong, HT 9) and links the small intestine meridian of hand Taiyang (See Fig. 5-8 p62).

5.2.3.6 The Small Intestine Meridian of Hand Taiyang

It originates from the tip of the ulnar side of the little finger (Shaoze, SP 1). Following the posterior border of lateral aspect of the dorsum and upper limbs, it runs and passes the cubital region, reaches the region posterior to the shoulder joint. After twisting in the scapular region it reaches the superior part of the shoulder (Dazhui, GV 14); then it runs forward to Quepen (ST 12) and enters the body cavity to connect with the heart, descends along the esophagus, passes through the diaphragm, reaches the stomach, and finally enters the small intestine, its belonging viscus.

Branch 1: Coming out from Quepen (ST 12), it ascends along the neck to the cheek. Arriving at the outer canthus, it then runs back and enters the ear (Tinggong, SP 19).

Branch 2: Arising from the cheek, it runs up to the infraorbital region, then reaches the inner canthus (Jingming, BL 1) to link with the bladder meridian of food Taiyang (See Fig. 5-9 p62).

5.2.3.7 The Bladder Meridian of Foot Taiyang

It originates from the inner canthus (Jingming, BL 1). Ascending to the forehead, it reaches the vertex (Baihui, GV 20) and meets its opposite meridian there.

Branch 1: Arising from the vertex, it runs to the region above the ear apex.

The straight portion: Starting from the vertex, it runs backward to the occipital region there it enters the cranial cavity to communicate with the brain. Returning, it descends to the nape (Tianzhu, BL 10), and further to Dazhui (GV 14), meeting its opposite meridian there. It then runs down along the medial aspect of the scapula and parallel with and 1.5 *cun* lateral to the vertebral column. Arriving at the lumbar region (Shenshu, BL 23), it enters the body cavity via the paravertebral muscles to connect with the kidney and join its belonging viscus, the bladder.

Branch 2: Branching out from the lumbar region, it descends alongside the vertebral column, and passes through the gluteal region. Then following posterior aspect of the thigh, it ends at the popliteal fossa (Weizhong, BL 40).

Branch 3: Starting from the nape (Tianzhu, BL 10), it descends along the medial aspect of the scapula. From Fufen (BL 41) it descends alongsode the vertebral column (3 *cun*) to the region of the greater trochanter. Then it runs down along the posterior aspect of the lateral side of the thigh to the popliteal fossa, where it meets the preceding branch. It further runs down and passes the musculus gastrocnemius. Passing by the posterior of the external malleolus, it runs along the lateral border of the dorsum of the foot and reaches the lateral side of the tip of the little toe (Zhiyin, BL 67), where it links the kidney meridian of foot Shaoyin (see Fig. 5-10 p63).

5.2.3.8 The Kidney Meridian of Foot Shaoyin

It originates from the inferior aspect of the little toe and runs obliquely through the center of the sole (Yongquan, KL 1). Emerging from the lower aspect of the tuberosity of the navicular bone, it runs behind the medial malleolus, branching out to enter the heel, ascends along the posterior border of the medial aspect of the leg to the medial side of the popliteal fossa, and runs further upwards along the posteromedial border of the thigh, entering the vertebral column (Changqiang, GV 1). Passing through the vertebral column, it enters the kidney, its belonging viscus, and connects with the bladder.

The straight portion: Starting from the kidney, it ascends and passes through the liver and diaphragm; then it enters the lung, and runs along the throat up to the tongue, ending on the two sides of it.

The branch: Arising from the lung, it connects with the heart and enters the chest to link the pericardium meridian of hand Jueyin (See Fig. 5-11 p64).

5.2.3.9 The Pericardium Meridian of Hand Jueyin

It originates from the inside of chest. Emerging, it enters its belonging viscus, the pericardium. Then it descends through the diaphragm to connect successively with the upper-middle-and lower-Jiao.

Branch 1: Arising from the chest, it runs along the inside of the chest and emerges superficially from the costal region at a point 3 *cun* below the anterior axillary fold (Tianchi, PC 1). Then it ascends to the axilla; following the midline of the medial aspect of the upper limb, it enters the cubital fossa, passes through the wrist, and enters the palm (Laogong. PC 8). It further runs along the radial aspect of the middle finger to its tip (Zhongchong, PC 9).

Branch 2: Coming out from the palm at Laogong (PC 8), it runs along the ulnar aspect of the ring finger to its tip (Guanchong, TE 1), and links the tri-Jiao meridian of hand Shaoyang (See Fig. 5-12 p65).

5.2.3.10 The Tri-Jiao Meridian of Hand Shaoyang

It originates from the end of ulnar aspect of the ring finger (Guanchong, TE 1). Ascending along the ulnar aspect of the ring finger to the dorsal aspect of the wrist, it runs upward between the radius and ulna. Passing through the olecranon and along the lateral aspect of the upper arm, it reaches the shoulder region. From there it runs forward and enters Quepen (ST 12) and further scatters over and connects with the pericardium. Passing through the diaphragm, it enters successively the upper-middle-and lower-Jiao, its belonging viscus.

Branch 1: Arising from the pericardium, it ascends and then emerges from Quepen (ST 12), and further runs to the shoulder region. Meeting its opposite meridian at the Dazhui (GV 14), it ascends to the nape, and runs by the posterior border of the ear (Yifeng, TE 7), running up directly to the region superior to the apex of the ear. Then it curves downward to the cheek and arrives at the infraorbital region.

Branch 2: Emerging from the retroauricular region, it enters the ear, comes out in front of the ear and passes by the area anterior to Shangguan point (GB 3), crossing the preceding branch at the cheek. It further runs to the outer canthus (Tongziliao, GB 1) to link the gallbladder meridian of foot Shaoyang (See Fig. 5-13 p66).

5.2.3.11 The Gallbladder Meridian of Foot Shaoyang

It originates from the outer canthus (Tongziliao, GB 1), and ascends to the corner of the forehead (Hanyan, GB 14). Then it turns downward to the retroauricular region (Wangu, GB 12); and turns back to re-ascend through the forehead to the superior region of the eyebrow (Yangbai, GB 14). Hereafter it returns and runs down to Fengchi point (GB 20), along the neck descends to the shoulder, meets its opposite meridian at Dazhui (GV 14), and finally reaches Quepen (ST 12).

Branch 1: Arising from the retroauricular region, it enters the ear, comes out and passes the preauricular region, and runs up to the posterior aspect of the outer canthus.

Branch 2: Emerging from the outer canthus (Tongziliao, GB 1), it descends to the Daying (ST 5) where it meets the branch of the tri-Jiao meridian of hand Shaoyang at the cheek, and arrives at the infraorbital region. Then it returns and runs down through the angle of the mandible (Jiache, ST 6) to the neck, meets the main meridian at Quepen (ST 12). From there it enters the body cavity, passes through the diaphragm to connect with the liver, and enters its belonging viscus, the gallbladder. Then it runs inside the hypochondriac region to the inguinal region. From there it emerges and runs superficially by the margin of the pubic hair and transversely runs into Huantiao point (GB 30) at the hip region.

The straight portion: Starting from the Quepen (ST 12), it runs downward to the axilla, further descends along the lateral aspect of the chest and through the floating ribs to Huantiao point (GB 30) where it meets the preceding branch. Then it again runs downward along the lateral aspect of the thigh and the lateral side of the knee joint. Going down in front of the fibula it directly reaches the lower end of the fibula. Coming out superficially at the anterior aspect of the external malleolus, finally it runs along the dorsum of the foot to the lateral aspect of the tip of the 4th toe (Foot-Qiaoyin, GB 44).

Branch 3: Branching out at the dorsum of the foot (Foot-Linqi, GB 41), it runs forward to the lateral aspect of the tip of the big toe. Returning, it passes through the nail and arrives at the hairy region of the big toe (Dadun, LV 1), where it links the liver meridian of foot Jueyn (See Fig. 5-14 p67).

5.2.3.12 The Liver Meridian of Foot Jueyin

It originates from the dorsal hairy region of the big toe, ascends along the dorsum of the foot to the region 1 *cun* anterior to the medial malleolus (Zhongfeng, LV 4). Then it runs upward along the medial border of the tibia to a site 8 *cun* above the medial malleolus. Where it crosses the spleen meridian of foot Taiyin and then runs by the medial side of the knee, and runs along the midline of the medial aspect of the thigh to the pubic hairy region. Curving round the external genitalia, it runs up to the lower abdomen and enters the abdominal cavity. It runs by the stomach, enters its belonging viscus, the liver, and connects with the gallbladder. After that, it continuously ascends through the diaphragm, branching out to spread over the costal and hypochondriac region. Then it ascends along the posterior aspect of the throat to the nasopharynx, and runs up to link the eye connector. Emerging from the forehead, it runs up to the vertex where it meets Du meridian at the Baihui (GV 20).

Branch 1: Arising from the eye connector, it descends, runs along the inside of the cheek, and curves round the inner surface of the lips.

Branch 2: Coming out from the liver, it ascends through the diaphragm and enters the lung to connect the lung meridian of hand Taiyin (See Fig. 5-15 p68).

5.3 Eight Extra Meridians

The eight extra meridians are the general term for Ren, Du, Dai, Yinwei, Yangwei, Yinqiao and Yangqiao meridians. Their distributions are not regular like the twelve meridians; they have no direct connection with and affiliation to the viscera, and also with no exterior-interior relations among themselves, being unlike the twelve meridians, so they are called extra meridians. Again they are of eight in number, therefore, called "eight extra meridians".

In the eight meridians, Ren meridian runs along the anterior mid-line; Du meridian runs along the posterior mid-line; Chong meridian runs in the abdomen, lower limb and front of the spinal column; Dai meridian runs transversely around the waist; Yinwei meridian runs in the medial aspect of the lower limb, abdomen and neck; Yangwei meridian runs in the lateral aspect of the lower limb, shoulder and nape; Yinqiao meridian runs in the medial aspect of the lower limb, abdomen, chest, head and eye; Yangqiao meridian runs in the lateral aspect of the lower limb, abdomen, posteriorlateral aspect of the chest, shoulder and head. Of which, except for Dai meridian, most of the meridians run from the lower to the upper, and no meridian distributes in the upper limb; the eight meridians not directly connect with or affiliate to the viscera, but they have close relations with the brain and womb. In addition, there is no exterior-interior relationship among the eight meridians; the running routes of every meridian are not like the twelve meridians, with no definite symmetrical relation on both right and left. Among them Ren, Du and Dai meridians are of only one route running singly.

The eight extra meridians run vertically, transversely, and crosswise among the twelve meridians; they have the functions to strengthen the communication among the meridians, and regulate qi-blood in the regular meridians. The functions of the eight extra meridians mainly present with the following aspects.

(1) Strengthening the communication among the twelve meridians: In the running and distributing process, the eight extra meridians not only criss-cross with the twelve meridians so as to strengthen the communication among the twelve meridians and supplement the shortage of them in distribution, but also play a classifying or grouping role. For example, Du meridian meets with the six yang meridians of both hand and foot at Dazhui (GV 14) point, thus is called "the sea of yang meridians"; Ren meridian meets the three yin meridians of foot at Guanyuan (CV 4) point, and the three yin meridians of foot connect with the three yin meridians of hand, so Ren meridian is called "the sea of yin meridans"; Chong meridian runs superiorly, inferiorly, anteriorly and posteriorly, communicating with three yin and three yang meridians, thus it is called "the sea of the twelve meridians"; Dai meridian binds all the meridians vertically run, communicates with the meridians run through the waist and abdomen; Yangwei meridians regulate all the yang meridians to link them with Du meridian; Yinwei meridians regulate all the yin meridians to link them with Ren meridian; and Yinqiao and Yangqiao meridians are in pair on the right and left, dominate yin and yang on both the right and left sides of the body respectively.

(2) Regulating qi-blood of the twelve meridians: The eight extra meridians, except for Ren and Du meridians, do not join the circulation of qi-blood of the fourteen meridians, but they possess the function to store and regulate qi-blood of the twelve meridians. When qi-blood of the twelve meridians gets over abundant, it will flow into the eight extra meridians for storage; as qi-blood of the twelve meridians gets deficient, the qi-blood stored in the extra meridians will flow out for compensation so as to keep a relatively constant state of qi-blood within the twelve meridians, being conducive to the demand for maintaining the physiological function of the body. This is the very meaning that ancient people compared the twelve meridians with "rivers" and extra meridians with "lakes". It can be thus seen that the functions of the extra meridians for the qi-blood of the twelve meridians are dual, or importation and exportation.

(3) Being closely related with some viscera: The eight extra meridians are not like the twelve meridians that have direct connecting and affiliating relationships with the viscera, however, in their running and distributing processes, they are relatively closely communicated with the brain, marrow and womb as well as kidney. For example, Du meridian "enters the cranial cavity to communicate with the brain", "runs along the inside of the spinal column"; and "joins the kidney"; Ren, Du and Chong meridians originate commonly from the womb, and communicate with each other.

5.3.1 Du Meridian

(1) Running route: Du meridian originates from the interior of the lower abdomen (womb). Descending, it emerges at the perineum. Then it ascends along the inside of the spinal column to Fengfu (GV 16) at the nape; there it enters the cranial cavity to communicate with the brain. It further runs following the midsagittal line of the head, via the vertex, forehead, nose and upper lip, and reaches at the frenulum of the upper lip (Yinjiao, GV 28).

Branch 1: Arising from the inside of the spinal column, it joins the kidney.

Branch 2: Starting from the interior of the lower abdomen, it straightly runs up along the inside of the abdomen. Passing through the center of the umbilicus and the heart, it arrives at the throat. It further ascends to the mandibular region, and curves round the lips, finally terminats at the center of the interior regions of the two eyes (See Fig. 5-16 p70).

(2) Function: Du here means governing or commanding. Du meridian, running in the back that belongs to yang, so it has the function to command qi-blood of the yang meridians in the whole body; and there are sayings of "general command of all the yang meridians" and "the sea of yang meridians". Du meridian runs along the midline of back; and its meridian qi several times meets qi of the three yang meridians of both hand and foot, Dazhui (GV 14) as their meeting point. Besides, Dai meridian comes out from the 2nd lumbar vertibra and and Yangwei meridian meets at Fengfu (GV 16) and Yamen (GV 15). Therefore the Du meridian qi communicates with qi of all the yang meridians. In addition, Du meridian runs along the inside of the spinal column, enters the brain, being closely related with the brain and spinal marrow. The life activity of the meridian qi is closely related with the brain. The viscera in the body cavities are controlled by the Du meridian qi through the Back-*Shu* points of the bladder meridian of foot Taiyang. So the functions of the viscera are related with Du meridian. Furthermore, Du meridian branches out to join the kidney. So, it also has a close relationship with the kidney. The kidney is the root of innateness, and governs reproduction. So physicians in ages believe the disorder of genital system like sterility with cold evil in the seminal vesicle is associated with Du meridian, and usually take the therapy to reinforce Du meridian.

5.3.2 Ren Meridian

(1) Running route: Ren meridian originates from the interior of the lower abdomen.

Descending, it emerges at the perineum. Then it ascends via the mons pubis and along the mid-line of the abdomen and chest to the throat. It further runs up to the mandibular region, curves round the lips, and passes through the cheek; it then bifurcates to arrive at the infraorbital regions.

The branch: Starting from the interior of the lower abdomen, it runs up, together with a branch of Chong meridian, in front of the spinal column (See Fig. 5-17 p70).

(2) Function: Ren here means assuming, undertaking. Ren meridian, running along the anterior midline of abdomen that belongs to yin; thus it has the function of controlling qi of all yin meridians in the body. So there are sayings "general control of all the yin meridians" and "the sea of yin meridians". Its meridian qi communicates with all the three yin meridians of both hand and foot. The three yin meridians of foot meet Ren meridian at Zhongji (CV 3) and Guanyuan (CV 4); Yinwei meridian meets Ren meridian at Tiantu (CV 22) and Lianquan (CV 23); and Chong meridian meets Ren meridian at Yinjiao (GV 28). The three yin meridians of foot ascend and meet the three yin meridians of hand. Therefore Ren meridian links with all the yin meridians. Ren meridian originates from the interior of the lower abdomen (or the womb for female), having a bearing with the conception and pregnancy. So, "Ren meridian is responsible for the origination and development of the fetus".

5.3.3 Chong Meridian

(1) Running route: Chong meridian originates from the interior of the lower abdomen (womb). Descending, it emerges at the perineum. Then it superficially bifurcates to reach the inguinal regions (Qijie, ST 30). Then it joins the kidney meridian of foot Shaoyin, ascends by the umbilicus, and spreads in the chest. Then it runs up through the throat and curving round the lips, terminating at the infraorbital region.

Branch 1: Comes out superficially at the inguinal regions, it runs down along the medial aspect of the thigh to the popliteal. Then it further descends along the medial side of the tibia to the sole. The branch of the area posterior to the medial malleolus runs forward and obliquely passes the dorsum of the foot, and enters the big toe.

Branch 2: Starting from the interior of the lower abdomen, it runs backward and connects Du meridian, running up in front of the spinal column.

(2) Function: Chong here means vital. Chong meridian runs upward to the head, and downward to the foot, posteriorly in the back and anteriorly in the abdomen and chest, running throughout the whole body. So, it is the communication hub to the circulation of qi and blood, and can regulate qi and blood of the twelve meridians. Ascending part of it runs up in front of the spinal column, opening into yang meridians; the descending part of it runs in the lower limb, opening into yin meridians. Therefore, it can receive and regulate qi-blood of the twelve meridians and the five *Zang*-viscera and six *Fu*-viscera, enjoying names of "the sea of the twelve meridians" and "the sea of the five *Zang*-viscera

and six *Fu*-viscera". In addition, the women's functions of menstruation and pregnancy all take blood as the basis. Chong meridian originates from the interior of the lower abdomen; its attribution is quite extensive. So it serves as "the sea of blood", and whether it functions powerfully or not is closely associated with the menstruation and pregnancy of women. Only when Chong and Ren meridians keep smooth and qi-blood are abundant, can the blood be poured downward into the womb, further discharged as menstrual flow or to nourish the fetus during the pregnancy. If qi-blood of Chong and Ren meridians get deficient or the meridians get impeded, then there may appear irregular menstruation, menopause or infertility. Therefore in clinical treatment of menstrual disorders and infertility, regulation of Chong and Ren meridians is usually taken as the focus.

5.3.4 Dai Meridian

(1) Running route: Dai meridian originates at the site inferior to the free end of the 12th rib, runs obliquely downward to points Daimai (GB 26), and then runs transversely around the body. Dai meridian in the surface of the abdomen runs down to the lateral aspects of the lower abdomen.

(2) Function: Dai here means belt. Because Dai meridian runs transversely around the waist and the abdomen, binds and controls the meridians, which run vertically, like a belt, hence the name of Dai. The twelve regular and extra meridians mostly run vertically, only Dai meridian runs around the waist so as to have the function of binding the meridians run vertically. It binds and controls the relative meridians to regulate qi of the meridians that so as to keep it free from obstruction. In addition, Dai meridian can control the white in women. So if Dai meridian gets insufficient and fails to control the meridians, there often appear leukorrhagia, soreness and weakness of the waist in women.

5.3.5 Yinqiao and Yangqiao Meridians

(1) Running route: Qiao meridians exist in pair on the left and right sides of the body. Both of Yinqiao and Yangqiao meridians originate from the site inferior to the malleoli.

Yinqiao meridian originates at Zhaohai point (KI 6) inferior to the medial malleolus and runs upward, via the posterior side of the medial malleolus and along the medial aspect of the lower limb, passing the external genitalia, ascending along the abdomen and chest to Quepen (ST 12). Running further upward by the area anterior to Renying (ST 9), it runs by the bridge of the nose to the inner canthu and meets with and Taiyang meridians of both hand and foot, and Yangqiao meridian.

Yangqiao meridian originates from Shenmai point (BL 62) inferior to the external malleolus, and runs upward via the posterior side of the external malleolus and along the posterior border of the fibular aspect of the thigh. Passing through the abdomen and along the posterolateral aspect of the chest, it runs up via the shoulder and lateral side of the neck to the angle of the mouth, reaching the inner canthus where it meets with

Taiyang meridians of both hand and foot, and Yinqiao meridian. Then it further ascends through the anterior hairline, turns down to the retroauricular region, and finally meets the gallbladder meridian of foot Shaoyang at the nape (Fengchi, GB 20)

(2) Function: Qiao here means heel and, forceful and nimble. Qiao meridians originate from the sites inferior to the malleoli, run up along the medial and lateral sides of the limb to the head and face, having the functions to communicate yin and yang qi of the whole body, and regulate the motion of the limbs and muscles; so that it can make lower limbs forceful and nimble in motion. Because Yinqiao and Yangqiao meridians meet at the inner canthus, enter the brain, and Yinqiao meridian and Yangqiao meridian respectively dominate yin and yang on both left and right sides of the body, so they also have the function of moistening the eyes, controlling the closing-opening of the eyelids and the motion of the lower limb.

5.3.6 Yinwei and Yangwei Meridians

(1) Running route: Yinwei meridian originates from the site at the medial side of the leg where the three yin meridians of foot meet, runs up along the medial side of the lower limb to the abdomen, then coinciding with the spleen meridian of foot Taiyin; arriving at the hypochondrium, it meets with the liver meridian of foot Jueyin. Then it ascends to the throat to meet with Ren meridian.

Yangwei meridian originates from the site inferior to the external malleolus. Coinciding with the gallbladder meridian of foot Shaoyang, it runs up along the lateral side of the lower limb, and posterolateral aspect of the trunk, passing through the posterior of the axilla to the shoulder. It further ascends via the neck and retroauricular region, and forward to the forehead, and then turns backward to the lateral side of the head and the back of the nape, where it communicates with Du meridian.

(2) Function: Wei here means regulating and connecting with. The major functions of Wei meridians are to regulate all the meridians of the body. Yinwei meridian in its course meets three yin meridians of foot and finally joins Ren meridian, so it is of the function to regulate and connect with yin meridians of the whole body. While Yangwei meridian in its course meets three yin meridians of foot and finally joins Du meridian, so it is of the function to regulate and connect with yang meridians of the whole body. Under the normal conditions, Yinwei and Yangwei meridians regulate commonly to play the role of importing and exporting qi-blood, but not to participate their circulation.

Appendix: Meridian Divergences, Divergent Collaterals, Meridian Musculatures and Skin Areas

(1) Meridian divergence: It is a regular meridian that runs divergently. The twelve meridian divergences are the important branching meridians arising respectively from the twelve meridians, running in the chest, abdomen and head.

Distribution regularity: The twelve meridian divergences branch out respectively from the regular meridians with the same names (called "leave"), run deep into the thoracic and abdominal cavities (called "enter"), then in the head and nape run out to the body surface (called "exit"), the divergences of the yang meridians join the regular meridians with the same names; the divergences of the yin regular meridians join the regular meridians with the exterior-interior relationships (called "join"). Each pair of divergences with the exterior-interior relationship respectively makes up "one join", altogether becoming "six joins".

Physiological functions: The twelve meridian divergences strengthen the communication in the interior between the two meridians in the twelve with exterior-interior relationship, and the communication among the viscera. It thus makes the communications between the twelve meridians and the all parts of the body more close, enlarges the scope of indications for the points of the twelve meridians.

(2) Divergent collaterals: Divergent collaterals are the larger ones in the collateral. Each of the twelve and, Ren and Du meridians give respectively one branch, plus additional large branch from the spleen meridian, totally they are of fifteen ones, known as "fifteen divergent collaterals" (If the larger collateral of the stomach meridian is counted, they are called "sixteen divergent collaterals"). The divergent collaterals control and dominate the "superficial collaterals" that run superficially and "minute collaterals" that are the tiniest and smallest ones.

Distribution regularity: The divergent collaterals of the twelve, after branching out respectively from the proper meridians at the sites below the elbow or knee join, all run onto the corresponding regular meridians with exterior-interior relationships to communicate with them. The divergence of Ren meridian branches out at Jiuwei (CV 15) point, hereafter it spreads over the abdomen. The divergence of Du meridian branches out at Changqiang (GV 1) point, hereafter it spreads over the head. The large collateral of spleen meridian branches out at Dabao (SP 21) point, hereafter it spreads over the chest and hypochondrium.

Physiological functions: The divergent collaterals of the twelve regular meridians strengthen the communication in the exterior between the two meridians in the twelve with exterior-interior relationship; with participation of all the divergent collaterals, they enhance the communication among the front, back and the lateral parts of the body, making the body a closely related whole; they command all the collaterals to form a close distributing network, so that they ooze qi-blood to nourish the tissues of the whole body.

(3) Meridian musculatures: They are tendon (muscle tendon and ligament), muscle and join systems that affiliated to the twelve meridians, being the parts for the twelve meridians to communicate with peripheral tissues. The functions of them depend upon the nourishment and regulation of meridian qi-blood.

Distribution regularity: The distributions of the twelve meridian musculatures are basically consistent with running routes of the twelve meridians in the body surface. The running routes are generally in the superficial parts, running from the ends of the limbs to the head or the trunk, in the body surface, converging and gathering in the join and skeleton. They generally do not enter the internal organs.

Physiological functions: The meridian musculatures can restrict and control the skeleton, being conducive to flexion and extension.

(4) Skin Areas: They are the regions in the body surface where the functions of the twelve meridians reflect, and also the regions where the qi of the regular meridians and their affiliated collaterals spread.

Distribution regularity: The twelve skin areas are the corresponding areas where the running routes in the body surface of the twelve meridians.

Physiological functions: The function of the skin areas is the same as the skin. They are of the action to protect the body and resist against exogenous pathogens. They can be used in diagnosis, and serve as the sites for practicing treatment.

5.4 Physiological Functions of the Meridian System

The functional activity is called "meridian qi". Its physiological functions play the very important role in maintenance of human body's normal life activity. Here the details are given as the following.

5.4.1 Communicating Superiorly, Inferiorly, Exteriorly and Interiorly, and Connecting All the Parts of the Body

The human body is made up of the five *Zang*-viscera, six *Fu*-viscera, four limbs, five sense organs, nine orifices, skin, muscles, tendons and bones. They have their own physiological function respectively; however, they again perform a common organic activity of the whole. In this way they keep coordination and unity of the body interiorly, exteriorly, superiorly and inferiorly to form an organic whole. This kind of organic coordination and mutual relationship is accomplished through communication and connection by the meridian system. The twelve meridians and their branches run criss-crossly, coming in and going out, ascending and descending, mutual affiliation to and connection with a pair of viscera; the eight extra meridians connect and communicate with the twelve regular meridians; the twelve meridian musculatures and the twelve skin areas connect and communicate with the skin, muscles, thus they commonly make every viscus and tissue of the body communicate organically, forming a unity in which all the parts exteriorly, interiorly, superiorly and inferiorly of the body relate to, coordinate and help one another. The communicating and connecting role of the meridian system are of multi-originations and multi-levels. The main ones are the following respects.

Connection between the viscera and the limbs and joins is accomplished mainly through the communication of the twelve meridians. The twelve meridians specially affiliate to and connect with the viscera interiorly, communicate with the tendons, muscles, joins and skin exteriorly. Thus the twelve meridians link the peripheral tissues of tendons, muscles, skin, limbs and joins with the internal organs.

Connection between the viscera and sense organs and orifices is also accomplished through the communication of the twelve meridians. The twelve meridians internally belong to the viscera; in the course of running and distribution, they also communicate with the sense organs and orifices such as mouth, eyes, nose, tongue, and two yin organs, closely related with them. For example, the hand Yangming meridians "runs by the mouth", the foot Yangming meridians "runs by the mouth, and curves around the lips", the hand Yangming meridian "crosses the philtrum to the site beside the opposite wing of the nose". In this way it makes the interior viscera communicate with the sense organs and orifices so as to form a whole.

Connection among the viscera is also closely related with the communication of the meridian system. Each of the twelve meridians affiliates to and connects with a *Zang*-viscus and a *Fu*-viscus, which is the major structural basis for the theory of pair-up of the viscera. For example, the lung meridian of hand Taiyin affiliates to the lung nad connects with the large intestine; and the large intestine meridian of hand Yangming affiliates to the large intestine and connects with the lung, etc.. Some of the meridians, besides affiliate to and connect with special viscera, again communicate with several other viscera. For example, the kidney meridian of foot Shaoyin not only affiliates to the kidney and connects with the bladder, but also passes through the liver, enters the lung, connects with the heart, and runs into the chest to join the pericardium. In addition, there are also the meridian divergences that supplement the shortcomings of the regular meridians. For example, the divergences of the foot Yangming, foot Shaoyang and foot Taiyang all pass by the heart. Thus it forms multiple communications among the viscera.

There is also close relation among the every part of the meridian system. The twelve meridians have certain regularity in connection and flow order of qi-blood. Besides communication from the head to the tail just like a cycle, there are also many crosses and meets. For example, the hand and foot yang meridians meet Du meridian at Dazhui (GV 14); the hand Shaoyin and the foot Jueyin meridians both connect with the eye connector. Amomg the twelve meridians, between the exterior-interior meridians, between the meridians with the same name, and between the meridians with different names there are all a relation in which the meridians communicate with each other, and qi-blood flows into each other, especially between the exterior-interior meridians. The twelve meridian divergences and the twelve collaterals strengthen the communication between the exterior-interior meridians respectively internally and externally. The twelve meridians and the eight extra meridians communicate with each other criss-crossly. The eight extra meridians, besides crossly communicate with the twelve meridians, communicate with each other among themselves too. For example, Yinwei meridian and Chong meridian meet in Ren meridian; Chong meridian joins Ren meridian in the chest and communicates with Du meridian in the back, all these presenting the relations among the extra meridians.

5.4.2 Conveying Qi-Blood to Nourish the Whole Body

Every viscus and tissue of the human body needs warming, nourishing and moistening by qi-blood so as to play their normal function. Qi-blood are the material basis for life activity of the body; however, they must depend upon the transportation and importation by the meridian so as to distribute over the whole body for warming, nourishing and moistening all the viscera and tissues, maintaining the normal function of the body. For example, nutritive qi harmoniously spreads into the five *Zang*-viscera and six *Fu*-viscera to provide the material conditions for their functional activities. Therefore, it is said the meridian system possesses the role to circulate qi-blood, regulate yin-yang and nourish the whole body.

5.4.3 Reaction and Conduction

The human's life activity is a very complex process. In the body, there are at all time exportation, exchange and transmission of life information. This must depends upon the reaction and to conduction of the meridian system to perform transmission of life information and communicate among every part. When a part of the human body is stimulated, through the meridian system this stimulation will import into the relative viscera within the body so as to make them produce the relative changes physiologically or pathologically. And all these changes again through the meridian are expressed in the body surface. The "arrival of qi" and "induction of qi" in acupuncture therapy are the complete embodiment of reaction and conduction of the meridian system. The functional activities of the internal organs and the information of the pathological changes may also be transmitted to the body surface via the meridian system, manifesting as different symptoms and signs.

5.4.4 Regulating Functional Balance for the Body

Under normal conditions, the meridian system can circulate qi-blood and coordinate yin-yang; on the condition of disease with disharmony of qi-blood and superiority or inferiority of yin or yang, the acupuncture and moxibustion therapies can be used to trigger the regulatory action of the meridian, by reducing what is excessive, or reinforcing what is deficient to regulate the body and maintain the equilibrium. Some experiences have proved acupuncture at the relative points of the meridian may produce the regulating role to visceral functions, and this is especially evident under the pathological conditions. For example, puncturing Zusanli (ST 36) point of the stomach meridian of foot Yangming can regulate the peristaltic and secreting functions of the stomach. When the stomach is in hypofunction, a mild stimulation given may strengthen the gastric contraction and increase the concentration of the gastric juice. As the stomach is in a hyperactive state, a strong stimulation given will cause inhibitory effect. Another example, puncturing Neiguan (PC 6) point of the pericardium meridian of hand Jueyin may both make the heart beat fast and, in some conditions, inhibit the heart throbbing. Therefore this point can clinically treat both bradycardia and tachycardia. It is thus can be seen that the regulatory action of the meridian may present with "adaptagen-like effect", or through its regulation there may occur inhibition for what is originally hyperactive, and excitement for what is originally inhibitory. This is the beneficial dual regulation, being of important significance in acupuncture, moxibustion and *Tuina* therapies.

5.5 Application of the Meridian Theory in Chinese Medicine

5.5.1 Expounding Pathological Changes

Under the normal conditions the meridian system possesses the functions to circulate qi-blood, reaction and conduction. As a disease occurs, it will become the passageway for transmit the pathogens and reflect pathological changes.

The meridians affiliate internally to the viscera, distribute externally in the body surface. So when the body surface is invaded by the pathogens, the pathogens may via the meridian system go from the exterior into the interior, from the shallow to the deep, gradually transmit inward even involve the viscera. The meridian system is the route for transmission of the exogenous pathogens from the skin and striea into the viscera. For example, as an exogenous pathogen invades the body surface, there at the beginning fever and aversion to cold, pain of the head and body, etc.; because the lung is associated with the skin and fine hair, if the pathogen in the exterior cannot be expelled, it will transmits inward into the lung after long, manifesting as symptoms of cough, chest distress, chest pain, etc.. The lung meridian and the large intestine meridian connect with each other, so there may appear accompanying disorder of the large intestine such as abdominal pain, diarrhea or constipation.

There is a close connection between the internal viscera and external constituents, sense organs and orifices, so the disorders of the viscera may be transmitted and reflected externally through the meridian. Clinically, the meridian theory may be used to expound the symptoms and signs of the special sites or the corresponding sense organs and orifices in the body surface that the disorders of the five *Zang*-viscera and six *Fu*-viscera show; and the thinking method of "understanding the internal condition by examining the internal" may be taken to examine the diseases. For example, the liver meridian of foot Jueyin curves round the external genitalia, descends to the lower abdomen, spreads its branches over the costal and hypochondriac region, and runs up to connect the eye connector; so stagnation of liver qi may show pains in the hypochondria and lower abdomen; up-flaming of liver fire may show redness of the eyes; dampness-heat in the liver meridian may show scrotal wetness and prurigo.

Mutual transmission of the visceral disorders may also be explained by the meridian theory. Since there are meridians among the viscera to connect, the disorder of a viscus may affect the other viscus through the meridians. For example, the liver meridian of foot Jueyin affiliates to the liver, runs by the stomach and enters the lung. So the disorder of the liver may affect the stomach, and the fire of liver may involve the lung. The kidney meridian of foot Shaoyin enters the lung and connects with the heart; so edema due to kidney insufficiency may "invade the heart" and "affect the lung". The spleen meridian of foot Taiyin enters the heart; so failure of the spleen in transformation and transportation may cause deficiency of heart blood.

5.5.2 Guiding Diagnosis and Treatment of Disease

5.5.2.1 Guiding Meridian Syndrome Differentiation

A meridian has certain running route and affiliation-connection of the viscera, and it may reflect the disorders of its related viscera; therefore clinically one can analyze the symptoms of a disease combining with the running route and the connected viscera of a meridian so as to diagnose what meridian the syndrome belongs to. For example, a pain in the hypochondria often indicates disease of the liver and gallbladder; a pain in the Quepen (the supiaclavicular fossa) usually means disorder of the lung. Another example, for headache, front headache relates generally to Yangming meridian; lateral headache to Jueyin meridian; occipital headache and nape pain to Taiyin meridian; and vertical headache to Jueyin meridian. In addition, during the process of disease in some meridian running routes or some points where the meridian qi gathers there often appear obvious tenderness, nodule or streak reaction; or morphologic or temperature or electric resistant changes, which are all conductive to diagnosis of disease. For example, for patients with abdominal carbuncle (suppurative appendicitis) there appears sometime tenderness in Shangjuxu (ST 37) point of the stomach meridian of foot Yangming; in real heart pain there is often pain at the left inframammary area in anterior pectoral region, even radiating to the left arm and little finger; in disorders of the spleen and stomach there usually abnormal changes at Pishu (BL 20) point; in irregular menstruation or nocturnal spermarrhea there is often tenderness at Henggu (KI 11) point; for patients with a prolonged indigestion there appear sometimes abnormal changes at Pishu (BL 20) point. Clinically some methods for detecting the changes on the meridian and point, such as examination along the meridian, examination at the point, meridian currency determination, etc. may be taken for reference to diagnosis.

There are also many applications of the meridian theory in diagnostics. For example, examination of the collateral, inspection of index finger veins in children, inspection of auricle, etc. all take the meridian theory as their theoretical basis. Examination of the meridian is also helpful to judge the cold, heat, deficiency and excess nature of disease.

5.5.2.2 Guiding Clinical Treatment

The meridian theory is widely used to guide the clinical treatment of diseases in various departments, being the theoretical basis for acumoxibustion, *Tuina*, pharmacotherapy, acupuncture anesthesia and ear acupuncture. We can use all the specialities of the meridian, through stimulating points by several ways like acumoxibustion, medicine, laser, ultrasonic wave to gain the therapeutic purpose of regulate the meridian system, qi-blood and yin-yang of the viscera so as to eliminating the pathogens and supplementing the vital. Points are the sites where qi-blood in circulation of the body gathers, and also the sites from where pathogens invade the body. So stimulating the points may treat the diseases of the viscera and the meridians. Thus it may be considered that the meridian system is the passageway for medicine to play its property, and for the body to sense the stimulations from mechanical, acoustic, optic, electric and magnetic agents. The actions of acumoxibustion mostly not directly aim at the pathogenic agents or pathological tissue; they are mainly through regulating the imbalanced yin-yang within the body to function. Acumoxibustion are a therapeutic means which can rectify the abnormal functional state, but do not disturb the normal physiological function.

Treatment of disease by acupuncture and moxibustion is through puncturing the point or applying burning moxa over the point to smooth meridian qi so as to restore the function of the meridian in regulating visceral qi-blood of the body, and thus to get the purpose of curing disease. Based on the network structure of the meridian system in distribution of the body, acumoxibustion in therapeutics are also of holistic feature. That is to say, acumoxibustion at the point may at the same time and at deferent levels act on normal or abnormal functions of several organs and systems. For example, during the process of a operation under the acupuncture anesthesia, acupuncture produces analgesic effect, at the same time it can regulate the functions of the relative systems in multiple aspects, so that during the operation the blood pressure and pulsation are kept stable, and the degree of post-operative pain in the incision becomes mild, complications like infection are reduced, and the post-operative recovery gets rapid. The regulation of acumoxibustion is of dual phases, or a treatment of acumoxibustion at the same point under the same condition, a regulatory function just opposite to the deviated function can be expected to get. For instance, in urinary retention and stress urinary incontinence resulting from diabetic cystipathy may both cause disorder of coordinative function between the detrusor urinae of bladder and sphincter urethrae. The former is because hyperglycemia results in injury of parasympathetic nerve dominating the detrusor urinae of bladder, leading to weak contractility of the detrusor urinae of bladder, with relative hyperactive function of sphincter urethrae; while the latter is just opposite, it is due to laxation of pelvic floor muscles and decrease of contraction of sphincter urithrae caused by various factors, thus the function of the detrusor urinae of bladder becomes relatively hyperactive. Acumoxibustion therapy can generally effectively rectify the disorder of coordinative function between the detrusor urinae of bladder and sphincter urethrae, making what hypo-contracts enhanced and what hyper-contracts inhibited. These all are the embodiment of the meridian theory in acumoxibustion therapy.

Pharmacotherapy is also taking the meridian as the way. Only it is through the conduction and transportation by the meridian system, can the medicine get to the focus to cure disease, playing its therapeutic effect. Through long and repeated practice, medical scholars found the medicinal theories on four natures, five flavors, as well as ascending, descending, floating and sinking actions. This is closely related to the meridian theory. A Chinese medicinal has a selective therapeutic effect to the illness of a certain meridian and its affiliated viscus, accordingly they founded the theory of "meridian-tropism of medicinal". The syndromes of cold, heat, deficiency and excess in diseases and syndromes of the twelve meridians are briefly summarized according to the meridians and their affiliated viscera, so that the four natures can be applied accordingly. The theory of five flavors is also under the guidance of meridian theory and visceral theory; it is a summarization of the law of medicinal treatment based on the clinical practice. In addition, the meridian theory is also the major basis for establishment of theory of ascending, descending, floating and sinking actions.

Clinically, single application of medicinal theories of four natures, five flavors, and ascending, descending, floating and sinking actions cannot fully guide medication. The diseases of every viscus and meridian are of special demand and selection to medication. For example, for the same cold syndrome there are difference between lung cold and stomach cold; for the same heat syndrome there are also difference between lung heat and stomach heat. The medicinals that can expel lung cold cannot definitely expel stomach cold, and vice versa. Application of meridian-tropism theory can more subtly distinguish the special effect of medicinal, thus it can more correctly guide clinical treatment of the complicated and changeable diseases. For example, Huanglian (*Rhizoma Coptidis*) reduces heart fire, Huangqin (*Radix Scutellariae*) reduces lung and large intestine fire, Chaihu (*Radix Bupleuri*) reduces liver, gallbladder and tri-Jiao fire, Baishao (*Radix Paeoniae Alba*) reduces spleen fire, Zhimu (*Rhizoma Anemarrhenae*) reduces kidney fire, Mutong (*Caulis Akebiae*) reduces heart and small intestine fire, Shigao (*Gypsum Fibrosum*) reduces stomach fire. Establishment of the meridian-tropism theory promoted the concrete application of the medicinals of meridian guider and herald. Meridian guider means some medicinals can direct the other medicinals selectively to treat the diseases of a certain viscera and meridians. Herald is drug guider, and different formulae need different drug guiders. Commonly used drug guiders are: medicated wine with action of activating blood, fresh ginger with action of relieving the exterior by means of diaphoresis, Dazao (*Fructus Jujubae*) with action of nourishing blood and strengthening the spleen, Longyanrou (*Arillus Longan*) with action of calming the heart, Dengxincao (*Medulla Junci*) with action of tranquilizing the mind, Congbai (*Bulbus Allii Fistulosi*) with action of expelling pathogens, Lianzi (*Semen Nelumbinis*) with action of clearing the heart, nourishing the stomach and harmonizing the spleen. The meridian tropism theory makes the application of medicinals more flexible and changeable, and some special laws in clinical usage of medicinals summarized.

The meridian theory is one of the main theories to guide the composition of formula. For example, Jiaotai Pill is composed of Huanglian (*Rhizoma Coptidis*) and Rougui (*Cortex Cinnamomi*). Viewing from analysis of the property only, Huanglian is bitter and cold, belonging to the medicine clearing heat and reducing fire; its major functions are to reduce fire and detoxify, clear heat and dry dampness. Rougui is acrid and sweat in flavor, great hot in nature, belonging to the medicine expelling cold; its major functions are to warm the kidney and invigorate yang, warm the meddle and expel cold. However because Huanglian is of tropism to the heart, spleen and stomach meridians, it can clear the heart to reduce the hyperactive fire, and because Rougui is of tropism to the kidney, liver and spleen meridians, combining with Huanglian it can guide the fire onto its root. Therefore combination of Huanglian and Rougui can communicate the heart with the kidney so as to treat insomnia resulting from disharmony between heart and kidney. Another example, in treatment of edema, because the disorders of the lung, spleen and kidney can all lead to edema, according to the etiology and pathomechanism, we can respectively select Baizhu (*Rhizoma Atractylodis*) that is of tropism to the spleen meridian, Zhuling (*Polyporus Agaric*) that is of tropism to the kidney meridian and Tongcao (*Medulla Tetrapanacis*) that is of tropism to the lung meridian. This shows that for the same disorder different medications can be given because of different etiologies and pathomechanisms. Taking sinking of spleen (qi) deficiency as another example, it may present with different diseases of proctoptosis, hysteroptosis and gastroptosis, for all of these diseases the medicinals that are of tropism to the spleen meridian such as Renshen (*Radix Ginseng*), Baizhu (*Rhizoma Atractylodis*), Huangqi (*Radix Astragali*), and Shengma (*Rhizoma Cimicifugae*) may be taken to compose the formula according to the principle for making up a formula. In clinical modification of a formula the meridian theory also plays a guiding role. For example, in a formula for treatment of headache, it may be modified according to the meridian distribution regions. Qianghuo (*Rhizoma Notopterygii*) is used for headache in Taiyang meridian region; Xixin (*Herba Asari*) for headache in Shaoyin meridian region; Baizhi (*Radix Angelicae*) for headache in Yangming meridian region; Chuanxiong (*Rhizoma Chuanxiong*) and Wuzhuyu (*Fructus Evodiae*) for headache in

Jueyin meridian region; Chaihu (*Radix Bupleuri*) for headache in Shaoyang meridian region. Briefly, both the changes in medicinal composition, and the modification of medicinals and their dosages need taking the condition of disease as the basis, and taking the meridian theory as the guide too; only then can we treat a complicated disorder by a properly changeable way and holding simple to drive in great number.

Review Questions

- What parts the meridian system is composed of?
- What are the regularities of the twelve meridians in running course and interconnection?
- What is the flow order of the twelve meridians?
- How many aspects do the physiological functions of the meridian system present?
- What are the eight extra meridians? And what are the physiological functions of them?

6 CONSTITUTIONAL THEORY

Constitution means the relatively constantly comprehensive characteristic in morphological structure, physiological function and mental activities, which is determined by hereditary and acquired factors in the life process of human individual. The constitutional theory, taking basic theories of Chinese medicine as guidance, is a doctrine which researches the concept, formation, feature, pattern, differential regulation of human constitution and its influence on the occurrence, development and evolution of disease, as well as guides the clinical diagnosis, prevention and treatment of disease. The constitutional theory thinks that the constitution is not only the differences in reaction and adaptation to stimuli from the outside under the physiological conditions, but also the internal important factor causing disease. It determines both the susceptibility to some pathogenic factors and the syndrome patterns of some disease. Therefore, emphasis of the research on the constitution can help not only to grasp the life characteristics of an individual from the whole, but also to analyze the law of occurrence, development and transmission of disease. It has an important guiding significance for the diagnosis, treatment, health maintenance, prevention and rehabilitation.

6.1 Formation of Constitution

6.1.1 Physiological Basis of Constitution

The human body is composed of tissue organs such as the viscera, meridians, body and orifices, and the basic substances such as essence, qi, blood, body fluid, which maintain the normal life activities. The difference in constitution expressed through tissue organs of human body is the actual reflection of deviant conditions of qi, blood, yin, and yang of the viscera and the difference of functional activity. In other words, the viscera, meridians, essence, qi, blood and body fluid are the physiological foundations for development of constitution. Research on constitution is actually the research from the difference in the viscera, meridians, essence, qi, blood and body fluid. The viscera are the center in constituting and maintaining the life activities of the human body. The physiological activities all depend upon the viscera. So the difference on constitution reflects partial or all characteristics of various essentials composing human body by taking the viscera as its center.

(1) Relation of constitution to the viscera and meridians: The morphological and functional characteristics of the viscera are the most basic factor composing and determining the difference on constitution. Under the interaction between the hereditary factor of the individual and the environmental factor, the different individual often shows the comparatively advantageous or disadvantageous tendency of a certain visceral manifestation system.

Among the five *Zang*-viscera, the kidney and spleen have more obvious effects on determining the constitution of the human body. On the basis of the innate endowments, the strong or weak constitution is determined by the waxing and waning of the kidney. Ample innate essence is the prerequisite for growing up healthily after birth and having powerful vitality. If the innate essence gets deficient, it will result in not only growth retardation, but also easy contraction of disease. Actually, the process of a person's growth, development and senility is the evolutionary process in which taking the essence-qi of the kidney as the basic material to trigger and propel the functions of viscera. The performance in each stage of the life process fully embodies the difference on constitution shaped in different stages of age, which is actually the result of waxing and waning changes of essence-qi in the kidney. The strength of the kidney will also cause the accompanying changes of the other viscera, thus showing the corresponding changes in physique, function and mental state.

The spleen and stomach are the key acquired factor in the formation of the constitution. Whether or not the diet is appropriate directly influences the functions of the spleen and stomach. As the same, whether or not their functions coordinate is closely related to the nutritive condition of human body, thus greatly influencing the constitution. So the strong or weak constitution is usually consistent with the strength of the function of the spleen and stomach. A person with a shortage of the innate endowment can improve his constitution with the aid of replenishment from foodstuffs. On the contrary, although with a good innate foundation, if a person is in lack of replenishment after birth, he can hardly maintain his health.

The meridians are affiliated to the viscera internally and connect the four limbs externally. They are the passages in which qi-blood circulate. The constitution is not only determined by the strong or weak functional activities of the viscera, but also dependent on their coordination. The meridians are exactly the structural foundation that communicate and coordinate the functions of the viscera. The viscera reside inside and their functions manifest outside. The constitution mainly shows through the exterior morphological characteristic. Because different individuals are of the differences in the waxing and waning of yin-yang in the viscera and in the condition of qi-blood in the meridians, their external manifestations are also different.

(2) Relation of constitution to essence, qi, blood and body fluid: The essence, qi, blood and body fluid are the important material foundation which determines the characteristic of constitution. They are the products of physiological activities of the viscera; they spread all over the body through the meridians as the material foundation of functional activities of the viscera, sensory organs and orifices so as to maintain the normal life activities. The waxing of essence-qi, amount of qi and blood, and abundance of body fluid and the conditions of their distribution and circulation all determine the strength of constitution and influence its type. The person with the deficiency of body fluid is predisposed to "the emaciated and dry-red constitution". The person with metabolic disorder of body fluid mostly presents with "the fat and damp-greasy constitution". The abundance or deficiency of essence also has something to do with the age. The constitution of the old is generally characterized by essence deficiency.

As a whole, structural and functional varieties of the viscera and meridians, the abundance and distribution of essence, qi, blood and body fluid are all the important factors to determine the constitution. The constitution reflects the deviant condition of the essence, qi, yin and yang of viscera through the differences in morphology, function, and mental state. Actually it is the comprehensive embodiment of intrinsic characters of the viscera, meridians, sensory organs and orifices.

6.1.2 Essential Component of Constitution

The essential component of constitution mainly includes three aspects of morphological structure, physiological function and psychological characteristic; among them, morphological structure and physiological function are the outstanding.

6.1.2.1 Morphological Structure

The difference in morphological structure is the important component of the characteristic of individual constitution, including the external and internal morphological structure. According to the cognitive method of "operating the exterior to surmise the interior", the internal morphological structure and external appearance are an organic whole. The external morphological structure is the external expression of constitution; the internal morphological structure is the internal foundation of constitution. Under the intact and harmonious foundation of internal structure, morphological structure mainly show through the external appearance, taking the physique as its foundation and having close relation with the visceral structure, so the constitutional characteristics present with the difference in external appearance first.

External appearance or appearance of the body surface, is the individual characteristic of the appearance in morphology, including the physique, somatotype, weight, sexual signs, posture, complexion, hair, tongue condition, pulse condition, etc.. The physique means the state which reflects the level of growth and development, the condition of nourishment and the degree of exercise. Generally it can be judged through observation and measurement of the size, shape and well-proportioned degree of every part of the body, as well as the weight, breadth of shoulders, chest circumference, pelvis width, skin and subcutaneous soft tissue, being the basic symbol reflecting the constitution. The somatotype means the morphological characteristic in proportion with each part of the body, also called the body type, it is the important index of measuring the constitution. Observation of the somatotype includes the difference of the obesity or emaciation and height of the shape, thickness and compact or flabby degree of the skin and flesh, and the color and elasticity of the skin. Among them, the obesity or emaciation is the most representative. Generally speaking, the relationship between the obesity or emaciation and the morbid constitution is that "the constitution of the fat person mostly consists with dampness and that of the thin person mostly with fire".

The morphological structure is the foundation of the physiological function. The different morphological characteristics of an individual determine the difference of physiological function and response to stimuli, but the individual characteristic of physiological function will influence its morphological structure, causing a series of corresponding changes. Therefore, the difference of physiological function is also the component of the individual constitutional characteristic.

6.1.2.2 Physiological Function

The physiological function is the reflection of integrity and harmony of its internal morphological structure, as well as the embodiment of normal functions of the viscera, meridians, essence, qi, blood and body fluid. Therefore, the difference in physiological function reflects the superiority or inferiority of visceral function, involving the functional difference of every aspect, i.e. digestion, respiration, blood circulation, metabolism, growth and development, reproduction, sensation and motion, consciousness and thought. The anti-disease ability, metabolic condition, self-regulating ability, and the basic state of being biased to excitation or inhibition, such as heart rate, rhythm, complexion, color of the lips, respiration, voice, appetite, taste, body temperature, pulse condition, tongue condition, preference for cold or heat, conditions of urine and feces, reproductive function, menstruation in women, moving condition of the body and its ability, condition of sleep, optesthesia, auditognosis, tactility, olfaction, threshold of pain, elasticity of skin and muscle, quantity and luster of hair, etc., all are the reflection of the physiological function of the viscera, meridians, essence, qi, blood, body fluid; and they are the important channel to understand the condition of constitution.

6.1.2.3 Psychological Character

The psychological state is the reflection of the objective thing in the brain, including sensation, consciousness, emotion, memory, thought, and character. It belongs to the category of "mind" in Chinese medicine. The Chinese medicine thinks that production of mind is closely related to the body and its existence depends upon the body, which is the material basis and residence of the mind; at the same time, it also believes that the mind dominates the body. Therefore, the views of human body, life and medicine based on unity of the body and mind determines that the physique of constitution includes the contents of both body and mind. The constitution is a comprehensive body of specific morphological structure, physiological function and the corresponding psychological condition. There is an intrinsic relationship among morphological structure, functional activity and psychological state. A certain particular morphological structure often manifests as a certain specific tendency in psychology. A different functional activity always shows a certain specific response of emotion and mood, as well as a cognitive activity. Because essence-qi of the viscera and their functions are different, the emotional activities expressed by each individual also have difference. For example, someone is easy to get angry, otherone is easy to get sorrowful, and still otherone is easy to get timid, But what should be pointed out is that the human psychological character not only has something to do with morphological structure, function, but also has an important relation with both the life experience and the social and cultural environment of individual. Even the people with the same morphological structure and physiological function can also present with the totally different psychological character. Certain morphological structure and physiological function are the foundations to produce psychological character, making the individual easily show a certain psychological characteristic, and the latter can reversely act on the morphological structure and physiological function, and shows the corresponding behavior characteristic. It is clear that, the structure, function and psychological state have close relationship in the component factor of constitution.

The difference of psychological characteristic mainly shows the difference of personality, temperament, and character. The personality means a synthesis of special and persistent psychological or behavioral characteristic of individual. It often determines the whole psychological feature, and is the core factor and symbol of the individual psychological and behavioral difference, and individulization. The temperament has difference in the modern psychology and the Chinese medicine. The temperament in modern psychology means the dynamic psychological characteristic of personality, that a person shows in mental activity or behavior pattern, i.e. the intensity, speed, stability, direction and flexibility. The temperament in Chinese medicine means the psychological characteristic of individual which gradually take shape after the birth, along with the growth of body and mature in physiology. The character in modern psychology means stable attitude to reality and habitual behavior pattern of individual.

6.1.3 Factors Affecting Constitution

The characteristic of constitution is determined by the strength and abundance of the viscera, meridians, essence, qi, blood and body fluid. Therefore, any factor that can affect their functional activities can influence the constitution.

6.1.3.1 Factor of Natural Endowment

The innate factor of constitution is mainly determined by parents. The initial state of an individual after birth is closely related with essence, mind, qi and blood of its parents. Everything of a filial generation is endowed by the parents. The filial generation inherits some characteristics of the parents, which constitute their foundation in constitution. Everything that the filial generation acquired from the parents before birth is generally called the natural endowment. The condition of natural endowment is closely related with the quality of reproductive essence of parents. The quality of reproductive essence of parents is related with many factors, such as their parents' constitutions, blood relative, age of reproduction, maternal conditions, and fetal nourishment during pregnancy.

(1) Constitution of the parents: The constitution of parents is the foundation producing offspring. Generally speaking, if the constitution of parents is strong, the constitution of filial generation is also strong. Whereas the constitution of parents is weak, the constitution of filial generation is also weak. The life of filial generation comes from essence-qi in the kidney of parents. Only when essence-qi in the kidney is abundant, can the filial generation acquire stronger vitality, having better constitution. Whether essence-qi in the kidney of parents is strong or weak is also determined by whether or not the whole functions of the viscera are healthy and vigorous. If the constitution of parents is strong and healthy, qi-blood of the viscera is prosperous, the kidney-essence is ample, and the mother gets pregnant and gives birth to a baby at this time, the constitution of filial generation will also be robust. If the constitution of parents is weak and poor, with deficient qi-blood of the viscera and shortage of the kidney essence, even the mother gets pregnant, the constitution of the filial generation will also be weak. Some hereditary diseases can be transmitted to the filial generation by the parents. Induced by a certain acquired factor, the filial generation will get the same disease as the parents, such as epilepsy and asthma.

(2) Blood relative of parents: Whether the blood relative of the parents is far or near is also one of the factors influencing the constitution of filial generation. The parents with consanguineous marriage will have seriously bad influence on the posterity. Among them, some make their filial generations present with teratism, some others make their filial generations present with serious constitution defect, or mental retardation, or being weak physique with predisposition to get disease.

(3) The marriage and child-bearing age of parents: The marriage and child-bearing age of parents is also a factor influencing the constitution of filial generation. The constitutional conditions of parents have something to do with their age. The constitution of a person changes with his age. This is a characteristic that the constitution is in a dynamic state. Therefore, the parents should marry and multiply during the best period of age so as to keep the constitution of filial generation strong. As a general rule, in the youth and prime of life the essence-qi of the kidney is abundant with the powerful vitality. At this time the parents give birth, and the constitution of filial generation is usually robust. If they bear child too early or lately, because essence-qi in the kidney is deficient, their offspring is often not strong. With essence gradual declines in old age, even they can bear child, the constitution of their offspring must be weak.

(4) Cultivating the fetus and pregnant diseases: Cultivating the fetus means that the pregnant woman should be given good care from pregnancy to delivery in her diet, daily living, mental state, work and rest. The waxing of essence-qi of parents in the kidney determines the basic hereditary factor of filial generation; however the developing condition of the fetus is also related to whether the advantage of parents' constitution can be fully embodied or not. In the meantime, the maternal health condition during pregnancy influences not only the growth and development of the fetus directly, but also the constitution after birth.

Maternal diseases during pregnancy can influence the development of the fetus and the constitution of filial generation. Therefore, the pregnant woman should avoid contracting diseases as far as possible, preventing invasion by the six exogenous factors for not impairing the fetus, and avoiding internal injuries by seven emotional factors and improper diet so as to make qi-blood abundant and vessels unobstructed, hence the fetus being cultivated.

The specific constitution built by the innate factor is usually deeply-rooted. Under the equal postnatal condition of cultivation, whether a person's constitution is strong or weak is mainly determined by the natural endowment. Inadequate natural endowment in childhood usually influences growth and development. The shortage of innate factor may also influence life span of the person.

6.1.3.2 Diet Factor

The food and drink is the source of the nourishing material of human body after birth, which is very important for the life activity. A rational and scientific dietary habit is an important guarantee in maintaining and improving the physique. However the living condition of people is not identical, the dietary habit is also different from each other, so people have developed different constitutions gradually.

(1) Over-hungry and over-eating: Over-hungry and over-eating mean imbalance of food intake. If the food is ample, the nourishment is well, the type of figure is full

and round, the constitution is better. If a person's food intake is short or he intentionally reduces his food intake, his nourishment will be worse, and his body will be weak and thin, then the constitution is inclined to be weak. If the person does not limit overeating or overeats delicious food, then his body may be large and firm-fleshed, but usually accompanied by many phlegm with exuberant physique and deficient qi, the constitution will be weak. When a person always eats the simple food, but with no hunger, then there is no production of phlegm-dampness, and his qi-blood is flowing smoothly, the constitution is better.

(2) Food partiality: Food partiality means that a person's dietary structure is not rational, and he excessively indulges in a certain food, or addicts to one of the five flavors, or to the cold or heat-natured food, or indulges in fatty and sweet food or fine wines. The production of qi, blood, yin and yang of the viscera depends on yin-yang harmony among the five flavors of food. If food partiality lasts for a long time, it may result in relative superiority or inferiority of yin, yang, qi and blood, further resulting in dysfunctions of the viscera. In the daily life, there are some people who are partial to sweet-flavored food, pungent-flavored food, salty and sour-flavored food, even warm and hot-natured or cold and cool-natured food for a long time. Indulging in the sweet which is helpful in producing phlegm and dampness easily develops the diathesis with exuberant phlegm-dampness. Indulging in the pungent which easily results in fire to consume body fluid may develop the yin deficiency diathesis accompanied by intense-fire. Indulging in the salty easily develops the diathesis with heart-qi deficiency due to impairment of both blood and heart. Eating warm and hot-natured food for a long time easily results in yin deficiency and yang exuberance. Often eating cold and cool-natured food easily results in yin exuberance and yang deficiency. Indulging in greasy and fat food, although may get a fat body with white complexion, but easily cause exuberant phlegm and dampness or generation of heat and fire internally. Indulging in fine wines, although may get s rosy complexion, but easily damage the liver and spleen due to dampness-heat in the middle-Jiao. So it can be seen from this, diet is closely related to a person's constitution.

6.1.3.3 Factor of Age

The life process of man is a developing and changing process of birth, growth, prime, aging, and death. In different stages of life, the human functional activityies of the viscera and the superiority or inferiority of qi, blood, yin, and yang vary. Therefore an individual's constitution may also change with the changes of age.

Childhood is the earlier period of growth and development, the characteristic of constitution is that the viscera have not matured and the body is tender. So children easily get deficient or excess syndrome as well as cold or heat syndrome in pathology. However they are full of vitality in the period of the growth and development, the constitution tends to strengthen gradually. Even if suffering from illness, he could be cured easily.

Youth and prime is the most prosperous period of the growth and development, the body is fully-matured with a strong physique, powerful function of the viscera, sufficient qi-blood and yin-yang, full of vitality, being competent to labor; so the constitution is strong and the person seldom suffers from disease.

Senility is the result of the physiological decline in the visceral functions. So the constitution of the old gradually declines. As the age increases, normal types of constitution get fewer and fewer, and abnormal types of constitution get more and more. In the meantime, abnormal constitution of the old is no longer as simple as that of the youth; it mostly takes a certain constitution as the main, accompanied by the characteristics of the others.

6.1.3.4 Factor of Sex

Because the male and female have difference in the hereditary character of gender, figure, visceral structure, etc., with the corresponding differences in physiological function and psychological characteristic. So there exists sexual difference in the constitution. Male pertains to yang, and female to yin. Comparative speeching, the male is endowed with manly temperament. The visceral function is stronger, with a sound physique, stronger explosive force, extroverted disposition, bold and unconstrained personality, being fond of moving, and broad-mindedness. The female is mostly endowed with gentle and quiet temperament. The visceral function is weaker, with a small and slender figure, stronger stamina, introverted disposition, subtle and refined personality, being fond of quieting, being sentimental and susceptible. A man has the kidney as his innateness, and essence-qi as his material basis. While a woman has the liver as her innateness, and yin-blood as her material basis. A man mostly utilizes qi in function, so he often suffers from qi-deficiency. While a woman mostly utilizes blood in function, so she often suffers from shortage of blood. The disease of male mostly shows the disorder of qi due to consumption of essence and qi; the disease of female mostly shows the disorder of blood due to consumption of blood. In addition, because women have special physiological conditions of menstruation, leukorrhea, pregnancy and parturition and nursing, they have the constitutional change during menstruation, gestational period and puerperium. During the menstruation, there is obvious periodic variety inside the body. Every system of the mother's body will produce a series of adaptation in the gestational period due to the need of fetus for development, and in puerperium because of laboring and nursing. So there is a saying "the pregnant woman is suitable for the cool; the puerperant woman is suitable for the warm". Comparing to female, the defect of constitution in male mainly expresses that men are more susceptible to pathogens, and more easily to contract diseases, often with more serious pathological changes and higher mortality.

6.1.3.5 Factor of Work and Rest

The proper manual labor or exercise can make bones and muscles strong, the movement of joint flexible, qi-blood coordinative, qi dynamic smooth, and the visceral function powerful. The full rest is helpful to eliminate fatigue, regain strength and intelligence, thus maintaining the normal life activity. A proper balance between work and rest is conducive to physicopsychic health, and profitable to maintain good constitution. The over-strain is easy to harm bones and muscles, as well as consume qi-blood to cause essence-qi shortage and hypofunction of the viscera, thus weak constitution develops. But over-ease, enjoying high position and living in comfort over a long time with less exercise will make the circulation of qi-blood unsmooth, muscles flabby, the spleen-stomach hypofunctional, thus fat and damp-greasy constitution develops.

6.1.3.6 Emotional Factor

Emotion is normal reaction of a person to the stimuli of objective things, as well as the adaptable and regulatory ability of the body to the variety of the natural and social environment. Creation and maintenance of emotional activity depend on the functional activity of the viscera, with qi-blood and yin-yang of the viscera as the material basis. The emotional changes can influence a person's constitution by affecting qi-blood variety of the viscera. So, the normal emotional activity consists in harmony. A harmonious emotional activity makes the circulation of qi-blood smooth, visceral function coordinated and the constitution strong. Contrarily, a drastical or prolonged emotional stimulus that once exceeds a person's physiological regulatory ability will cause impairment of qi-blood and dysfunction of the viscera, resulting in negative influence on the constitution. The qi-depressed constitution which is commonly seen in clinical is mostly caused by this. Qi-depression can also accumulate heat to cause fire, as well as impair yin and consume the body fluid, then leading to the yang heat diathesis or yin deficiency diathesis. Qi stagnation can produce the blood-stasis constitution. The changes of constitution caused by emotional changes also have a particular relation with the onset of some diseases. The person with "wood-fire constitution" who easily gets sulky and irritable will be susceptible to vertigo and stroke. The person with "liver depression constitution" who easily gets persistent anxiety and depression will be predisposed to blood stasis and abdominal mass. Therefore keeping good mental state is very beneficial to constitutional health.

6.1.3.7 Geographical Factors

Prevention and treatment of disease should follow the principle of "treatment according to the local condition", namely, considering that the constitution is different in population of different region. The difference in region determines multiple differences, such as property of water and soil, climatic type, habits and customs of people. There is a saying "in each region people there have their own special characteristics". The dissimilarity of region would undoubtedly produce direct or indirect influence on the constitution.

In the developing process of geology, the distribution of chemical elements in earth's surface gradually form variety, which controls and influences the growth of world-wide mankind, animals and plants to a certain extent, thus resulting in the ecological differences of the creatures in regions. The continent in China has a vast territory; there are greatly differences in the geographic condition and climatic characters in different regions. These factors make people in different regions adaptable to their long-lived residence. People in different regions have a different life habit. Among them, the dietary habit has the biggest influence. The structure of constitution has obvious difference in the population of different geographic regions, such as the number of people with yang deficiency diathesis in north is much more than that in the south, and the number of people with yin deficiency diathesis in the south is much more than that in the north. People with phlegm and blood-stasis constitution are commonly seen in Qinghai-Tibet plateau and southeast along the coast.

6.1.3.8 Social Factors

Generally speaking, a person feels helpless to social environment. As a result people usually have no choice to bear some social influence. Along with the development of science and technology, industry and commerce, as well as the urbanized and individualized social life, the rhythm of people's life correspondingly speed up, interpersonal relationship becomes complicated further, and living incidents correspondingly increase. These all may become social factors influencing the constitution.

(1) Economic life: In economic life, over wealth or over poverty all can make people's constitution descend. The flying development of modern industry brings on serious environmental pollution and quicker living rhythm; further more the enriched material life is followed by bad life style. All these injure the health of mankind from the body and mind, and make people's constitution descend continuously.

(2) Social status: Particular outlook on life and values urge people to pay more attention to their social status. The vicissitudes of social status caused by various reasons can obviously influence individual constitution.

(3) Occupation: People with different occupations have their own corresponding work environment, labor intensity, economic income, social status and economy position. That can also become one of the factors which influence various constitution types.

(4) War: The environmental damage, the epidemic of diseases and stress caused by war can often lead to general constitution decline of population in the war region.

6.1.3.9 Disease, Acupuncture, Medicine and the Other Factors

A disease can accelerate the change of constitution. If the damages caused by some diseases could not recover quickly, then the impairment of qi-blood and yin-yang could become the factor influencing the constitution. Particularly some chronic wasting diseases and dystrophic diseases have strong influence on the constitution.

Under general circumstances, changes of constitution caused by disease mostly develop in an unfavorable direction. For example, a serious illness or prolonged illness often makes the constitution weak. Some chronic diseases lasting for a long time are apt to make the constitution present a certain particularity easily. However after being affected by a given disease, human body will have corresponding immunity and not be affected by this disease again in the rest life. In addition, a disease can cause the change of constitution, and the type of constitution can also altered with the development of disease. For example, the patients with chronic hepatic disease mostly present with the diathesis of qi-stagnation in the early stage of disease, and then the constitution may change into the different types of constitution, such as the blood-stasis or yin deficiency diathesis in the middle and last stage. It is clear that constitution and disease are usually of relationship of cause and effect.

The nature and flavor of medicine or reinforcement and reduction by acupuncture and moxibustion can all adjust waxing and waning of visceral qi-blood and yin-yang and the biased conditions of meridian qi-blood. Proper application of them can attain the effect of rectifying a deviation and correcting an error. But an inappropriate use will aggravate the damage of constitution, resulting in bias or waxing and waning of qi-blood and yin-yang.

In addition to above factors, there are other factors influencing the constitution such as marriage-delivery and exercise. The marriage and delivery are normal physiological activities of mankind, but sexual activity and conception all should be restrained. Indulging in sensual pleasures and fecundity can all damage essence-qi and result in decline of constitution or premature senility, hence influencing life span. Physical exercise is the activity by which the mankind actively transforms the constitution, being advantageous to enhancement of the physique, promotion of the physicopsychic health. So a prolonged lack of physical exercise will make the constitution decrease.

6.2 Classification of Constitution

In Chinese medicine, the classification of constitution is mainly based on the basic theory of Chinese medicine to ascertain the constitution dissimilarity of different individuals in population. There are many methods of classifying the constitution. The traditional classification and modern classification will be introduced in this section.

6.2.1 Traditional Classification

The traditional classifications are various. Here yin-yang classification and five elements classification are mainly introduced.

6.2.1.1 Yin and Yang Classification

Viewing from the whole, the healthy population should keep the relative equilibrium between yin and yang. But in regard to specific persons, there exists difference among different individuals. Constitution of some people inclines to yang (yang as the dominant aspect), that of some other people inclines to yin (yin as the dominant aspect), and that of again some other people get around the balance of yin and yang. The yin-yang in the constitution type mainly refers to yin-qi and yang-qi, which take opposition-restriction as the principle and mostly present with being inclined to cold or heat and motion or stillness. Other constitution types are usually derived from and developed on the basis of yin or yang inclined constitution. The normal constitution of human body is divided into three categories, i.e. the yin-yang balanced constitution, yang inclined constitution and yin inclined constitution.

(1) Yin-yang balanced constitution: The yin-yang balanced constitution is the more harmonious constitution category in both body and mind. The constitutional features are: strong physique, moderate build, adaptation to the change of cold and heat, lustrous skin, bright and ruddy complexion, bright and piercing light in eyes, optimistic character, open-mindedness and tolerant attitude, moderate intake of food, smooth urination and defecation, good sleeping, being full of energy, quick reaction, agile mind, big potentiality of work, stronger self-adjustment and adaptability, pink and moist tongue, even and moderate pulse with vitality.

The persons consistent with the characteristic of yin-yang balanced constitution are hardly affected by exogenous pathogenic factors, and seldom falling ill. Even suffering from an illness, they may mostly present with an exterior and excess syndrome, mild condition of the disease, being easily cured, quickly recovering from illness, and often getting self-recovery. If they get proper cultivation after birth, no accident injury and no unhealthy addiction, their constitutions are stable and not easily changed, hence mostly having longevity.

(2) Yang inclined constitution: The yang inclined constitution means a constitutional type which has characteristics of being more excited, inclined to heat and excessive movement. The constitutional features are: moderate or biased lean build but being fairly sturdy, slightly red or black complexion, or greasy and glossy skin, extroverted personality, being fond of moving, being eager to do well in everything, being irritable easily, poor self-control, bigger intake of food, robust digestion and absorption, usually dry stools and dark-colored urine, intolerance of heat and preference for the cool ordinarily, or higher body temperature, easily perspiration while moving, preference for cold drinking, energetic and quick action, nimble reaction, stronger sexual desire, slightly red lips and tongue with thin yellow coating, slightly rapid pulse.

The persons conforming to the characteristic of the yang inclined constitution have stronger susceptibility to yang pathogen such as wind, summer-heat, dryness and heat. After affected by yang pathogen, they may usually present with a heat and excess syndrome, with a tendency of yin impairment and production of dryness. For internal injury a syndrome of intense fire, hyperactive yang or accompanied by yin deficiency may often develop, manifested by vertigo, headache, palpitation, insomnia and bleeding. And furuncle, prickly heat, carbuncle, nail-like furuncle and boil, herpes simplex of the skin and muscles are also mostly common. Since the persons are in a condition of yang-qi superiority, excessive movement and less stillness, after a considerable period of time they will have a worry of consumption of yin. If the persons get improper nursing, excessively hard work, worry constantly, indulge in sensual pleasure with loss of essence or indulge in smoking and drinking, or hot spicy food. It must accelerate impairment of yin, and then they will develop the pathological constitutions of hyperactive yang, yin deficiency, and phlegm-fire.

(3) Yin inclined constitution: Yin inclined constitution means a constitutional type which has characteristics of being more inhibited, inclined to cold and stillness. The constitutional features are: moderate or biased fat build, but being fairly weaker and easily tired, slightly white but little lustrous complexion, introverted personality, being fond of stillness and little moving, or timidness and being easily frightened, little intake of food, generally weaker digestion and absorption, ordinarily intolerance of cold and preference for warmth, or lower body temperature, shortage of energy, sluggish action, slower reaction, frigidity, pale lips and tongue, enlarged tongue body with tooth-prints, slightly slow and weak pulse.

The persons conforming to yin inclined constitution have stronger susceptibility to yin pathogen such as cold, dampness. After affected by yin pathogen, they may usually present with a cold and deficiency syndrome, and the superficial pathogen can easily transmit from the exterior to the interior of the body, or cold pathogen can directly attack the viscera. For the internal injury a syndrome of yin predominance and yang deficiency often develops, manifested by retention of dampness, edema, diarrhea, fluid retention, and blood stasis. A chilblain often occurs in winter. Since the persons are in a condition of yang inferiority, after a considerable period of development, they may get deficiency of yang-qi, hypofunction of the viscera, internal production of water-dampness; and then they will develop the pathological constitutions of yang deficiency, phlegm and dampness, water pathogen.

It should be pointed out the terms used in classifying the constitution, i.e. biased yang, biased yin, hyperactive yang, predominant yin, phlegm and fluid retention, blood stasis, are both different and related with the names of syndrome. The syndrome is an analysis and generalization of pathological nature of a disease at a certain stage or in a certain type; while the constitution reflects a kind of the individual particularities existing in physiological scope. The constitution is the internal factor that the disease occurs and develops, so the constitutional type and its syndrome pattern have intrinsic relativity, too.

6.2.1.2 Five Elements Classification

Five elements classification is to conclude and summarize five different kinds of constitutional types, i.e. wood, fire, earth, metal and water, according to the characteristics of the color of the skin, shape, disposition, attitude and adaptability.

(1) Person with wood pattern: The constitutional characteristics of persons with wood pattern are: greenish skin, small head with a long face, broad shoulder, straight waist and back, short and weak stature, agile movement of hand and foot, being capable and experienced, acute mentality, less physical strength, being more worried, diligence in work. To the changes of the seasons, the person likes the warmth of spring and summer, and can hardly endure the cold of autumn and winter. If the persons contract the cold-dampness pathogen, they will get sick easily.

(2) Person with fire pattern: The constitutional characteristics of persons with fire pattern are: reddish skin, small head with a pointed chin, thick and broad back, well-balanced stature, small hands and feet, even and slow step, shaking shoulders while walking, full-muscled back, stronger insight, agile mind, thinking of more morality and less wealth, lack of self-confidence, being more worried, being keen on good-looking, irritable temperament. To the changes of the seasons, the person likes the warmth of spring and summer, can hardly endure the cold of autumn and winter. If the persons are invaded by the cold-dampness pathogen, they will get sick easily.

(3) Person with earth pattern: The constitutional characteristics of persons with earth pattern are: yellowish skin, big head with a round face, broad shoulders and thick back, pot-belliedness, sound and firm thigh and calf, smaller hands and feet, full musculature, well-balanced stature, even and slow step, graceful gait, calm-heartedness, taking pleasure in helping others and fond of making friends. To the changes of the seasons, the person likes the cool of autumn and winter, and can hardly endure heat of spring and summer. If the persons contract the heat pathogen, they will get sick easily.

(4) Person with metal pattern: The constitutional characteristics of persons with metal pattern are: whitish skin, small head with a square jaw, narrow shoulders and back, small-belliedness, small hands and feet, bigger and thicker heel as if the bone is outside heel, brisk action, honest and upright disposition, irritable and firm temperament, handling affair seriously, resolute and agile action, being adept in making a decision. To the changes of the seasons, the person likes the cold of autumn and winter, and can hardly endure heat of spring and summer. If the persons contract the heat pathogen, they will get sick easily.

(5) Person with water pattern: The constitutional characteristics of persons with water pattern are: blackish skin, big head with a wrinkled face, being hollow-cheeked, narrow shoulder, pot-belliedness, being fond of moving, shaking body while walking,

the upper body being longer than the lower body, respect tess and dauntless disposition, intelligence, lack of honesty and trustworthiness. To the changes of the seasons, the person likes the cool of autumn and winter, and can hardly endure heat of spring and summer. If the persons are invaded by the heat pathogen, they will get sick easily.

6.2.2 Modern Classification

With the aid of means of investigation and research in epidemiology, and mathematical statistics, more modern classifications of constitutions in recent years have been achieved. According to the present status of the population, the constitution is classified into the following seven categories with this method.

6.2.2.1 Strong and Excited Constitution

The persons with strong and excited constitution are characterized by more sturdy build compared with normal persons, and hyperfunction. The concrete manifestations are being vivacious and fond of moving, quick and powerful action, warm body, tolerance of cold and cool, preference for cold-natured food, facial acne, greasy skin, loss of hair easily, hyper-sexual desire, poor self-control, excessive consumption due to hyper-metabolism with a tendency of consuming yin and impairing vital qi. It may easily evolve into the hot and asthenic-hyperactive constitution after a considerable period of time.

6.2.2.2 Weak and Tired Constitution

The persons with weak and tired constitution are characterized by being weaker body compared with normal persons, and hypofunction. The concrete manifestations are dispiritedness, less desire for movement and polylogia, being easily tired, lassitude on little exertion, lusterless or sallow complexion, intolerance of cold and heat, catching cold easily, suffering from an illness with little fever and hardly be cured. Because of hypo-metabolism, it may easily evolve into the cold and slowly-acting constitution after a considerable period of time.

6.2.2.3 Hot and Asthenic-hyperactive Constitution

The persons with hot and asthenic-hyperactive constitution are characterized by being leaner build compared with normal persons, and asthenic-hyperfunction. The concrete manifestations are usually feverish sensation in the palms and soles, perspiration in the palms, a burst of hot sensation in the face and flushed cheeks, thirst with a desire for cold drinks, restlessness and short temper, irritability and anxiousness, emotional upset, usually insomnia, occasionally constipation, slightly dark urine. The persons are easily contracted by yang-heat pathogen. Because of production of dryness due to impairment of yin after suffering from an illness, it may easily evolve into the emaciated and dry-red constitution after a considerable period of time.

6.2.2.4 Cold and Slowly-Acting Constitution

The persons with cold and slowly-acting constitution are characterized by being moderate or fatter build with whiter skin compared with normal persons, and hypofunction. The concrete manifestations are slightly lower body temperature, cold limbs, intolerance of cold, preference for hot food, slow action, sluggish reaction and even dullness, bradycardia, pale complexion, dark purplish, even grayish purple lips and tongue, loose stools, diarrhea easily induced by abdominal pain, obviously low metabolism. The persons are easily affected by cold-damp pathogen; and cold conversion or dampness conversion commonly occur during the course of disease. This constitution, the weak and tired constitution, the fat and damp-greasy constitution, and the dark and stagnated constitution can transform into one another after a considerable period of time.

6.2.2.5 Fat and Damp-Greasy Constitution

The persons with fat and damp-greasy constitution are characterized by being fatter and tender build compared with normal persons, and disorder of function. The concrete manifestations are heavy sensation of the whole body, reluctance of motion, being qualified to ordinary labor but with a slow reaction, potbelliedness at the middle age, epigastric stuffiness and fullness, sweet sensation in the mouth with no desire to drink, thick and greasy tongue coating. The persons are predisposed to edematous diseases, diarrhea, chest qi-blockage and apoplexy. The youth and middle aged women usually get irregular menstruation, leukorrhagia, even sterility. The persons are easily affected by cold-damp pathogen. During the course of disease yang-qi is predisposed to be damaged, and cold conversion or dampness conversion may occur. This constitution can transform into the cold and slowly-acting constitution after a considerable period of time.

6.2.2.6 Emaciated and Dry-Red Constitution

The persons with emaciated and dry-red constitution are characterized by being obviously thinner build compared with normal persons, hypofunction or asthenic hyperfunction, and deficiency of yin-fluid. The concrete manifestations are rough and old features of face, dark-brown, dry, rough and hard skin; thirst with no desire for drinks, physical asthenia, preference for activity but hardly lasting long; difficult defecation, once every several days, with the feces in hard dry balls; dark-red lips and tongue with little coating or without coating. This constitution usually develops from the hot and deficiency-hyperactive constitution.

6.2.2.7 Dark and Stagnated-Obstructed Constitution

The persons with dark and stagnated constitution are characterized by being the same body as or thinner body compared with normal persons, functional disorder, and stagnation of qi and blood. The concrete manifestations are dull complexion, blackish color of the area around the eye sockets, dark purple lips and tongue; thick and bluish-purplish tip of fingers, rough skin, even squamous dandruff, or being red-streaked and vascular spider; pain especially in winter. The persons have obvious obstacle in metabolism. If the persons contract a disease, the disease is usually lasts long and is hardly cured; and the patients easily suffer from abdominal masses after a considerable period of time.

Among the above-mentioned types of constitution, it is found in the investigation that the most commonly seen types of constitution are the weak and tired constitution, cold and slowly-acting constitution, hot and asthenic-hyperactive constitution, and fat and damp-greasy constitution, which have a large proportion especially in the old and the weak people. The weak and tired constitution is the most common. The fat and damp-greasy constitution prevails among urban residents, especially in the eastern coastal towns. Although the emaciated and dry-red constitution and the dark and stagnated constitution are less seen, they are of larger threat to the healthy.

Review Questions

- Why are the viscera, meridians, essence, qi, blood and body fluid said to be the physiological basis for constitutional formation?
- What are the constitutional characteristics in childhood, the youth-prime of life, and old age respectively?
- What is the dissimilarity of the male and the female on the constitution?
- What constitutional changes could bad diet habit cause?
- What influences would rest-work and emotion produce on the constitution?
- What are the constitutional and pathogenic characteristics in yin-yang balanced constitution?

7 ETIOLOGY AND PATHOMECHANISM

The human body maintains a relative dynamic balance among viscera and tissues, and between the body and its external environment, in which contradictions constantly occur and are resolved. In such a manner, the body maintains normal physiological activities. Whenever this dynamic balance gets disharmonious due to some factors and cannot recover by self-regulation, illness will immediately ensue.

Factors that cause disharmony of the relative balance and lead to disease are the causes of disease, or known as pathogenic factors. Pathogenic factors are many and varied, such as abnormal climatic changes, pestilence infection, emotional stimulation, improper diet, overstrain and stress, traumatic injuries, and insect or animal bites. In the course of a disease, cause and effect are often inter-active. An effect in a pathological stage may be a cause in another pathological stage. Examples are phlegm-stagnant-fluid and stagnant blood, which are pathological outcomes of a disturbance of the functions of viscera, qi and blood, may become pathological factors causing disease.

The patho-mechanisms means the mechanism causing pathological changes because various pathogenic factors act on the body, namely, the occurrence, development and changes of disease. Diseases are many and varied, and the pathological mechanisms involved are complicated. Different diseases have their own pathological characters. However, general laws exist in different pathological changes of quite different diseases caused by various pathogenic factors. These general laws can effectively guide syndrome differentiation, treatment, and allow the practitioner to recognize more profoundly the nature of a disease.

7.1 Etiology

There are many factors that can cause diseases, including the six climatic pathogens, seven emotional factors, improper diet, overstrain and over ease. In order to further understand the nature and pathogenic character of pathogenic factors, ancient practitioners of Chinese medicine had classified pathogenic factors. For example, *Huáng Dì Nèi Jīng* (*Huangdi's Inner Classic of Medicine*) classified them into two kinds, yin and yang. Chen Wuze of the Song Dynasty put forth "the doctrine of three causes", i.e., exogenous pathogens are invasion by the six climatic pathogens, endogenous pathogens are internal injury of the five *Zang*-viscera by emotional factors, and non-exo-endogenous pathogens are injury due to improper diet, overstrain, traumatic wound, and insect or animal bites. All of these etiological classifications by ancient practitioners of Chinese medicine in combining pathogenic factors with and the way of disease occurrence have a certain guiding significance in clinical syndrome differentiation.

Chinese medicine holds that there is no syndrome without cause. Any syndrome is a disharmonious reflection of the body under the influence and action of some factors. Chinese medicine studies the cause of a disease, besides by understanding objective conditions that may become pathogenic factors according to the clinical manifestations of the disease, mainly through analysis of symptoms and signs of the disease to infer its cause. This process or method gives a basis for treatment and prescription, which is called "referring the cause by syndrome differentiation." Therefore, etiology in Chinese medicine not only studies the nature and pathogenic characters of pathogenic factors, but also probes into clinical manifestations they cause. Thus, it can play a good role in clinical diagnosis and treatment. In this chapter the causes are divided into four categories of exogenous pathogens, endogenous pathogens, pathogens from pathological products and miscellaneous pathogens according to the ways of attack and the development of disease.

7.1.1 Exogenous Pathogens

Exogenous pathogens means the pathogens that invade the human body to cause disease from the outside via the surface of the body, or/and mouth and nose. Disease caused by exegenous pathogens are dallecl excgenous diseases, They are generally acute in onset, and manifested early by aversion to cold, fever, superficial pulse, soreness of the bones and joints, etc.. They include six climatic pathogens and pestilent pathogens.

7.1.1.1 The Six Climatic Pathogens

The six climatic pathogens are a collective term used for six kinds of exogenous pathogens of wind, cold, summer-heat, dampness, dryness and fire. Under normal conditions, wind, cold, summer-heat, dampness, dryness and fire as "six climatic factors," are normal climatic changes in nature. Normally the six climatic factors do not cause disease. Only when the climatic change is sharp or the resistance of the body becomes weak, the six climatic factors will become pathogens, causing the body to fall ill. The six climatic factors are then called the six climatic pathogens. Since the six climatic pathogens are abnormal, they also refer to as the "six evils", and are causes of exogenous diseases.

Generally, the pathogenic characters of the six climatic pathogens are as follows:
① The pathogenesis of the six climatic pathogens is often connected with seasons and environmental conditions. For example, wind-disease often occurs in spring; summer-

heat-disease in summer, dampness-disease in late summer, dryness-disease in autumn, and cold-disease in winter. In addition, prolonged stay in a damp environment may contribute to the invasion of dampness; a high-temperature may contribute to the invasion of dryness-heat or fire. ② Each of the six climatic pathogens may cause disease alone or in mixture with another. For example, wind and cold can invade the body and cause a common cold, dampness and heat can cause diarrhea, and wind, cold and dampness can cause "*Bi*" (arthralgia) syndrome. ③ In the pathological process, the nature of a syndrome caused by the six climatic pathogens may change under certain conditions. For example, cold may turn into heat after entering the interior of the body. After long stay in the body, summer-heat-dampness may change into dryness to consume yin. ④ The six climatic pathogens usually invade the body through the body surface, or the mouth and nose, or through both simultaneously. Therefore, diseases caused by them are known as "exogenous diseases".

Viewing from clinical practice, the pathogenesis of the six climatic pathogens, include not only climatic factors, but also pathological changes caused by several kinds of biological pathogenic factors (bacteria, virus, etc.), physics and chemical factors that act on the body.

(1) Wind: Wind prevails in spring, but it may occur in any season. While invasion by wind pathogen may often occur in spring, it is not limited to spring. Wind pathogen mostly invades the body from the body surface to cause exogenous diseases. Chinese medicine holds that wind pathogen is a very important pathogenic factor in causing exogenous diseases.

The nature and pathogenic character of wind pathogen are as follows: ① Wind is a yang pathogen, and is characterized by dispersing. Wind pathogen tends to move constantly, possessing a nature of dispersal, upward and outward movement; and thus belongs to yang. The dispersal means that when it invades the body, it tends to loosen the striae of the skin and muscles, and open the pores. Wind pathogen is apt to invade the upper portion of the body (head and face) and body surface, and thus results in headache, sweating, and aversion to wind. ② Wind is characterized by constant movement and rapid change. "Constant movement" implies that the diseases caused by wind pathogen possess the feature of migration. For example, in a *Bi* (arthralgia) syndrome caused by invasion of wind, cold and dampness, if the arthralgia is migratory, and on and off, it is a case in which wind pathogen prevails. It is thus called "*Xing bi*" (migratory arthralgia) or "*Feng Bi*" (wind arthralgia). "Rapid change" denotes that disease caused by wind pathogen is characterized by sudden attack and quick transformation. For instance, the urticaria is characterized by cutaneous pruritus changeable in location and rising one after another. In addition, exogenous diseases caused mainly by wind pathogen are generally abrupt in onset and rapid changing. ③ Wind is the first and foremost factor in the cause of disease. Wind, a leading exopathic factor, is the precursor of exogenous pathogens causing disease, and other pathogens usually follow wind to invade the body. For example, wind-cold, wind-heat, and wind-dampness may attack the body exogenously.

(2) Cold: Cold is prevalent in winter. There is a difference between exogenous cold and endogenous cold in disease. Exogenous cold means that cold pathogen attacks the body from outside. In diseases caused by exogenous cold, there is a difference between cold-attack and cold-stroke. A case in which cold pathogen attacks the body surface and depresses the defensive-yang is known as a "cold-attack"; while a case in which cold pathogen directly invades the interior and damages the visceral yang-qi is called "cold-stroke". Endogenous cold is the pathological state resulting from the failure of yang-qi to warm the body due to its deficiency. While exogenous cold is different from endogenous cold, they are mutually influence and related to each other. A patient with endogenous cold due to deficiency of yang is predisposed to an invasion of exogenous cold pathogen. Whereas exogenous cold pathogen invading and staying in the body for a long period is likely to damage yang-qi, and thus lead to endogenous cold.

The nature and pathogenic character of cold pathogen are as the following: ① Cold is a yin pathogen, and apt to damage yang-qi. Cold is an expression of excessive Yin-qi, belonging to yin. Invasion of cold pathogen is thus apt to damage yang-qi of the body. For example, as cold pathogen attacks the exterior, defensive-yang will get depressed, marked by aversion to cold. If cold directly invades the spleen and stomach, it can damage spleen-yang and result in epigastric pain with a cold feeling, vomiting, and diarrhea. ② Cold is characterized by stagnation, condensation, and obstruction. Invasion of the body by cold pathogen may cause stagnation of qi and blood in the meridians, thus giving rise to various kinds of pain. ③ Cold is characterized by contraction, traction, and constriction. When cold pathogen invades the body it may depress qi dynamic, and constrict and tighten the striae, meridians and tendons. If cold pathogen attacks the body surface, it may make the pores and striae close up and result in depression of defensive-yang. Thus chills, fever, and anhidrosis occur. If cold pathogen invades and stays at the blood vessel, the flow of qi and blood will stagnate, the vessels will contract. Therefore, pain in the head and trunk, with a tense pulse might appear. If cold pathogen invades the meridians and joints, the meridians and tendons will tighten and contract, there may appear spasm and pain of the limbs and joints and impaired movement.

(3) Summer-heat: Summer-heat prevails in summer; it comes from transformation of fire and heat. It is remarkable in that it only appears in summer. Summer-heat is a pure exogenous pathogen, and there is no such thing as endogenous summer-heat.

The nature and pathogenic character of summer-heat pathogen are as follows: ① Summer-heat is a yang pathogen characterized by burning heat. Summer-heat comes from transformation of the fiery hotness of summer. As fiery hotness belongs to yang, summer-heat is a yang pathogen. Invasion of the body by summer-heat pathogen often results in high fever, fidgets and thirst, flushed face, and a surging pulse. ② Summer-heat is characterized by rising and dispersion, and apt to consume qi and body fluid. Invasion of the body by summer-heat tends to make the striae of the skin and the muscles open, resulting in heavy sweating. Too much sweating consumes body fluid, and a shortage of body fluid may in turn lead to thirst, deep yellow and scanty urine. When heavy sweating occurs, qi will escape with release of body fluid, resulting in qi deficiency. This may then lead to shortness of breath, lassitude, collapse, or loss of consciousness. ③ Summer-heat often combines with dampness. In summer, it is often rainy and is moist. Heat evaporates dampness, increasing the level of humidity. Invasion of summer-heat, therefore, often combines with dampness pathogen to attack the body. Besides fidget and thirst, there usually appear lassitude with a heavy sensation of the limbs, chest distress, nausea, vomiting, and sticky and loose stools.

(4) Dampness: Dampness is prevalent in late summer. The period when summer is changing into autumn is the time of a year with the most humidity. There is a difference between exogenous dampness and endogenous dampness in disease. Exogenous dampness is a pathogenic factor invading the body from outside because of damp climate, being caught in rain, or living in a damp condition. Endogenous dampness is a pathological state when water-dampness accumulates internally, which is usually caused by failure of the spleen in transportation. Exogenous dampness and endogenous dampness are different, but they often influence each other in onset of disease. Exogenous dampness that invades the body from outside usually affects the spleen, making the spleen fail in transportation, and thus causes formation of dampness internally. However, a patient with retention of water-dampness internally due to deficiency of spleen yang is predisposed to invasion of exogenous dampness.

The nature and pathogenic character of dampness pathogen are as follows: ① Dampness is a yin pathogen, apt to damage yang-qi and hinder the qi dynamic. The nature of dampness is similar to that of water, and thus it is a yin pathogen. When invading the body, dampness pathogen is most likely to damage yang-qi. When dampness pathogen invades the spleen and makes the spleen-yang hypoactive, leading to failure in transformation and transportation, it will give rise to diarrhea, oliguria, and edema. When attacking the body and staying in the viscera and meridians, dampness pathogen is apt to depress the qi dynamic, leading to disharmony of qi in ascending and descending, and obstruction of the meridians; there will appear chest distress, epigastric distention, dysuria with scanty urine, and dyschesia with mucosa in the stool. ② Dampness is characterized by heaviness-turbidity, and sinking downward. Heaviness means a disease caused by dampness pathogen usually has symptoms of a heavy sensation in the head, general lassitude, aching and a heavy feeling in the limbs. Turbidity means that diseases caused by dampness pathogen present with filthy and foul discharges or secretions, such as a dirty complexion with hypersecretion in the eyes, pus, bloody stools, turbid urine, massive leukorrhea in female, or eczema with filthy purulent fluid. Sinking downward means the symptoms caused by dampness pathogen mostly appear in the lower part of the body, such as leukorrhea, stranguria with turbid urine, and diarrhea or dysentery. ③ Dampness is characterized by viscosity and stagnation. This appears in two ways. First, in symptoms, invasion by dampness pathogen mostly leads to sticky and greasy discharges and secretions. Next in course, a disease caused by dampness pathogen usually has a long course, relapses repeatedly, and is lingering and difficult to cure. Dampness *Bi* (arthralgia), eczema, and dampness-warm disease are the examples.

(5) Dryness: Dryness is prevalent in autumn. The climate in autumn is dry, and the atmosphere is lacking in moisture. As a result, dryness-diseases often occur. Dryness invades the body mostly via the mouth and nose to attack the lung-defense. There are differences between warm-dryness and cool-dryness. In early autumn, summer heat lingers, and dryness combines with warm-heat to invade the body, leading to a warm-dryness disease. In late autumn, early winter cold appears, dryness and cold usually associate with each other to attack the body, and thus leading to cool-dryness disease.

The nature and pathogenic character of dryness pathogen are as follows: ① Dryness is yang pathogen, and characterized by aridity. Exogenous dryness pathogen invading the body is most likely to consume body fluid, resulting in various dry symptoms and signs, such as dry mouth and nose, thirst, dry, rough and chapped skin, dry hair, scanty urine, and constipation. ② Dryness is prone to impair the lung. The lung is a "delicate organ" with a desire for moisture and an aversion to dryness. The lung governs qi and controls respiration. It relates externally to the skin and hair, and opens into the nose. Therefore, a dryness pathogen invading the body via the mouth and nose is most likely to consume lung-fluid, making the lungs fail in diffusing and descending with such symptoms as a dry cough with little sputum, or sticky sputum that is difficult to be coughed out, blood-tinged sputum, asthma, and chest pain.

(6) Fire: Fire and heat both belong to yang in nature and may be collectively called fire-heat. Though they are similar, yet there are still differences. Heat is the lesser of fire, and strong heat results in fire. Heat is mostly from the outside, such as wind-heat, summer-heat, and dampness-heat, while fire usually generates inside, such as flaring up of the heat-fire, hyperactivity of liver-fire, and transverse invasion of gallbladder-fire.

There is difference between exogenous and endogenous diseases caused by fire and heat. Exogenous diseases mainly originate from a direct invasion of a warm-heat pathogen exogenously. Endogenous diseases often develop from hyperactivity of yang-qi due to disturbance of visceral yin-yang and qi-blood. In addition, invasion of the body by wind, cold, summer-heat, dampness, dryness, or emotional stimulation may all give rise to fire under certain conditions. It is thus said that the "five climatic pathogens generate fire" and "five emotional pathogens generate fire."

The nature and pathogenic character of fire pathogen are as follows: ① Fire is a yang pathogen characterized by burning heat. Yang is characterized by restlessness and upward going. Fire (heat) burns and leaps up, and thus fire is a yang pathogen. Therefore, invasion of the body by fire often leads to high fever, aversion to heat, fidgets, thirst, sweating, and a surging and rapid pulse. ② Fire is characterized by flaring up. Diseases caused by fire pathogen mostly have symptoms in the upper part of the body, such as in the head and face. Fire pathogen invading the body often goes upward to disturb the heart-spirit, marked by fidgets with insomnia, mania, and even coma and delirium. If heart-fire flares up, it will lead to a red tongue tip, and mouth or tongue ulcers. If stomach-fire is flaring, it will cause toothache with swelling gums. If liver-fire flares up, it will result in red eyes with swelling and pain. ③ Fire is likely to consume qi and fluid. Fire pathogen invading the body is most likely to result in a loss of fluid and consumption of yin-fluid, thus symptoms of thirst with a desire for drink, dryness in the throat and tongue, deep yellow urine scanty in volume, and constipation appear. Fire pathogen consumes vital qi. So diseases caused by fire pathogen may have the symptoms of shortness of breath, reluctance to talk, and general weakness. ④ Fire is apt to stir up wind and cause bleeding. Fire pathogen invading the body often burns the liver meridian to consume yin-fluid, which in turn deprives the tendons of nourishment. As a result, it leads to an internal stirring of liver-wind, called " extreme heat results in wind". It is marked by high fever, coma, and delirium, convulsive limbs, upward staring of the eyes, rigid neck, and opisthotonos. At the same time, fire pathogen may accelerate blood circulation, burn the vessels, force blood to flow out of the vessels and lead to bleeding such as hematemesis, epistaxis, hemafecia, hematuria, ecchymosis, and uterine bleeding. ⑤ Fire is likely to cause pyogenic infection. Invasion of fire pathogen into the blood level may accumulate in a local area, corrode the muscles and putrefy blood, and thus result in carbuncles and abscesses marked by redness, swelling, hotness and pain, even pyogenesis, and ulceration.

In addition, fire corresponds with the heart. The heart governs blood and houses spirit. Flaring fire may give rise to, besides blood-heat and bleeding, a disturbing sign of the heart by fire pathogen including restlessness, fidgets, delirium, mania or coma.

7.1.1.2 Pestilent Pathogens

Pestilent pathogens are a kind of exogenous pathogens with a strong infectivity.

In Chinese medical literature for pestilent pathogens recorded there some other names such as pestilentiol agents, toxic qi, and special pathogens.

Diseases caused by pestilent pathogens have the features of abrupt attack, serious condition, similar symptoms, and intense infectivity and epidemicity. Pestilent pathogens may be transmitted through air or contagious infection, and often invade the body through the mouth and nose.

Diseases caused by pestilent pathogens may occur sporadically or pandemically. The examples are erysipelas of the face, mumps, fulminate dysentery, diphtheria, scarlatina, smallpox, cholera and plague. In fact, these actually include many infectious and intense infectious diseases in term of modern medicine.

The occurrence and epidemic of pestilential diseases usually involve the following factors: ① Natural climatic factors: Abnormal changes in the climate including prolonged drought, flooding, burning heat, bad fog, and natural disasters such as earthquakes. ② Environmental and dietary factors: For example, air, water and food pollution. ③ Social factors: Warfare or germ warfare, conditions of poverty, and social turbulence, as well as bad habit of health may all lead to epidemics of pestilential diseases. ④ Prevention and isolation are not well conducted..

7.1.2 Endogenous Pathogens

7.1.2.1 The Seven Emotions

The seven emotions refer to joy, anger, worry, thinking, sorrow, fear and fright. They are the psychological states of the body and different reflections of the body to objective things. Under normal conditions, they generally do not cause diseases. Sudden, intense or prolonged emotional stimulation beyond the regulatory range of physiological activities of the body can cause disturbances of qi dynamic, disorders of yin-yang and qi-blood of the viscera, thus giving rise to the onset of disease. As they are one of the major pathogenic factors causing endogenous diseases, they are also known as the "endogenous seven affects."

(1) Relations of the seven emotions to qi-blood and viscera: Chinese medicine theory holds that emotional activities are closely related to the viscera, and functional activities of the viscera depend on the driving and warming actions of qi, and the nourishment of blood. A *Zang*-viscus relates generally with an emotion, i e., the heart is associated with joy, the liver with anger, the spleen with thinking, the lung with worry, and the kidneys with fear. Joy, anger, thinking, worry and fear are collectively known as the "five emotions." Different emotional changes have different impacts on the viscera, and changes in qi-blood and the viscera also influences emotional changes.

(2) Pathogenic character of the seven emotions: There are differences between the seven emotions and six climatic pathogens in their pathogenicity. The six climatic pathogens invade the body through the skin or mouth and nose. At the early stage, the disease shows an exterior syndrome. An endogenous injury by the seven emotions however, directly affects the relative viscus, causing a disorder of qi dynamic in the viscus, a disturbance of qi-blood, and thus resulting in a variety of diseases. ① Direct injury to the viscus. Rage hurts the liver, over joy hurts the heart, over thinking hurts the spleen, grief hurts the lungs and great fear hurts the kidneys. Since the heart governs the spirit, it is the master of five *Zang*- and six *Fu*-viscera. If the heart-spirit is damaged, it will involve other viscera. The heart governs blood and houses the spirit. The liver is

in charge of free flow of qi, and stores blood. The spleen governs transformation and transportation, being located in the middle-Jiao as the hub of qi dynamic in ascending and descending, and is the source for generation of qi and blood. The diseases and syndromes caused by emotional pathogens, therefore, are common in the heart, liver and spleen, and in disturbances of qi-blood. For example, over thinking and overstrain of mind often harm the heart and spleen, leading to a deficiency of both qi and blood in the heart and spleen, marked as a disorder of the heart-spirit and failure of the spleen in transformation and transportation. Emotional depression and rage harm the liver, rage causes qi to go upward, and blood follows adverse rise of qi, and thus there may occur hypochondriac distension and sighing due to qi stagnation in the liver meridian; or hypochondriac pain, menorrhagia, amenorrheain in women, or abdominal masses due to qi stagnation with blood stasis. In addition, endogenous injury by emotional pathogens may also cause formation of fire, or "five emotions generate fire." This may lead to flaming up of fire with yin-deficiency, or stagnation of dampness, foodstuffs and phlegm. ② Influence on qi dynamic of the viscera: Because differences of stimulating factors, different emotional changes may cause their own special changes of qi dynamic of the viscera. Namely, "rage causes qi to go upward, over joy causes qi to relax, grief causes qi to be consumed, great fear causes qi to sink, great fright causes qi to get disordered, over-thinking causes qi to depress."

Rage causes qi to go upward. Rage may cause liver qi to go adversely upward, and blood follows. Clinically flushed face with congested eyes, hematemesis, and even syncope may occur.

Over joy causes qi to relax. There are two conditions. Under normal conditions, joy can relax mental tension, making the circulation of qi and blood smooth and putting the mind at ease. However, too much joy will make heart qi sluggish, and the spirit will be unable to rest, manifesting as absent-mindedness, and mental confusion.

Grief causes qi to be consumed. Great sorrow will result in depression and consumption of lung qi, marked by despondency, listlessness, shortness of breath, and lassitude.

Great fear causes qi to sink. Great fear will make kidney qi unconsolidated and sink downward. Clinically there might be incontinence of urine and feces, soreness and weakness of the bone, and spermatorrhea due to damage to the essence by prolonged fear.

Great fright causes qi to be disordered. Sudden fright may make the heart spirit lose its house, with presentations of hesitation and panic.

Over-thinking causes qi to depress. Over-thinking and anxiety may make spleen qi stagnated. Over-thinking may also cause the consumption of heart-blood and result in loss of nourishment for heart spirit, manifesting as palpitation, amnesia, insomnia, and dreaminess. Qi stagnation may cause the spleen to fail in transformation and transportation, and the stomach to fail in receiving and digestion. Thus loss of appetite, abdominal distention, and loose stool may occur.

Emotional upset may aggravate the patient's condition or rapidly exacerbate it. For example, if a patient with a history of dizziness becomes enraged, liver yang will suddenly rise. This can result in vertigo, or even sudden coma, hemiplegia, and deviation of the eye and mouth. The condition of a patient with heart disease can be aggravated by emotional upset.

7.1.2.2 Improper Diet

Food and drink are essential materials for the body to get nourishment and maintain its vital activities. However, an immoderate, insanitary or imbalanced diet may be important pathogens leading to disease. Food and drink mainly depend on the digestion of the spleen and stomach. So dietary ignorance mainly damages the spleen and stomach, leading to disorders of ascending and descending of qi, and accumulation of dampness, production of phlegm, generation of heat, or other disorders.

(1) Immoderate Diet: It is good to be moderate in eating and drinking. Starvation or overeating may result in disease. Starvation may lead to a reduction of the source of production of qi and blood due to shortage of food. After a long period, it will result in deficiency of qi and blood and cause disease. Meanwhile, because of deficient qi and blood, the vital qi becomes weak, and the resistance decreases. The body will then be subject to invasion by exopathic pathogens and other diseases. Overeating and fullness may cause stagnation of food and drink and harm the spleen and stomach. As a result, epigastric or abdominal distention with pain, foul belching and acid regurgitation, anorexia, vomiting, and diarrhea with foul and stinking stools will occur. Children with weak spleens and stomachs are likely to get this kind of disease, because they generally cannot control their intake.

(2) Insanitary Diet: Intake of dirty food may cause a variety of gastrointestinal diseases, marked by abdominal pain, vomiting, diarrhea, and dysentery. Some parasitic diseases caused by roundworm, hookworm, and tapeworm are marked by a sallow complexion with emaciation, parorexia, and abdominal pain. If the roundworm enters the biliary tract, it will result in "*Hui Jue*" (colic syndrome caused by roundworm) with symptoms of acute paroxysmal epigastric pain, cold limbs, and even vomit of roundworm. If one takes in poisonous or stale food, it will often lead to acute abdominal pain, vomit, diarrhea, or in severe cases even coma and death.

(3) Particular diet: Diet should be reasonably arranged and only in this manner can it supply the nutrition demanded by the body. An improper diet easily results in a deficiency of nutrients, or superiority or inferiority of either yin or yang, and hence disease. For example, rickets and night blindness are the outcome of malnutrition. Excessive intake of raw or cold foods may easily damage spleen yang, leading to a formation of internal cold dampness, and thus resulting in abdominal pain, and diarrhea. Over intake of greasy or spicy foods or indulgence in alcohol may lead to the formation of dampness heat, phlegm, stagnation of qi

and blood, and thus, bleeding, hemorrhoids, carbuncles and sores may occur.

7.1.2.3 Maladjustment of Work and Leisure

Improper work and leisure include over-strain and over-ease. Appropriate work and physical exercise are helpful in maintaining the proper circulation of qi and blood, and at the same time build up the physique. Suitable rest can dispel tiredness and restore the energy of both body and mind. Prolonged over-work or over-ease may cause disease.

(1) Over-work includes three aspects: physical over strain, mental over strain and sexual over strain

Physical overstrain refers to a long period of physical over-work leading to disease. Overstrain of the body consumes qi, leading to a deficiency of qi over a long period. Manifestations are feebleness, lassitude, reluctance to talk, listlessness, shortness of breath, panting and sweating on exertion.

Mental over strain refers to over thinking and mental work that harm the spleen and heart. Mental over strain consumes heart blood and harms spleen qi, and leads to the heart spirit losing its nourishment. This condition can manifest palpitation, amnesia, insomnia and dream disturbed sleep. In addition, it may also lead to a failure of the splan in transport and transformation, manifesting as poor appetite, abdominal distention, and loose stools.

Sexual over-strain implies intemperance in sexual activities or excess sexual intercourse. It consumes kidney-essence, resulting in aching and weakness of the lower back and knee joints, dizziness, tinnitus, lassitude and listlessness, spermatorrhea, premature ejaculation, impotence, menstrual disorders and leukorrhea.

(2) Over-ease: Over-ease includes lack of work and exercise. The human body needs suitable physical exercise everyday for good circulation of qi and blood. Over-ease may cause stagnation of qi and blood, flaccid tendons, weak bones, and hypofunction of the spleen and stomach manifesting with listlessness, general weakness, poor appetite, palpitation, dyspnea and sweating on just a little exertion, obesity, weak resistance against disease, and being subject to invasion of exopathic pathogens.

7.1.3 Pathogens from Pathological Products

A disease is a complicated pathological process with a given form caused by pathological factors. In the process, every stage has its own special pathological changes and clinical manifestations. Phlegm, stagnant fluid, and stagnant blood are the pathological outcome in the course of disease due to pathogenic factors. Once they form, they may disturb directly or indirectly the viscera and tissues, resulting in new disorders. Hence, they belong to one of the secondary pathogenic factors.

7.1.3.1 Phlegm and Stagnant Fluid

(1) Meanings of phlegm and stagnant fluid: Phlegm and stagnant fluid are the

pathological products of a water metabolism disorder. Generally, phlegm is thick and turbid, and stagnant fluid is thin and clear.

Phlegm not only implies sputum that is coughed up and visible, but also includes turbid phlegm that is in scrofula, subcutaneous nodules, or stagnating in the viscera and tissues that cannot be discharged. The latter can be determined by the syndrome caused by it, and is known as "invisible phlegm."

Stagnant fluid implies body fluid accumulation in a certain area of the body. According to the place where it accumulates and the symptoms it causes, it has different names such as "gastrointestinal fluid retention," "suspended fluid retention," "spilling fluid retention" and "propping fluid retention".

(2) Formation of phlegm and stagnant fluids: Phlegm and stagnant fluid form as body fluid stagnates because of water metabolism disturbances due to dysfunctions of the lungs, spleen, kidneys and tri-Jiao in qi transformation. This condition is usually caused by an exogenous invasion of the body by the six climatic pathogens, by endogenous injury of the body by dietary ignorance or the seven emotions. The retained water may become phlegm when it is simmered by yang-qi, and may condense into stagnant fluid when it meets yin-qi. After formation, stagnant fluid usually stays in the stomach, intestines, hypochondrium, chest, and subcutaneous areas; while phlegm follows the ascending and descending of qi to go into the viscera internally, and tendons, bones, skin and muscles externally, leading to a variety of disorders.

(3) Characters of disorders caused by phlegm and stagnant fluid: ① Blocking circulation of qi and blood: Phlegm and stagnant fluid are substantial pathological products. When they block meridians, they may adversely influence the circulation of qi and blood. When stagnating in the viscera, they may influence the functions of the viscera and the ascending-descending movement of qi. ② Influencing the metabolism of water: When phlegm and stagnant fluid stagnate in the viscera, they may influence the functions of the viscera to cause disorder of metabolism of water. ③ Being prone to disturb spirit: Heart spirit should keep clear to maintain its normal function. If the turbid-phlegm rises upward, it may confuse the heart and disturb the spirit. ④ Causing various and changeable diseases: Phlegm and stagnant fluid may go to every part of the body, inward to the viscera and outward to subcutaneous tissues, resulting in many disorders. Diseases caused by phlegm and stagnant fluid are characterized by both variety and changeableness.

7.1.3.2 Stagnant Blood

(1) Meaning of stagnant blood: Stagnant blood refers to stagnated blood held within the body. It includes extravagated blood and sluggish or stagnated blood. Stagnant blood is the pathological outcome in the progression of a disease. It is also a pathogenic factor for some diseases.

(2) Formation of stagnant blood: There are two main aspects involved in the

formation of stagnant blood. One type of stagnant blood is due to circulatory retardation caused by various factors including qi deficiency, qi stagnation, blood-cold and blood-heat. Qi is the commander of blood, and deficient or stagnate qi cannot properly circulate blood. Other causes for stagnant blood include a cold pathogen invading the blood vessels, making the vessels contract and spasm; and a heat pathogen invading the blood vessels and mingling with blood. Secondly, extravasated blood held in the body caused by various traumas, a deficient qi tailing to control blood, and wild flow of blood due to heat in it.

(3) Characters of disorders caused by stagnant blood: ① Blocking the flow of qi and blood: Blood can convey qi. As stagnant blood forms, it will lead to disorder of qi dynamic. Qi can circulate blood. As qi dynamic is disordered, it will lead to obstructed flow of blood. ② Influencing formation of new blood: As the stagnant blood blocks in the interior, it will cause disturbance of circulation of qi and blood, thus the viscera will dysfunction due to losing their nourishment. This may influence the formation of new blood. ③ Fixed location of disease with many and varied patterns: When stagnant blood stays in a certain part of the body, it will not easily to be dispelled; so the location of disease is relatively fixed. The different locations of stagnant blood stay are of different causes of formation; therefore, their pathological manifestations are also different. As a result, there will appear clinical feature of many and varied patterns.

7.1.4 Other pathogens

The reasons leading to diseases, besides exogenous pathogens, endogenous pathogens and pathogens from pathological products, include fetal transmission factor, parasite, and traumatic injuries.

7.1.4.1 Fetal Transmission Factors

Fetal transmission factors refers to the factors that form during the developing process of the fetus or inherited from the parents and cause diseases after birth. It may also be called congenital factors.

Fetal transmission may be due to shortage of parents' essence-qi; or during the pregnancy, the mother has disorders in emotion, diet and life style to influence normal growth and development of the fetus, leading to occurrence of various diseases after birth. The commonly seen are five flaccidities (flabby head and nape, flabby mouth, flabby hands, flabby feet, and flabby muscles), five retardations (standing retardation, walking retardation, tooth-erupting retardation, hair-growing retardation, and speaking retardation), infantile metopism, bayberysore, convulsion of newborn, newborn cold, and newborn heat.

7.1.4.2 Parasite

Taking in the food contaminated by parasitic ovum or contacting with polluted water, or earth may allow the parasite (or ovum) to enter the body, lodging in the viscera of the body to cause various diseases. Therefore, the parasites pertain to the category of pathogenic factors. The commonly seen are roundworm, hookworm, tapeworm, pinworm and schistosome.

The parasites mostly exist in the intestinal tract. Invasion of them presents generally with abdominal pain, parorexia, sallow complexion with emaciation. There are differences in infectious way and the part invaded by the parasites, so the clinical manifestations are also different. For example, in ascariasis, there is epigastric and abdominal pain; in ascriasis of biliary tract, there are acute pain of the abdomen and extreme cold of the limbs; in oxyuria, there is often itching of the anus. Besides, hookworm and schistosome mainly invade directly the body via the skin, stay in the viscera to cause functional disorders of the viscera, hence the diseases.

7.1.4.3 Traumatic Injuries

These refer to traumatic wounds, burns and scalds, frostbite, struck by lightening, drowning, and injuries by insect or animal.

Traumatic wounds include gunshot wounds, incised wounds, injuries from falls, fractures, contusions and strains, injuries by heavy loads, traffic accidents. All these can directly damage the skin, muscles, tendons, bones and internal organs.

Burns and scalds are mainly caused by burning and scorching from things with high temperature, fire, or fire device. They pertain to the attack by fire-toxin. The areas of the body invaded by them may immediately present with bubble in the local, brown skin and pain.

Frostbite refers to a general or local injury due to invasion of the body by low temperature. Generally, the lower the temperature is, the longer the time of exposure to cold, the more severe the frostbite. It includes general frostbite and local frostbite. Local frostbite often occurs in the hands, feet, auricles, nasal tip, and cheeks.

Struck by lightening refer to the damage to the body by thunders and lightening.

Drowning is sinking into the water caused by various reasons. It may cause one to get asphyxia, or even death.

Injuries by insect or animal include bites by poisonous snakes, beasts of prey, and mad dogs; or stings by scorpions and wasps. Injuries by insect or anima may cause damage to the skin and muscles in mild cases, injure the internal organs, or lead to death in sever cases.

7.2 Pathomechanism

Patho-mechanism is the mechanism of onset, development and change of a disease. The onset, development and change of disease are associated with the strength and physique of the patient and the nature of the pathogenic factors. Patho-mechanism includes three aspects of pathogenesis, types of attack and basic patho-mechanism.

7.2.1 Pathogenesis

Under normal conditions, the viscera and meridians of the body function well physiologically and qi-blood and yin-yang are in a harmonious balance. This state is known as "sound yin and firm yang". When the body is invaded by pathological factors, the physiological functions of the viscera and the meridians become disordered, and the harmonious balance of qi-blood and yin-yang are broken down, leading to an "imbalance of yin and yang" manifested by various clinical symptoms, hence the onset of a disease.

7.2.1.1 The Onset of a Disease Concerns Vital Qi and Pathogenic Qi

Vital qi, also known as "the vital", refers to functional activities (including the functions of the viscera, meridians, qi and blood) and the resistance and recovery capacity of the body. Pathogenic qi generally refers to various pathogens causing disease, and it is known as "the pathogen". The onset and change is a reflection of the struggle between the vital and pathogens in a certain condition.

(1) A deficiency of vital qi is the inner basis of pathogenesis. Chinese medicine attaches a great importance to vital qi. It is believed that when vital qi is vigorous, qi and blood are abundant, external defensive power is strong, the pathogenic qi cannot invade the body, and disease will not occur. Only when vital qi becomes relatively weak, the defensive power externally unconsolidated, resistance is not sound, can the pathogenic qi invade the body, leading to disease.

(2) The invasion of pathogenic qi is the important condition of pathogenesis. Chinese medicine attaches importance to the vital qi. However at the same time of emphasizing the leading role of the vita, Chinese medicine does not rule out important role of the pathogenic qi in the onset of disease The pathogenic qi is the important condition for the onset of disease; and under a certain conditions, it even plays a leading role. The diseases caused by pestilent pathogens or traumatic injury are the examples. Therefore, when talking about prevention of various infectious diseases, *Sù Wèn* (*Plain Questions*) put forth that in addition to the importance of maintaining vigorous vital qi, one must also strive to "keep away from the toxic."

7.2.1.2 The Situation of Struggle between Vital and the Pathogen Determines Whether a Disease Occurs or Not

The struggle between vital qi and pathogenic qi not only involves the onset of a disease, but also governs the development and prognosis of the disease.

(1) No disease occurs as the vital can defeat the pathogen. In the process of the struggle between the vital and the pathogen, if the vital qi is vigorous and strongly fights

against the pathogen, the latter will fail in invading the body, or the invading pathogen will be promptly eliminated by the vital qi. Thus, no pathologic change occurs and no disease appears. For example, in nature various pathogenic qi exist, but not everyone exposed to them becomes ill. This is the outcome that the vital defeats the pathogen.

(2) Disease occurs as the pathogen defeats the vital. In the process of struggle between the vital and the pathogen, if the pathogenic qi is superior in strength to the vital qi, the pathogen will defeat the vital, leading to an imbalance of yin-yang and qi-blood of the viscera, disorders of qi dynamic, and hence a disease occurs.

After the onset of a disease, different patterns of disease may appear because of differences in the strength of vital qi, the nature and quantity of the invading pathogen, and the depth of location of the pathogen.

The relation of disease to the strength of vital qi: As vital qi is vigorous; the fight between the vital and the pathogen will be intense, which is usually marked as an excessive syndrome. While if the vital qi gets deficient, it will fight weakly against the pathogen, which often manifests as a deficient syndrome or a mixed syndrome of deficiency and excess.

The relation of disease to the nature of the invading pathogen: Generally speaking, a yang-pathogen invasion is apt to lead to an exuberance of yang and consumption of yin, resulting in an excess-heat syndrome; while a yin-pathogen invasion is likely to cause an exuberance of yin and damage to yang, leading to a cold-excess syndrome.

The relation of disease to the quantity of the invading pathogen: Generally, the less the pathogen is, the milder the disease is; and the more the pathogenicis, the severer the disease is.

The relation of disease to the location of the invading pathogen: As the pathogen may invade the tendons, bones, meridians, or viscera; so the disease patterns will be different.

7.2.1.3 Various Factors Influencing Vital Qi

Chinese medicine holds that pathogenic factors (pathogens) are the significant condition in the onset of a disease, and deficiency or relative deficiency of vital qi is the internal ground in the onset of a disease. The major factors that influence vital qi are the constitution and psychological state of a person.

(1) Relation between the constitution and the vital qi: A person with a strong constitution has sound functions of the viscera, abundant essence, qi, blood and body fluid, and then he has a strong vital qi. A person with a weak constitution has weak functions of the viscera, deficient essence, qi, blood and body fluid, and then he has a weak vital qi.

The constitution of an individual depends upon the innate endowment, dietary nutrition, and physical training. Generally, one with an ample endowment from her or his parents enjoys a strong physique while one with a deficient endowment has a weak physique. A reasonable diet and proper nutrition are essential for a person to grow and develop. Lack of food and or malnutrition will decrease the formation of qi and blood and in turn lead to a weak physique. Eating and drinking too much will damage the spleen and stomach. A particular diet will cause an imbalance in nutrition and adversely influence the physique. Physical training and work may maintain the smooth circulation of qi and blood and at the same time keep one fit. Over-ease and a lack of exercise will harm the circulation of qi and blood, reduce the functions of the spleen and stomach and ultimately result in a weak physique.

(2) Relation of psychological state to vital qi: The psychological state of an individual is directly influenced by emotional pathogens. A relaxed mind and happy feeling contribute to a smooth movement of qi, harmony of qi and blood, and cooperative functions of the viscera, thus, the vital qi will be vigorous. Conversely, an uneasy mind and depressed feeling may cause disturbances of qi dynamic, imbalances of yin-yang and qi-blood, and dysfunctions of the viscera, thus the vital qi will decline. Therefore, when one pays attention to mental hygiene, keeps an easy mind, and has no strong desires, then the genuine qi will be harmonious and the individual will be full of go.

Briefly, deficiency of vital qi is the internal basis of the onset of a disease. The constitution and psychological state concern the strength of the vital qi. A strong constitution and happy mood contribute to sound vital qi with strong resistance, then the pathogenic qi cannot invade the body, or the invading pathogen is easily to be eliminated, thus disease will not develop. If the constitution is weak and the mood is unhappy, the vital qi will be deficient, with weak resistance, and thus the body will be easily invaded by the pathogenic qi to cause disease.

7.2.2 Type of Attack

The natures, quantities and passages of the invading pathogens are different, so are individual constitutions and strengths of vital-qi. Therefore, there may appear differences in type of attack. To sum up, there are five types of attack: immediate attack, latent attack, slow attack, secondary attack and relapse.

7.2.2.1 Immediate attack

Immediate attack, being also called "sudden attack" or "instant attack", refers to that a disease immediately occurs after contraction of a pathogen. Clinically, it is a common type. It includes the following aspects. The first is newly contraction of exogenous pathogens. Invasion by six climatic pathogens is mostly an exogenous disease that occurs immediately after contraction. The second is invasion by pestilent pathogens. Some pestilent pathogens have strong pathogenicity and infectivity. Therefore, their invasion will lead to sudden attack, and the condition is more critical. The third is sudden emotional disturbance. For example, acute emotional changes such as great rage and heavy grief may make disordered flow of qi-blood to cause sudden attack. The fourth is poisoning. If one has wrongly taken in the poisonous food, drugs and inhales poisonous gases, or bites by poisonous insects or snakes, he may quickly get an illness with a toxic reaction, or even die. The fifth are acute traumas such as incised wound, gunshot, falls down, sprains and strains, burns and scalds, frostbite and struck by electricity, directly resulting in diseases.

7.2.2.2 Slow attack

It is opposite to immediate attack. It is closely associated to nature of the pathogen, and the constitutional factor of the patient. For example, the dampness pathogen is characterized by stagnation and viscosity, so, most of exogenous diseases caused by it slowly occur, with a long course. For some old patients whose vital-qi has already gotten deficient, if they are affected by exogenous pathogens, the disease often slowly occurs. This is due to low response of the body. In endogenous disease, pensiveness, great sorrow, indulgence in sexual life, addiction to alcohol, and preference for eating fat food with thick flavors may cause pathological changes that progressively develop day by day, and result in obvious clinical symptoms and sign after a long period.

7.2.2.3 Latent attack

It is also called attack by latent pathogen, indicating that after a pathogen invades the body, it hides in a part of the body, after a period of time or under the action of a certain inducing factors, a disease occurs. The examples are tetanus, rabies, AIDS and warm-disease caused by latent pathogen in Chinese medicine. As for the mechanism of pathogenesis by latent pathogen, ancient physicians believed that, because the quantity of the invading pathogen is little and the vital qi is deficient, the disease would not immediately appear; however, the pathogen can take the advantage of the deficient vital qi to hide in the body, and to cause disease later. In endogenous diseases, the cases caused by the latent pathogens are also common. For example, apoplexy with hemiplegia duo to blockage of collaterals by wind-phlegm, which is usually due to a long period of internal retention of phlegm and stagnant fluid, and the contribution of inducing factor like emotional disturbance.

7.2.2.4 Secondary attack

A new disorder occurring based on the primary disease is called secondary attack. Secondary disease must take primary disease as its prerequisite. So, there are closely pathological relations between them. For example, hypochondriac pain and jaundice in liver disease, if not to be treated in time and appropriately, after a long period, they may develop secondarily abdominal mass and tympanite. Another example, repeated attack of malaria tertian may secondarily result in splenomegaly. A prolonged indigestion with insufficiency of the spleen and stomach of intestinal parasitosis in children can produce malnutrition with accumulation.

7.2.2.5 Relapse

Relapse Refers to attack once more or repeatedly of the primary disease. This is a special type of attack, and a reflection of struggle between the vital and the pathogen under a certain conditions.

(1) The characters of relapse: The relapse of disease has the following characters: First relapse of any disease is the representation of the basic pathological changes and major pathological features of the primary disease. Secondly, relapse of disease mostly is of severer condition than the original, and the more times of relapse, the more complicated the condition. The last, relapse of disease mostly has a certain inducing factors.

(2) The factors of relapse: The factors of relapse are mainly as the following: ① Relapse due to improper diet: At the beginning of recovery, a reasonable diet is conducive to the recovery of the health. If one eats too much or takes in the food that is not easily digested, then it will hinder the recovery of his vital qi. In addition, it again helps the residual pathogen by stagnated foodstuffs and heat induced by alcohol. Thus, the disease may relapse. ② Relapse due to overstrain: When a disease has just been cured, appropriate rest and adjustment can help recovery of the vital qi of the body. Too early work will consume qi; or indulgence in sexual life makes the essence damaged; or metal overstrain injures qi and blood. All these can lead to disharmony of yin-yang, and disorder of qi-blood, and jury of the vital qi. Then the residual pathogen may get rampant again to cause relapse. For example, such endogenous diseases as edema, fluid retention and asthma often relapse repeatedly due to injury of the vital qi by overstrain or re-contraction of exogenous pathogens. ③ Relapse due to abuse of medicine: As a disease tends to be cured, some medicinal regulation as the subsidiary can serve as the important mean to promote recovery of the vital qi. The principle for medication should be to strengthen the vital but not help the pathogen, and to eliminate the pathogen but not damage the vital. If the regulating medicinal regimen is not proper, tonics are in abuse taken, or too early or too drastically the tonics are given, it will lead to lingering of the pathogen, and thus relapse occurs. ④ Relapse by new affection: When a disease is in the period of getting well, re-contraction of exogenous pathogens may also be a factor to cause relapse. For example, after a primary disease goes through a developing stage, it is in a silent period, but the residual pathogen does not be removed, and the vital qi does not recover yet, with a lower resistance. At this moment, it is most easily to catch new pathogen and induce the relapse of the primary disease. ⑤ Relapse by other factors: Relapse of disease is also related to some other factors such as metal factor, geographic and environmental factors, and improper medical care. If the emotional disturbance is too large, or suddenly one gets strong psychological stimuli, then it not only influences

the recovery of the vital qi, but also can make reverse flow of qi-blood, and thus relapse occurs. ⑥ Spontaneous relapse: It mainly refers to a case that, during the early recovery, the disease spontaneously relapses, without any reasons such overstrain, improper diet, medication and turbulent emotion, as well as exogenous contraction of new pathogen. This is mostly due to insufficiency of the vital qi and internal stay of the residual pathogen.

7.2.3 Basic Patho-mechanism

The basis pathomechanism means the fundamental mechanisms of the onset, development and change of disease.

The onset, development and change of a disease are related to the strength of constitution of the patient and the nature of pathogenic qi. When a pathogenic factor invades the body, vital qi will go up to fight against the pathogen, and thus leading to a struggle between the vital and the pathogen. This in turn leads to breakdown of the relative balance of yin and yang in the body, disorders of the ascending and descending of qi dynamic of the viscera, and disturbance of qi and blood. As a result, a series of pathological changes occur. Therefore, diseases are complex and changeable, but their pathological processes generally fall under the general laws of struggle between the vital and the pathogen, and imbalances of yin and yang.

7.2.3.1 Superiority or Inferiority of the Vital or the Pathogen

The struggle between the vital and the pathogen not only concerns the onset of a disease, but also governs the development and conversion of the disease. Meanwhile, it also directly influences the deficient or excessive change of a disease pattern. Thus in a sense, the processes of many diseases are the processes of the struggle between the vital and the pathogen.

(1) The relations of struggle between the vital and the pathogen to deficient or the excessive changes: The strengths of two sides of the vital and the pathogen are oppositely changeable during the process of their fight. In general, as the vital grows the pathogen declines, and as the pathogen grows the vital declines. Following the outcome of the growth and decline of the vital and the pathogen, the patient will present with pathologies and patterns of deficiency and excess. There is a saying in *Sù Wèn* (*Plain Questions*): "Superiority of pathogenic qi leads to an excess and inferiority of essential qi leads to a deficiency".

Excess in this case means that the pathogenic qi is excessive. It is a pathological reflection indicating that excessive pathogenic qi is the principal aspect of the contradiction. The pathological features are as follows: Pathogenic qi is excessive and the vital qi is not decline but strong enough to fight against the pathogenic qi, thus the struggle between the vital and the pathogen is acute. Clinically this condition is an excess syndrome with an intense reaction. It is often seen in the early or middle stages of exogenous diseases, and in disorders caused by stagnation of phlegm, foodstuffs, blood or water. For example, such clinical symptoms as high fever, mania, speaking lustily, coarse breathing, abdominal pain aggravated by pressure, retention of urine and stool, and forceful pulse, all come under the category of excess syndrome.

Deficiency implies that the vital qi is deficient. This condition is a pathological reflection of deficient vital qi as the principal aspect in the contradiction. The pathological features are as follows. The vital qi gets deficient and fails to fight against pathogenic qi, with no presentations of intense pathological reaction, and clinically there are a series of hypoactive and weak syndromes. Deficient syndromes usually occur in patients with a weak physique, or in the late stage of a disease, or in a chronic disease. For example, all may cause deficiency of vital qi with hypo-function such as consumption of essential qi in a serious or protracted disease; or consumption of qi, blood, body fluid due to polyhidrosis, profuse vomiting or diarrhea, or heavy bleeding. The manifestations are listlessness, lassitude, wan and thin appearance, palpitation, shortness of breath, spontaneous or night sweating, dysphoria with a feverish sensation in the palms and soles, aversion to cold with cold limbs, and feeble pulse.

The struggle between the vital and the pathogen can determine deficiently or excessively pathological changes. In some long and complicated diseases, it can also lead to a mixture of deficiency and excess. This is often caused by injury of the vital qi due to long say of the pathogen, or originally the vital qi is weak and fails to drive the pathogen, thus leading to stagnation and blockage of phlegm, foodstuffs, blood and water. As a result, it makes the excess pathogens accumulated to block the meridians so that qi and blood cannot flow smoothly, hence a case of real excess with pseudo-deficiency; or it gives a rise to shortage of visceral qi and blood with hypofunctions of the viscera, hence a case of real deficiency with pseudo-excess.

(2) The relations of struggle between the vital and the pathogen to conversion of disease: In the course of a disease, the struggle between the vital and the pathogen may result in either a superiority of the vital with a decline of the pathogen or a superiority of the pathogen with a deficiency of the vital. In the former, the disease takes a turn to better and gets well; and in the latter, the disease gets deteriorated or the patient dies. If the vital and the pathogen are evenly matched in strength, then it will result in a situation known as "the vital and the pathogen in a stalemate."

Superiority of the vital with decline of the pathogen: In the struggle between the vital and the pathogen, if the vital qi is sufficient with a strong resistance, then the pathogenic qi will have difficulty in growing, and the effects of the pathogen on the body will disappear or stop. In turn, the viscera and the meridians with pathological injury will gradually recuperate, the essence, qi, blood and body fluid consumed will gradually be replenished, the dynamic balance between yin and yang will be restored, and the disease cured. For example, in exogenous diseases, the pathogenic qi invades the body via the skin, hair, mouth and nose. When the vital qi is sufficient to fight against the pathogen, it will not only confine the disorder to the body surface or meridians, but also drive the pathogen out quickly. Through diaphoresis, which can relieve the exterior and eliminate pathogens, the defensive and the nutritive qi will become harmonized, and hence the disease will be cured.

Superiority of the pathogen with deficiency of the vital: In the struggle between the vital and the pathogen, should the pathogenic qi be excessive and vital qi deficient, the resistance would become more and more insufficient, and might not check the growth of pathogenic qi. This condition will result in the injury of the body pathologically and will become more and more serious. Hence, the condition of the patient will tend to deteriorate. If the vital qi collapses and pathogenic qi gets rampant, the physiological functions of qi-blood, viscera and meridians will become insufficient, and yin and yang will separate. Thus, the vital activities of the body will stop and the patient will die. Examples of this are the "depletion of yin" and "depletion of yang" in the progress of exogenous febrile diseases.

In addition, in the struggle between the vital and the pathogen, if the two sides are evenly matched in strength, the vital and the pathogen will be at a stalemate, or the vital is deficient while the pathogen lingers, or the pathogen is eliminated while the vital is not yet restored. Under these conditions, the disease can develop from acute to chronic, or leave some sequelae, or become retractable.

7.2.3.2 Imbalance of Yin-yang

The imbalance of yin and yang is a pathological state in which either yin fails to check yang or yang fails to check yin when a superiority or inferiority of either yin or yang results from a loss of their relative balance due to action of pathogenic qi on the body. An imbalance of yin and yang is also a generalization of the disharmonious interrelations in viscera, meridians, qi-blood, nutritive-defensive qi, and a disorder of qi in ascending and descending. Since various pathogenic qi acting on the body such as the six climatic pathogens, seven emotions, improper diet, and overstrain must lead to an imbalance of yin and yang in the body so as to cause disease, the imbalance of yin and yang is again the inner basis of the onset and development of a disease.

Though the pathological changes caused in an imbalance of yin and yang are very complicated, their manifestations, however, all come under the aspects of superiority of yin or yang, inferiority of yin or yang, mutual affection of yin and yang, blockage of yin or yang, and depletion of yin or yang.

(1) Superiority of yin or yang: This mainly refers to an excess syndrome because "exuberance of pathogenic qi leads to excess". An invading pathogen is bound to associate its kind alike. In other words, a yang-pathogen invading the body may cause a superiority of yang and a yin-pathogen invading the body may cause a superiority of yin.

Yin and yang have an inter-restrictive relationship. Yang is bound to wane as yin is waxing, and yin is bound to wane as yang is waxing. A superiority of yang will certainly check yin and cause a yin deficiency. A superiority of yin will also check yang and cause a yang deficiency.

The superiority of yang is a pathological state, during the process of a disease, presenting with exuberance of yang qi, hyperactive functions and surplus heat. The pathological feature is an excess-heat syndrome resulting from exuberant yang without yin deficiency. The causative factors for a superiority of yang are mostly invasions by warm-heat pathogens of a yang nature, invasions by yin pathogens that turn into heat by later joining yang, fire production transformed from extreme emotions, and or heat from qi stagnation, blood stasis, or food retention. Yang is characterized by heat, dynamic and dryness. Thus, a superiority of yang will cause an excess-heat syndrome manifesting as a high fever, flushed face, red eyes, restlessness, red tongue with yellow and dry coating, abdominal distending pain which is aggravated by pressure, tidal fever, and delirium. Predominating yang makes yin suffer, so in a syndrome of yang superiority, the accompanying symptoms of yin deficient such as thirst with a desire for cold drink, constipation, and scanty urine might also appear.

The superiority of yin is a pathological state occurring during the process of a disease in which yin-qi is prevailing with hypoactive functions, a decrease in thermogenesis, and an accumulation of pathological products metabolized. The main pathological feature is an excess-cold syndrome resulting from exuberant yin without yang deficiency. The causative factors for a superiority of yin mostly include an invasion by a cold-dampness pathogen of a yin nature, or an excess intake of raw and cold food resulting in retention of cold-dampness in the middle-Jiao, which in turn leads to a failure of yang in checking yin and yin then becomes excessive. Yin is characterized by cold, stillness and dampness. A superiority of yin often manifests as a cold-excessive syndrome with symptoms of cold body and limbs, pale tongue, abdominal pain with a cold feeling aggravated by pressure, and loose stools. Since predominating yin makes yang suffer, in a case of yin superiority, yang deficiency symptoms of aversion to cold, listlessness, and lying with in the body curled up might appear.

(2) Inferiority of yin or yang: This is a deficient syndrome because "despoliation of essential qi leads to deficiency". When reduction of substance or a decrease of function in either side of yin or yang occurs, it will lead to a relative exuberance of the counterpart. Then the following pathological changes appear: A yang deficiency leads to superiority of yin and a yang deficiency results in cold (deficiency-cold); a yin deficiency leads to hyperactivity of yang and a yin deficiency results in heat (deficiency-heat).

The inferiority of yang is a pathological state developed during the process of a disease with yang qi deficiency, and hypofunction and shortage of thermogenesis. The main pathological feature is a deficiency-cold syndrome resulting from a relative exuberance of yin due to a failure of deficient yang in checking yin. The causative factors are congenital defects, dietary ignorance, overstrain, or damage of yang-qi due to a protracted disease. An inferiority of yang leads to cold. Clinically it often shows a deficiency-cold syndrome manifesting as aversion to cold, cold limbs, restlessness, lying with the body curled up, abdominal pain responsive to warmth and pressure, loose stools, clear and profuse urine, and slow and forceless pulse.

The inferiority of yin is a pathological state that results in the process of a disease with consumption of essence, blood and body fluid, and hyperfunction of a deficient nature due to relative hyperactivity of yang because failure of yin to check yang. The pathological feature is a deficiency-heat syndrome resulting from relative exuberance of yang due to decreased action of yin-fluid in nourishing, calming and restricting yang-heat. The inferiority of yin is mostly caused by damage of yin by yang-pathogens, consumption of yin by fire resulting from extreme emotional changes, or injury of yin due to a protracted disease. An inferiority of yin leads to heat. Clinically it usually presents with a deficiency-heat syndrome. The manifestations are dysphoria with a feverish feeling in the five centers, tidal fever as if spreading out from steaming bones, flushed face, emaciation, night sweating, dry throat and mouth, red tongue with little coating, and thready, rapid forceless pulse.

(3) Mutual affection of yin and yang: The mutual affection of yin and yang means that in a prerequisite of deficiency of either yin or yang, illness progresses to involve the counterpart, resulting in a pathological state of deficiency of both yin and yang.

Involvement of yang by yin deficiency: This implies that, because of shortage of yin-fluid, the illness involves yang-qi, leading to dyspoiesis or escape of yang qi due to shortage of what it depends on. Hence, based on yin deficiency, there appears yang deficiency, forming a pathological state of deficiency of both yin and yang, but with yin deficiency being more serious. For instance, in deficiency of kidney-yin, there is dizziness and vertigo, and soreness and weakness in the lower back and knees. Once the production of kidney-yang is affected, it may lead to kidney-yang deficiency manifested as impotence or cold limbs. The illness might then turn into a deficiency of both yin and yang due to involvement of yang by yin deficiency.

Involvement of yin by yang deficiency: This means that, because deficiency of yang-qi makes the generation of yin-fluid short. As a result, based on yang deficiency, yin deficiency appears, forming a pathological state of deficiency of both yin and yang, with yang deficiency standing out. For instance, in edema due to yang deficiency once the production of yin-essence is harmed, there will appear accompanying symptoms of yin deficiency such as emaciation, dysphoria, or chronic convulsion. It thus becomes a deficiency of both yin and yang due to involvement of yin by yang deficiency.

(4) Blockage of yin or yang: This is a kind of special pathological changes in the imbalance of yin and yang. It includes two respects: Exuberant yin blocks yang and

exuberant yang blocks yin. The mechanism of blockage of yin or yang is that yin or yang becomes so extreme that it condenses internally and rejects its counterpart externally, rendering a condition that yin and yang are unable to hold together. Thus there appears the pathological phenomenon of a real cold with pseudo-heat or a real heat with pseudo-cold.

Exuberant yin blocks yang: This is a pathological state because exuberant yin-cold pathogens accumulate internally and force yang qi to go outside, and thus yin qi and yang qi fail to connect with each other. In this case, the exuberance of yin-cold internally is the essence of the disease; but the yang is rejected outside, so there appear the signs of red complexion, heat with dysphoria, thirsty and large pulse. So, it is called a real cold syndrome with pseudo-heat symptoms.

Exuberant yang blocks yin: This is a pathological state because excess yang heat accumulates deeply and internally, yang-qi fails to go externally to the limbs and rejects yin externally. The exuberance of yang-heat inside is the essence of the disease. However, because yin is blocked externally, clinically there appear the signs of pseudo-cold such as cold limbs, and deep and hidden pulse. Therefore, it is called a real heat syndrome with pseudo-cold symptoms.

(5) Depletion of yin or yang: Depletion of yin or yang is a pathological state of critical illness caused by a sudden massive loss of yin-fluid or yang-qi of the body.

Depletion of yang is a pathological state of the sudden failure of bodily functions caused by a sudden exhaustion of yang-qi. The commonly causes for depletion of yang may be invasion of excessive pathogens, which defeat the vital and lead to a sudden exhaustion of yang-qi; or ordinarily yang deficiency with a weak vital qi, and over consumption of qi by overstrain, or improperly or excessively use of diaphoresis, emesis, and purgation which lead to a massive loss of body fluid with consequent exhaustion of yang-qi, or outside escape of deficient yang in a chronic consumptive disease. It is clinically a critical syndrome with manifestations of profuse sweating, cold skin and limbs, listlessness, and faint pulse hardly felt.

Depletion of yin is a pathological state of collapse of the functions of the entire body caused by a sudden and massive loss or consumption of yin-fluid. The causative factors are too much heat pathogen, or protracted detention of heat pathogen that greatly consume yin fluid, or a massive consumption of yin-fluid due to other factors. The clinical manifestations of this critical syndrome are short and rapid breathing, thirst, warm limbs, and hyper-hidrosis with a tendency to collapse.

Depletion of yin and depletion of yang are different in both pathomechanism and manifestations, However, because of the interdependence of yin and yang, yin depletion will make yang lose its attachment and escape; and yang depletion will make yin loss its basis for production and exhausts. Therefore, a depletion of yin and a depletion of yang usually occur in succession, and finally lead to a "separation of yin and yang," hence the end of life.

7.2.3.3 Disorders of Qi and Blood

Disorders of qi and blood are pathological states that occur during the process of a disease because either of struggle between the vital and the pathogen, or disturbance of visceral functions, including deficiency of qi or blood, disturbance in circulation or physiological function of qi or blood, and disturbance in relationship between qi and blood.

(1) Disorders of qi: Disorders of qi mainly refer to qi deficiency due to dyspoiesis or over consumption of qi, and functional insufficiency of qi; and disturbance of qi dynamic as well,

Qi deficiency: It is a pathological state of qi shortage because of dyspoiesis or over consumption of qi, in which there appear hypofunctions of the viscera and tissues and weak resistance. The causative factors for deficiency of qi include shortage of inborn essence due to defect of natural endowment; or reduction of production due to malnutrition after birth; or too much consumption of qi in a protracted disease; or dyspoiesis of qi due to functional disturbance of the lung, spleen and kidney.

Qi has the functions to drive, control and transform. Therefore, the common disorders of qi deficiency are anomalies in failure of qi to drive, control and transform. The manifestations are lassitude and listlessness, spontaneous sweating, being apt to catch cold. As it further develops, it may lead to short production and slow circulation of essence, blood and body fluid, or loss of them due to failure of them to be controlled,

Disturbance of qi dynamic: It is a pathological change of qi in ascent, descent, exit and entrance resulting from disturbance by the pathogens, or functional disorders of the viscera. The condition may be summarized into five respects of stagnancy of qi, regurgitation of qi, sinking of qi, blockage of qi and exhaustion of qi.

Stagnancy of qi: This is a pathological state of hindered flow and stagnation of qi. It is mainly caused by emotional depression or retention of excess pathogens such as phlegm-dampness, foodstuff accumulation, stagnant blood; or obstruction of qi dynamic by invading exogenous pathogens; or functional disorders of the viscera. These conditions influence the normal flow of qi, and cause hindering or blockage of qi dynamic in a local part or the whole body. The stagnancy of qi in different parts has its own concrete patho-mechanism and clinical manifestations. For example, an invasion of exogenous pathogens makes the lung fail to diffuse and descend, the upper-Jiao is blocked in qi dynamic, then there often appear panting, cough, and chest distress. A dietary injury leads to qi stagnancy in the intestine and stomach, then their dredging and descending functions fail, there usually occur abdominal distension, and pain that is on and off, and relieved by either passing flatus or belching. However there are a common feature for qi stagnancy everywhere; and stuffiness, distension and pain are the common clinical manifestations.

Regurgitation of qi: It is a pathological state of adversely rising of qi due to hyper-ascending and hypo-descending. It is mostly caused by emotional injury; or improper diet in food temperature; or invasion by exogenous pathogens; or retention of turbid phlegm. The disorders of qi regurgitation mostly occur in the lung, stomach and liver. For example, exogenous pathogens invade the lung or turbid phlegm blocks the lung, it will make the lung qi fail in purification and descent and cause qi to go adversely upward; then there may occur panting and shortage of breath. An improper diet in food temperature or foodstuff accumulation with indigestion may lead to failure of stomach qi in harmonious descent or adverse rising of qi dynamic; then there will appear nausea, vomiting, hiccup and eructation. An emotional injury by anger may cause qi to go upward adversely, or lead to generation of fire because the liver qi gets depressed; or qi-blood will adversely rise because the liver qi hyperactively ascends and moves; then there may occur flushed face, red eyes, distention and pain in the head, irritability, or oven hematemesis, and syncope.

Sinking of qi: This refers to a pathological state characterized by powerless lifting of qi based on qi deficiency. It belongs to disorder of ascending and descending of qi. Since the spleen and stomach are located in the middle-Jiao, being the origin for production of qi-blood; and spleen qi is in charge of descending and stomach qi is in charge of descending, being the hub for ascending and descending of qi dynamic. Therefore, the disorder of qi sinking is closely related with the qi deficiency of the spleen and stomach. Generally sinking of qi is called "sinking of the middle qi" or "sinking of the spleen qi". It is mainly caused by weak physique in a prolonged disease, or in elderly people, or protracted diarrhea, or too many times of childbearing in women, which make qi too deficient to keep lifting power. Owing to deficiency of the spleen qi, it fails to send up the clear; thus, no enough foodstuff essence can be transported upward to the head and eyes, then there occurs shortage of the upper qi manifested as dizziness and vertigo, tinnitus, and deafness. Because the spleen qi is short of lifting power there even occur prolepses of the internal organs with the manifestations of down-bearing sensation of lower abdomen, frequent desires for defecation, or proctoptosis, hysteroptosis, and gastroptosis,

Blockage of qi: This is a pathological change of depression and blockage of qi dynamic, and obstruction of qi to go out. It is a pathological state of sudden syncope. It is mostly due to extreme emotional changes which make the liver fail to keep flow of qi and thus yang qi cannot go externally and being depressed internally in the heart; or blockage of exogenous pathogens with accumulation of turbid-phlegm which causes lung qi blocked and obstruction of gas tract. Therefore the disorders of blockage of qi are mostly acute, presenting with sudden syncope or comma, unconsciousness, non-warmness of the limbs, dyspnea, and cyonoses of the face and lips.

Exhaustion of qi: This is a pathological change of extreme qi deficiency with a critical tendency of collapse. It is a pathological state of general functional failure mostly caused by failure of the vital qi to fight against the pathogen, or outside escape of qi due to prolonged deficiency of qi to the extreme. Exhaustion of qi is the major patho-mechanism of various disorders of faintness. The causative factors are too rampancy of the pathogens and failure of the vital qi to fight against them; or extreme deficiency of qi due to a long period of consumption of qi in chronic diseases; or exhaustion of qi following exhaustion of blood, or great loss of body fluid resulting from massive bleeding or profuse sweating. Because qi looses greatly, there occur serious deficiency of qi generally, and thus the functional activities become declined. So clinically, the patient with exhaustion of qi has a critical signs of pale complexion, continuously sweating, open mouth, closed eyes, general flaccid paralysis, flaccid hands, incontinence of urine and stool.

(2) Disorders of blood: Disorders of blood mainly refer to the pathological states of deficiency of blood caused by dyshematopoiesis or over consumption of blood, hypofunction of blood in nourishing and disordered circulation of blood

Deficiency of blood: This is a pathological state of shortage f blood or hypofunction of blood. The liver stores blood and the heart governs blood. Therefore, deficiency of blood mostly occurs in the two viscera. The causative factors for blood deficiency are mainly of three aspects: One is massive loss of blood and no new blood can be promptly replenished. Next is shortage of production such as that, the spleen and stomach get insufficient and fail in transformation and transportation, then the production of blood gets reduced; or kidney essence gets short, thus the essence-marrow will be not enough to transform into blood. The last is gradual consumption of nutritive-blood due to a prolonged illness.

All the tissue organs of the body rely on nourishing function of blood, and blood can convey qi. As blood gets short, qi in it will be deficient. Furthermore blood is also the material basis of mental activity, so as blood gets deficient, and its nourishing function gets declined, there will appear a serious general or local asthenic presentations of pale and un-lustrous complexion, lips and nails, dizziness, amnesia, listlessness, lassitude, emaciation, palpitation, insomnia, dry and discomfort feeling of eyes, and blurred vision.

Disorder of blood flow: This means a pathological change of blood stasis, or accelerating flow of blood, or bleeding due to frenzied flow of blood. Its causative factors are the influence of some invading pathogens or functional disturbance of the viscera during the course of a disease.

Blood stasis: Blood stasis imports a pathological state that circulation of blood is sluggish or obstructed, even stagnates and stops. The common reasons for blood stasis are as follows: impeded blood flow due to stagnation of qi; sluggish flow of blood due to lack of driving power resulting from deficiency of qi; coagulation of blood caused by invasion of cold pathogen; boiled down of blood on account of invasion by heat pathogen; obstruction of the vessels by turbid phlegm; and "involvement of the collaterals due to a prolonged illness". When blood stagnates in the viscera, meridians or a local part, it will cause local pain being fixed (hindrance goes before pain), or even formation of abdominal mass. If sluggish blood flow occurs generally, there may appear darkness and cyonoses of face, lips, tongue, nails and skin.

Acceleration of blood flow: This refers to a pathological state that blood is forced to flow quickly and looses its calm nature under the actions of some pathogenic factors. Development of this condition is mostly caused by invasion of heat into blood level due to exogenous contraction of pathogens of yang-heat nature, fire transformed from depressed emotions, or heat transformed from some yin pathogens like phlegm-dampness as they have been long depressed. It may also be caused by turbulence of blood qi resulting from hyperactivity of a viscus like the liver. As blood looses its calmness and gets turbulent, it will inevitably lead to acceleration of blood flow, or even damage to the vessels, thus blood will be forced to go frenziedly. At the same time, blood and mind are closely related, as blood gets turbulent, the mind will also become turbulent, leading to restlessness of the mind. So the common presentations of the condition are flushed complexion, red tongue, rapid pulse, dysphoria, even bleeding, and comma.

Bleeding: This means blood does not circulate along the normal tract and escapes out of the vessels during the course of a disease. The causes for bleeding are of many. The common ones are: invasion of blood level by exogenous pathogens of yang-heat nature that forces blood to flow frenziedly or damages the vessels; failure of deficient qi in controlling that leads to escape of blood; break-down of the vessels due to various traumatic injuries; adversely rising of qi-blood due to hyperactivity of yang qi of some viscera; or break-down of the vessels due to obstruction of phlegm and stagnant blood. Bleeding mainly includes hematemesis, hemoptysis, hemefecia, hemeturia, hypermenorrhea, epistaxis, gingival bleeding, and hematohidrosis. Since the causes leading to bleeding are different, the manifestations of bleeding are also different. The bleeding due to frenzied flow of blood forced by fire-heat or breakdown of the vessels by traumas is acute, with bright red color, and massive. The bleeding due to failure of deficient qi in controlling is of a long course, with pale red color, and scanty volume; and the focus is generally in the lower part of the body. The bleeding due to breakdown of the vessels resulting from blockage of stagnant blood is of dark purplish color or with clots.

(3) Disorders of qi and blood simultaneously: This refers to a pathological state resulting from destruction of the mutually dependent relationship between qi and blood.

Qi stagnancy with blood stasis: It is a pathological state in which stagnancy of qi and blood stasis co-exist. Obstruction of qi flow may lead to disturbance of blood flow, and blood stasis will definitely deteriorate the qi stagnancy. Since the liver is in charge of free flow of qi and sores blood. The liver plays a key role in the freedom of qi dynamic, concerning the flow of qi-blood of the whole body. Therefore, the condition is closely associated with the functions of the liver. Because the heart governs blood circulation, the lung connects with vessels and governs qi of the whole body. Therefore, functional disorders of the heart and lung may also lead to qi stagnancy with blood stasis.

Failure of qi to control blood: It imports a pathological state of various bleeding due to qi deficiency with hypofunction in controlling blood, leading escape of blood out of the vessels. The spleen controls blood. If the spleen qi gets deficient and fails to control blood, it will lead to escape of blood out of the normal tract, or even the middle-qi fails in lifting up, and thus blood sinks along with qi. This disorder of failure of qi to control blood is mostly ascribed to deficiency of spleen qi..

Qi deficiency with blood stasis: It is a pathological state that qi in deficiency fails to drive blood to circulate, resulting in blood stasis. This disorder takes qi deficiency as its basis.

Deficiency of both qi and blood: This is a pathological state in which qi deficiency and blood deficiency coexist. It is mostly caused by gradual injury of both qi and blood due to consumption in a prolonged illness; or lack of source for blood production because qi deficiency firstly.

Qi exhaustion following blood: It implies a pathological state that qi escapes following the loss of blood at the same time of massive bleeding. Qi exhaustion following blood takes massive bleeding as the prerequisite, such as traumatic hemorrhage, metrorrhagia or massive postpartum hemorrhage in women. Since blood is the mother of qi, and conveys qi, a large amount bleeding will make qi loose its attachment, and thus qi will escape and deplete accordingly.

Failure of qi-blood to nourish meridian: This refers to a pathological state of motor disorders or abnormal sensation of the muscles and limbs resulting from decrease of nourishing functions of qi-blood to the meridians, tendons, muscles, and skin due to deficiency of qi and blood or disharmony of qi and blood.

7.2.3.4 Disorders of Metabolism of Body Fluid

Disorder of metabolism of body fluid refers to a pathological change of shortage of body fluid or retention of fluid in the body because the formation, distribution and excretion of body fluid are disordered.

(1) Shortage of body fluid: Shortage of body fluid implies a pathological state that there appear a series of dry and puckery symptoms because the viscera, sense organs and orifices cannot be sufficiently moistened and nourished due to shortage of body fluid. It is mostly due to consumption and burning of body fluid caused by exogenously invading pathogens of yang heat nature, or fire transformed from emotional disturbance; or due to consumption of body fluid cause by profuse sweating, serious vomiting and diarrhea, polyuria, heavy bleeding of over administration of acrid and dry remedies.

There are differences between *Jin* (thin fluid) and *Ye* (thick fluid) in quality, distribution and physiological function. Therefore, there are some differences between shortage of *Jin* and *Ye* in patho-mechanism and pathological manifestations. *Jin* is lucid and thin with more fluidity. It moistens the blood vessels and nourishes the viscera internally; and moistens the skin, hair, and orifices externally. It is apt to be consumed and to escape, but it is also easily to be replenished. For example, in summer with scorching sun, there are often polyhidrosis, oliguria, or high fever with a strong desire for drinking; or there are dry mouth, nose and skin caused by dry climate. All the cases take consumption of *Jin* as its main mechanism. *Ye* is turbid and thick with less fluidity. It moistens the viscera, replenishes the bone marrow, brain marrow and spinal marrow, and lubricates the joins. It is not likely to be consumed, but once it is consumed, it cannot be rapidly replenished. For example, during the late stage of exogenous febrile disease, or in a case of yin consumption in a long illness, there appear emaciation just like a figure of only skin and bone, glossy and red tongue without coating, tremors of the hands and feet. All the cases take exhaustion of *Ye* as its main mechanism. Consumption of *Jin* and exhaustion of *Ye* are different in both the mechanism and manifestation. However, the two are originally as an integrity, they promote and depend on each other physiologically; and mutually influence pathologically. Consumption of *Jin* is not definitely accompanied by exhaustion of *Ye,* but exhaustion of *Ye* is definitely mixed by consumption of *Jin.*

(2) Retention of water: This is a pathological summarization of retention of water-dampness-phlegm-stagnant-fluid resulting from the disturbance of body fluid in distribution and excretion. The disturbance of body fluid in distribution and excretion is mainly associated with the functional disorders of the lung, spleen, kidney, urinary bladder and tri-Jiao, and it is influenced by the failure of the liver in keeping free flow of qi. If the spleen fails to soundly transport, the flow of the body fluid will be sluggish, the clear qi fail to rise, and water-dampness generate internally. If the lung fails to diffuse and ascend, the water passage will be unsmooth, the body fluid flow sluggishly. If the kidney yang gets deficient, qi transformation will fail in function, then the clear cannot ascend and the turbid cannot descend, and water will stagnate internally. If qi dynamic of the tri-Jiao is obstructed, the water passage will be unsmooth, and thus the distribution of body fluid will be disordered. If the qi transformation of the urinary bladder gets disturbed, the clear qi cannot descend, and water will not flow down. If the liver fails in governing free flow of qi, the qi dynamic will be hindered, then water will stagnate because of qi stagnancy, influencing circulation of water in tri-Jiao.

Sweat and urine are the important ways for discharge of metabolized water. So excretory disturbance of sweat and urine are the manifestations of functional disturbance of the internal viscera; but they are also the link most easily to cause internal production of water-dampness due to retention of body fluid. Transformation of body fluid into sweat mainly depends upon the diffusing and dispersing actions of the lung. The process the body fluid transforms into urine and excretes out of the body mainly relies on the steaming and qi transforming actions of kidney yang, and the closing-opening action of the urinary bladder. Therefore, hypofunctions of the lung, kidney and urinary bladder influence not only the distribution of body fluid, but also obviously the excreting process of body fluid. Of which the steaming and qi transforming actions of kidney yang run through the whole process of fluid metabolism, playing a dominating role in the excreting process of body fluid. As the lung qi fail to diffuse and disperse, the striae will close, and then the excretion of sweat is disordered. However, the waste fluid after fluid metabolism can change into urine to discharge out of the body. However if the qi transforming action of kidney yang is declined, it will cause disturbance of production and excretion of urine, thus it definitely result in illness with retention of water.

(3) Disorders of body fluid and qi and blood simultaneously: The production, distribution and excretion of body fluid depend upon the qi dynamic of the viscera, while qi takes body fluid as its carrier to flow superiorly, inferiorly, exteriorly and interiorly to the whole body. The functional coordination between body fluid and qi-blood is an important factor for guaranteeing the normal physiological activity of the body. Once the relationship is disordered, there may appear the following several pathological changes.

Water retention with qi stagnancy: This is a pathological state that water stagnates and accumulates in the body to block qi dynamic. The pathological presentations vary with the location where fluid-qi accumulate. For example, if phlegm and stagnant fluid stagnate in the lung, the lung-qi will stagnate and fail to diffuse and descend, there may appear chest fullness, cough, and inability to lie flat with dyspnea. If water-dampness stay in the middle-Jiao and block qi dynamic of both the spleen and stomach, it may lead to failure of the clear-qi to ascend and failure of turbid-qi to descend, with manifestations of distension and fullness in the epigastrium and abdomen, belching, and poor appetite. If water-fluid overflow to the limbs, it may block qi dynamic in the meridians, with the presentations of heaviness, and distending pain in the limbs.

Qi exhaustion following fluid: It is a pathological state of sudden exhaustion of yang-qi because massive loss of body fluid and thus qi escapes out of the body along with the fluid. It is mostly caused by burning of fluid by high fever, or consumption of fluid due to profuse sweat, serious vomiting and diarrhea, and polyuria, leading to qi exhaustion following fluid loss. For example, invasion of summer-heat may force the body fluid to discharge out and induce polyhidrosis, then there appear not only the symptoms of injury of fluid such as thirst with a desire for drinking, scanty and yellow urine, and dry stool; but also the presentation of consumption of qi such as lassitude, shortness of breath and reluctance to speak. Because fluid can convey qi, at the same time of great loss of fluid due to vomiting and diarrhea, there must appear the presentation of injury of qi. Thus it will lead to deficiency of both fluid and qi in a mild case; and exhaustion of both fluid and qi in a severe case.

Fluid exhaustion with blood dryness: This is a pathological state that body fluid and blood become deficient at the same time. Fluid and blood come from the same origin. Moreover, body fluid is the important component of blood. Therefore, injury of fluid may lead to deficit of blood, and loss of blood may lead to shortage of fluid. For example, high fever, polyhidrosis, heavy vomiting and serious diarrhea may greatly consume fluid, at the same time, they may also lead to shortage of blood to a given degree; thus there develops a case of fluid exhaustion with blood dryness, with common presentations of restlessness, dry and squamous skin with itching feeling.

Fluid shortage with blood stasis: It is a pathological state of obstructing circulation of blood due to shortage of body fluid. Body fluid is the important component of blood; so as body fluid is sufficient, blood circulation will be smooth. If body fluid is consumed massively due to high fever, burns and scalds in large areas, or severe vomiting, diarrhea and sweat, it will cause shortage of blood volume and thick quality of blood with a resultant sluggish flow of blood. Thus on the basis of shortage of fluid, there appears disorder of blood stasis. Besides the symptoms of fluid shortage, there may occur the manifestations of blood stasis such as dark purplish complexion, ecchymoses in the skin, dark purplish tongue, or with petechiae and ecchymoses.

7.2.3.5 Five Endogenous Pathogens

They refer to the five pathologic changes similar to those caused by exogenous wind, clod, dampness, dryness and hire (heat), resulting from disorders of yin-yang of the viscera, and abnormal metabolism of qi, blood and body fluid during the process of a disease. Because the disorders occur internally, so they are respectively called endogenous wind, endogenous cold, endogenous dampness, endogenous dryness, and endogenous fire (heat). Five endogenous pathogens are not patholoaenic qi but the comprehensively pathological changes caused by disorders of yin-yang of the viscera, and anomalies of qi, blood and body fluid

(1) Stirring of wind internally: This is also called endogenous wind. It is a pathological state forming due to hyperactivity and adverse rising of yang qi in the body. Owing to that stirring of wind internally is mostly a series of pathological phenomena resulting from failure of the liver in governing free flow of qi. Therefore, it is called liver wind or stirring of liver wind internally. According to different pathogeneses and clinical characters, it may be classified into four kinds of production of wind from liver yang, generation of wind with extreme heat, stirring of wind with yin deficiency, and stirring of wind with blood deficiency.

Production of wind from liver yang: This is a pathological state resulting from failure of water to nourish wood with yin deficiency and yang hyperactivity, which is mostly caused by emotional injuries and mental overstrain that consume yin of the liver and kidney, and thus lead to undersupply of nourishment for the tendon and vessels. Its clinical manifestations are, in a mild case, numbness of the limbs, tremor, vertigo with a tendency to fall down, or wry mouth with distorted eyes, or hemiplegia; or in a severe case, sudden coma and unconsciousness.

Generation of wind with extreme heat: This is common in the stage of rampant heat in exogenous febrile diseases. It is a pathological state of generation of wind caused by exuberant yang heat. This is mostly invasion of rampant pathogenic heat that can burn body fluid, affect nutritive-blood and scorch the liver meridian, and thus lead to undersupply of nourishment for the tendon and vessels. The major patho-mechanism for generation of wind with extreme heat is rampancy of pathogenic heat; it is an excess illness. Therefore, its clinical manifestations are high fever, coma, delirium, spasm of the limbs, staring eyes straightly upward, and opisthotonus.

Stirring of wind with yin deficiency: This is a pathological state caused by exhaustion of yin-fluid, which fails to nourish and thus lead to undersupply of nourishment for the tendon and vessels. The causative factors of this condition are commonly yin-fluid deficient in the late state of a febrile disease, or consumption of yin-fluid in a chronic or prolonged illness. The pathological essence pertains to deficiency, so the wind symptoms are usually mild and chronic, such as peristalses of the hand and feet.

Stirring of wind with blood deficiency: This is a pathological state caused by shortage of blood, which fails to nourish the tendons and vessels, or fails to nourish the collaterals. It is commonly caused by heavy bleeding, or less production of blood, or consumption of yin-blood in a prolonged illness, or shortage of essence-blood in the elderly people, leading to shortage of liver blood. The pathological essence is deficient, so its symptoms are also mild and chronic. The common presentations are numbness of the limbs, tremor of the tendons and muscles, constriction of the hand and feet.

(2) Production of cold internally: This is endogenous cold. It is a pathological state that deficiency-cold is produced internally or yin-cold spreads all over the body, which is caused by decline of yang-qi with hypofunction of warming and qi transforming. The development of endogenous clod is mostly associated with yang qi decline of the spleen and kidney.

Deficiency of yang qi leads to internal production of deficiency-cold. There are mainly three respects of manifestations in pathological changes: First, yang qi has declined and failed to warm the body, such as intolerance of cold with cold limbs. Secondly, the function of qi transformation decreases, thus it leads to disturbance of fluid metabolism with accumulation of pathological products such as phlegm, stagnant fluid, and water-dampness. Thirdly, yang-qi fails to steam and vaporize yin, thus body fluid cannot be transformed into qi, with such symptoms as frequent urination with lucid and profuse urine, and lucid sputum and slobber.

Production of cold internally and exogenous contraction of pathogenic cold are both different and related. "Endogenous cold" is mainly a case of yang deficiency with yin superiority; it presents mainly with insufficiency of the vital, belonging to deficiency-cold. While "exogenous cold" is invasion of the body by pathogenic cold, it has also the pathological changes of damage to yang by cold pathogen, but it is mainly a case of pathogen-excess, pertaining to excess-cold. The major relation of them: When cold pathogen invades the body, it will definitely damage yang-qi, and thus the condition may lead to yang deficiency. While if a person has a constitution of yang deficiency, he will be predisposed to contraction of cold pathogen because of his lower resistance against exogenous pathogens.

(3) Internal generation of turbid-dampness: This is endogenous dampness. It is a pathological state of internal generation and accumulation of water, dampness, phlegm and stagnant fluid, which is caused by disturbance of distribution and excretion of body fluid. The key of patho-mechanism of the endogenous dampness lies in disorder of the spleen in transformation and transportation.

The major manifestations of this condition in pathological change are of two respects: First, the dampness is characterized by heaviness, turbidity, and viscosity, and apt to hinder qi dynamic; thus, there may appear chest distress, abdominal distention, and discomfort defecation. Secondly, dampness is a turbid-yin material, internal blockage of dampness pathogen may further affect the functional activities of the lung, spleen and kidney. For example, if dampness blocks the lung, the lung qi will fail to diffuse and descend; and thus chest distress, cough and expectoration may occur. If the turbid-dampness accumulates long and further damages yang-qi of the spleen and kidney, it may lead to a morbid case of yang deficiency with excess of dampness. Any part of the upper-, meddle- and lower-Jiao of the body, the turbid-dampness may block, nevertheless, the commonly seen case is blockage of the middle-Jiao by dampness and spleen insufficiency with dampness harassment.

Exogenous contraction of dampness and endogenous production of dampness are both different and related. "Exogenous dampness" is invasion of the body by pathogenic dampness, it is mainly a case of injury of body surface and tendons and bones by dampness pathogen. While "endogenous dampness" is a case of production of dampness from water retention due to functional disturbance of the lung, spleen and kidney, especially failure of the spleen in sound transformation and transportation. The relation of them is that an invasion of exogenous dampness tends to damage the spleen, and if the dampness blocks the spleen and damages yang, it is likely to cause generation of endogenous dampness because of failure of the spleen in sound transformation and transportation. While a person who has an insufficient spleen failing to transport with excess of dampness ordinarily is subject to invasion by exogenous dampness.

(4) Generation of dryness from fluid consumption: This is endogenous dryness. It is a pathological state of a series of dry and astringing symptoms because the tissue organs of the body loose their moisture, which is caused by shortage of fluid in the body.

The development of endogenous dryness is mostly due to consumption of yin-fluid in a prolonged illness, or shortage of yin-fluid resulting from heavy sweating, serious vomiting, or diarrhea, or massive loss of blood and essence, consumption of fluid by exuberant heat in the process of some exogenous febrile diseases. Since the fluid is short, it fails to irrigate the viscera internally, and moisten the skin, sense organs and orifices, externally and then there appear a series of dry symptoms such as dry skin, dry mouth and throat, dry stools with constipation. The essence of the endogenous dryness is deficit of fluid in the body. Therefore, the disorders of endogenous dryness may occur in any tissues and organs, but they mostly occur in the lung, stomach and large intestine.

(5) Generation of fire-heat internally: This is endogenous fire or endogenous heat. It is a pathological state of internal harass of fire with hyperactive function of the body, which is caused by exuberance of yang, or yin deficiency with yang hyperactivity, or transformation of fire from emotional disturbance. Generation of fire-heat internally is of difference in deficiency and excess. The patho-mechanisms are as follows.

Fire transforming from exuberance of yang-qi: Under normal conditions, human's yang-qi has the action to warm the viscera and tissues; and it is called "minor fire". However, under the pathological conditions, if yang-qi gets too hyperactive, it will transform into fire to make abnormal excitement of functional activity. This pathological hyperactivity of yang is named "hyperactive fire".

Fire produced from stagnation of pathogens: This includes two sides. One is that the invading pathogenic wind, cold, dampness and dryness make generation of fire through a long period of stagnation during the pathological process. For example, cold pathogen leads to production of fire and production of fire by stagnation of dampness. The other is that the pathological products such as phlegm-dampness, stagnant blood, and foodstuff retention make generation of fire by a long period of stagnation.

Fire produced by extreme emotions: This is a pathological state of generation of fire resulting from yang exuberance, or a long period of depression of qi dynamic, which is caused by abnormal psychological and emotional stimuli that affect qi-blood and yin-yang of the viscera.

Hyperactive fire with yin deficiency: This is a pathological state of internal production of deficiency-fire, which is caused by yang hyperactivity with failure of deficient yin to restrict yang due to great injury of yin-fluid. It is most common among the persons with either chronic or prolonged illness. For example, gingival swelling and pain, sore throat, steaming sensation of the bones, and flushed cheek due to yin deficiency are all the outcome of flaring of deficiency-fire.

Review Questions

- What are the natures and pathogenic characters of wind, cold, summer-heat, dampness, dryness and fire?
- What are the pathogenic characters of the seven emotions?
- What are the common characteristics of disorders caused by stagnant blood?
- Please describe the patho-mechanism for imbalance of yin and yang.
- What are the patho-mechanism and clinical presentation of endogenous Cold?

8 PRINCIPLES FOR PREVENTION AND TREATMENT OF DISEASE

8.1 Principles for Prevention of Disease

Prevention means taking a certain measure in advance to stop the occurrence and development of disease.

Huáng Dì Nèi Jīng (*Huangdi's Inner Classic of Medicine*) puts forward the concept of "treating the undiseased", which emphasizes that one should nip a disease in the bud. This includes two respects of prevention before a disease occurs and treatment before a disease develops.

8.1.1 Prevention before a Disease Occurs

This implies that before a disease occurs, various measures should be taken to prevent its occurrence.

The onset of a disease has close relationship with vital qi and pathogenic qi. Vital qi indicates functional activities (including the functions of the viscera, meridians, qi and blood) and the resistance and recovery capacity of the body. Pathogenic qi indicates various causes resulting in disease. When vital qi is abundant, the resistance of the body against disease will be strong, pathogenic qi cannot invade the body; even though pathogenic qi invades the body, vital qi can repel it outside the body, and disease will not occur. Therefore, a deficiency of vital qi is the root cause in the onset of a disease. In some special conditions, the invasion of pathogenic qi plays a decisive role in the onset of a disease, so pathogenic qi is an important requirement for the onset of disease. For prevention of disease, on one hand, the vital qi should be enhanced to increase the resistance against disease; and on the other hand, the invasion of pathogenic qi should be avoided.

8.1.1.1 Increasing Resistance against Disease

(1) Taking good care of body: Taking good care of body can build up one's health and increase resistance against disease, thus reducing or preventing the occurrence of disease. One should understand the laws of nature, and adapt to environmental changes in

order to keep fit, maintain a high spirit, and prolong life. One should lead a regular life, have a proper diet, and work regularly but not over strain. By this way one can maintain vigorous vital qi so as to prevent disease. Contrarily, if one leads an irregular life and is not careful about his diet, work and rest, it will weaken his resistance against disease, affect health, and lead to the occurrence of disease.

Life rests upon exercises, which determines health. Life is the highest form of substantial movement, and physical health is the reflection of normal progress of life activity. It is proved in practice that abundant vigor consists in sound body, and a healthy physique often results from proper work and unremitting physical exercise. Therefore, regular physical exercise can build up one's constitution, thus reducing or preventing the occurrence of disease.

Famous doctor Hua Tuo of the Han dynasty created the five mimic-animal exercises according to the law of "running water never gets stale, and a door hinge is never worm eaten". Among them the exercise mimicking tiger helps to boost up physical strength; the exercise mimicking deer helps to stretch bones and muscles; the exercise mimicking bear helps to relieve the syndrome of excess in the upper and deficiency in the lower; the exercise mimicking ape helps to smooth joints; and the exercise mimicking crane helps to enhance breathing function, smooth qi-blood, and dredge the meridian. By doing some physical exercises and proper work, one can both improve blood circulation to make the joints flexible, and make qi dynamic free, so that he can strengthen the resistance against disease, improve healthy level, and prevent and reduce the occurrence of disease. At the same time, these also have a certain therapeutic function for some diseases.

(2) Training mental health: Chinese medicine not only attaches importance to taking good care of body, but also especially pay attention to taking good care of mind to make the spirit high and optimistic. It is of important signification to reduce mental stimulation and excessive emotional alteration for preventing or reducing the occurrence of emotional disease.

Whether the mental activity is normal or not has an important impact to the physiological activity and pathological changes; for mental and emotional activities take essence, qi, blood and body fluid as their substantial foundation, and they are closely related to visceral functions. Spiritual, conscious and thinking activities may have both active or enhancing function, and negative or reducing function to the body. Active and enhancing function can improve body's motion. For example, amused emotion may make flow of qi and blood smooth, and function hyperactive. While negative and reducing function can decrease body's motion. For example, depressed emotion may lead to qi stagnation and blood stasis, dysfunction, decrease of resistance, and consequently lead to the occurrence of disease.

The ancient people emphasize taking good care of mind internally. This means one should carefully pay attention to volitional exercise and emotional stabilization, build up volition and resolution for overcoming disease, and try to have a breadth of mind and scanty desire, and as such, he can prevent and decrease emotional stimulation so as to gain the aim of reducing disease and prolonging life. Therefore, to emphasize mental training, one must keep "a peaceful and happy mood, humility and few desires thus to have a vigorous vital qi internally", so that he can attain the aim of "being full of go, and never suffering from disease" in preserving health.

(3) Having a proper diet: Diet is one of indispensable conditions for life of human being. Weather the diet is normal and regular or not directly affects one's health. Foodstuff essence coming from diet are the substantial foundation for production of qi and blood, and the necessary condition for maintaining growth and development, achieving various physiological functions, assuring survival and health. Having a proper diet means the diet should be appropriate and regular. Improper diet will lead to the occurrence of disease. So one should cultivate a good dietetic habit, having his diet in relatively fixed times and with relatively fixed quantity, neither starvation nor over-fullness, especially not overeating richly fatty and sweet foodstuffs. One should also pay attention to regulation of the nature and flavor to make heat and cold harmonized, and five flavors balanced. In addition, one should pay attention to dietetic sanitation to prevent "disease from the mouth".

(4) Medicinal prevention: There is a record in the *Sù Wèn* (*Plain Questions*) that "taking *Xiaojin* pellets can keep pestilence away". As early as in the 16th century the "human variolation" was created to prevent smallpox in ancient China. This method was the forerunner of immunocology in the world. Furthermore, Chinese medicine uses certain medical herbs for disinfection, such as Cangzhu (*Rhizoma Atractylodis*) and Xionghuang (*Realgar*). In recent year, herbs have been used to prevent diseases, which has been paid more and more attention in medical field worldwide, and has been greatly developed. For instance, Guanzhong (*Rhizoma Dryopteris Crassirhizomae*), Banlangen (*Radiz Isatidis*) or Daqingye (*Folium Isatidis*), etc. are taken to prevent flu; Yinchen (*Herba Artemesiae Scopariae*) *Herba Artemesiae Scopariae*; and *Zhizi* (*Fructus Gardeniaei*) to prevent hepatitis; Machixian (*Herba Portulacae*) to prevent dysentery.

8.1.1.2 Avoiding Invasion by Pathogens

Pathogenic qi are an important condition in onset of disease. In a certain special condition, pathogenic qi can play the leading role. For example, high temperature, high voltage electricity, Chemical poison, gunshot, insect and animal injury, may damage the body and lead to the occurrence of disease even if the vital qi is strong. Pestilential qi often becomes a decisive factor for the occurrence of disease in some special conditions. Therefore, avoiding invasion by pathogenic qi is also an important measure for preventing disease.

8.1.2 Treatment before a Disease Develops

Prevention before a disease occurs is the ideal preventative measure. However, once a disease already occurs, one should strive for an early diagnosis and treatment so to stop the disease from further development and transmission. Therefore, practitioners should, according to the developing law and transforming way of disease, strive for an early diagnosis and an effective treatment to stop the progress of the difsease. In clinical treatment of a liver disease, the method of strengthening the spleen and normalizing the stomach is often taken as an auxiliary method. This is an application of the principle of treatment before a disease develops. Ye Tianshi, a famous physician of the Qing dynasty, believed such a law that after stomach yin is injured in warm-heat diseases, the kidney yin will often be involved. So he advocated herbs salty and cold in nature and with action of nourishing the kidney should be added into the prescriptions for treating syndrome of stomach yin deficiency by sweet and cold natured herbs. In this way of nourishing kidney yin, the involvement of the kidney yin due to a prolonged shortage of stomach yin can be prevented. And he also put forth the principle of prevention and treatment, i.e., "the part that has not been invaded by the pathogens must be treated first". This is an example of idiographic application of the principle for treatment before a disease develops.

8.2 Principles for Treatment

In Chinese medical clinic, in a long term of medical practice, a suit of theories and methods for differentiation of syndrome and treatment has developed based on deep recognition of the occurring and developing law of disease and through accumulation and summarization of rich clinical experiences by medical experts through ages. Differentiation of syndrome and treatment of disease is not only to correctly make a diagnosis of the disease condition by distinguishing and analyzing the various clinical presentations according to the theory of Chinese medicine, what is more, to establish a correct therapeutic principle, apply a proper therapeutic method on the basis of the result of syndrome differentiation, so as to use a reasonable remedy or effective therapeutic measure for curing the disease. In the process of treatment, establishment of therapeutic principle and choice of therapeutic methods are of very important signification.

The therapeutic principle is the rule for treating disease. It is formulated under the guidance of the holism and treatment determination based on syndrome differentiation. It is a universal guiding principle for determination of methods, formula and medicinals clinically.

The therapeutic method is the concrete method for treating disease. It is different from therapeutic principle. The therapeutic principle is the general rule aiming at the clinical disorder and guiding the method; while the therapeutic method is the concrete method aiming at a concrete syndrome (or a type of syndrome), being the concrete embodiment of the principle. Therefore, any concrete method always belongs to a certain therapeutic principle. For example, viewing pathogenic qi and vital qi, all diseases are governed by the struggle between the vital and the pathogen. It is therefore a general rule in treatment to strengthen the vital and eliminate the pathogen. Under the guidance of the general rule, the methods of replenishing qi, supplementing yin, nourishing blood, and strengthening yang are the concrete methods to strengthen the vital; while the methods of diaphoresis, emesis, purgation and clearing are the concrete methods to eliminate the pathogen. It is obvious that the therapeutic principle and methods are both strictly different and closely related internally.

Disease syndromes are varied with complicated pathological changes. The condition of disease may be mild or severe, chronic or acute. Furthermore, the time, place and individual may all exert different influences on disease. So a practitioner must be adept at grasping the essential aspects of a disease in the complicated and changeable manifestations and give a treatment aiming at its root aspect; determine treatment by examining the root cause, take a relevant measure, to regulate yin and yang so as to newly resume the relatively balance of yin-yang, thus a satisfactory effect can be achieved. The therapeutic principles include treatment aiming at the root of a disease, strengthening the vital and dispelling the pathogen, attaching importance to the whole, harmonizing yin-yang, regulating viscera, harmonizing qi-blood, and determining treatment suitable to the difference

8.2.1 Treatment Aiming at the Root of a Disease

Disease is a complicated process of conflicting between the vital and the pathogen, in which there are several contradictions within the body, and both true and false clinical manifestations. For example, in majority of diseases the external phenomena are consistent with the internal essence, but in some of diseases there may be non-consistence between the external phenomena and internal essence (such as true or false heat or cold syndrome, true or false excess or deficiency syndrome). Therefore, a practitioner must distinguish between the primary and secondary contradictions of disease, see through the phenomena into the essence of disease, and as such he can resolve the disease by using appropriate treatment.

Treatment aiming at the root aspect of a disease means, when treating a disease, one must seek for its root cause and give a treatment directing to the root. This is a cardinal principle for treatment determination based on syndrome differentiation.

"Emergency or chronicity of the root or the branch", and "routine treatment and contrary treatment" embody this basic therapeutic principle.

8.2.1.1 Emergency or chronicity of the root or the branch

The root is judged by comparing it with the branch. In the course of occurrence and development of any disease, there are primary contradiction and secondary contradiction.

"The root" means the primary contradiction or the primary aspect of a contradiction in a disease, playing the leading decisive role; "the branch" means the secondary contradiction or the secondary aspect of a contradiction, being in the secondary position. Therefore, the root and the branch are relative concepts with multiple meanings. They may be used to explain the primary and the secondary relation in various contradictions in the course of a disease. For instance, viewing the two sides of the vital and the pathogen, vital qi is the root and pathogenic qi is the branch. In terms of cause and symptom, the cause is the root and the symptom is the branch. Considering the order of diseases, the old or primary disease is the root while the new or secondary disease is the branch.

The onset and development of any disease always present some symptoms, but these symptoms are only the phenomena of the disease, not the essence of the disease. Only by synthetically analyzing on the basis of fully collecting and understanding all kinds of information, can one see through the phenomenon to grasp the essence, finding out the root cause of disease, and then to choose an appropriate therapeutic method. For example, headache can be caused by many reasons, such as exo-pathologic factors, blood deficiency, phlegm-dampness, stagnated blood, hyperactivity of liver yang, etc.. Therefore, on treatment, one cannot simply take the symptomatic therapy of analgesia, and should synthetically analyze to find the pathogenic causes, and as such, he can respectively apply dispelling exo-pathologic factors, nourishing blood, drying dampness and resolving phlegm, activating blood to remove stasis, and soothing the liver to subdue yang, so that a satisfactory effect can be achieved.

There are treatments of the branch for emergency, the root for chronicity and both the branch and the root simultaneously about the concretely use of "treatment aiming at the root of a disease".

(1) Treating the branch for emergency: In general, the primary contradiction or the primary aspect of a contradiction in a disease is the root rather than the branch, "treatment aiming at the root of the disease" is a radical principle. However, for a complicated disease there should be divisions of the acute first and the chronic second in treatment because of the difference of the branch and the root or the primary and the secondary. When the branch aspect of the condition is very serious and becomes the principal aspect of a disease, if not treated promptly, it will endanger the life of the patient or influence treatment of the root condition; then the principle of "treatment of the branch for emergency" should be taken to handle the branch condition first and the root condition second. For example, a patient with massive bleeding, no matter what kind, emergency measures should be taken first to stop the bleeding for the branch. Then after the bleeding stops, the root condition is treated. Another example, some patients suffering from chronic disease with original old disease contract again exogenous pathogens and get new disease, when the new disease is emergent, the exogenous contraction should be treated first, and then the old disease is treated after the new disease is cured. It can thus

be found that treatment of the branch in an emergency is an expedient measure to create a favorable condition for treating the root. The final goal is still aiming at a better treatment for the root. However, the method of treating the branch can be temporally used but should not be used long; otherwise it will damage the vital qi.

(2) Treatment of the root in chronicity: This means, under the general conditions, the essence of a disease should be grasped and the root cause of the disease should be treated so as to resolve the radical contradiction. For example, for a phthisis in a stage of yin deficiency leading to internal heat, and deficient-fire burning the lung, the manifestations are cough, low fever, dryness in the mouth and throat, dysphoria with hot feeling in the five hearts, flushed cheek, and night sweat. In this condition the symptoms like cough are the branch, and yin deficiency is the root. So the treatment should be to nourish the yin to moisten the lungs for treating the root instead of relieving the cough and dispelling phlegm for treating the branch. Only when the body's disease-resisting ability is improved, can the phthisis be cured.

(3) Treating the branch and the root simultaneously: When both the branch and the root conditions are either acute or chronic, the branch and the root should be treated at the same time. For example, for an exogenous heat disease, when the heat pathogen gets into the interior to cause a serious injury to yin fluid, it may present with a syndrome of deficiency of the vital and excess of the pathogen, and emergency of both the branch and root, with manifestations such as abdominal fullness, hardness and pain, constipation, fever, dry mouth with cracked lips, charred and dry tongue coating. On treatment, both the branch and root of the disease should be treated at the same time, i.e., clearing and purging the excess heat for treating the branch and nourishing yin to produce fluid for treating the root. If only the purgation is used, the body fluid will be consumed further; if only the yin is nourished, the internal excess heat cannot be cleared. While if the two methods are taken simultaneously, they can supplement each other, so that the aim of dispelling the pathogen and resuming the fluid can be got. Take dysentery as another example, it may present with abdominal pain, tenesmus, diarrhea with purulence and blood, yellow greasy tongue coating, slippery and rapid pulse. The cause for dysentery is dampness-heat as its root, so the treatment should be to clear dampness-heat for treating its root to sooth the intestines and to smooth qi in order to relieve the emergency of abdominal pain and tenesmus. This is also embodiment of treating the branch and root simultaneously. Again an example is a patient who has an interior syndrome already, and again gets contraction of exterior pathogen to have an exterior syndrome, or whose exterior syndrome is not relieved yet, but an interior syndrome develops, thus the patient has disorders of both exterior and interior. For this case the therapy of releasing both the exterior and interior should be taken, which also belongs to the category of treating the branch and the root simultaneously.

It should be pointed out the principle of treatment of the branch for emergency and treatment of the root for chronicity can not be absolutely used in clinical practice. The root might also be treated in the emergency. For example, yang depletion is treated by restoring yang from collapse in emergency; and qi collapse following massive hemorrhage is treated by replenishing qi to save patient from collapse, all the two cases are the treatment of root. In the same way, the branch might also be treated in chronicity which may sometime be in favor of treating the root. In conclusion, no matter of the branch and the root, treatment of the emergent one should be an essential principle. Practitioners should distinguish the transformation of the condition and grasp the primary contradiction or the primary aspect of a contradiction in clinical practice, and achieve the goal of treatment aiming at the root.

8.2.1.2 Routine Treatment and Contrary Treatment

Sù Wèn (*Plain Questions*) points out two therapeutic principles of "routine treatment for the counter, contrary treatment for the consistent". However both are concrete application of the essential principle of treatment aiming at the root of a disease viewing from the essence.

(1) Routine treatment: This means to differentiate the disease nature of cold, heat, excess, deficiency by analyzing clinical symptoms and signs, and then to apply respectively the different methods of heating what is cold, cooling what is hot, notifying what is deficient, and reducing what is excessive in treatment. This is a commonly used therapeutic method which goes against the essence of a disease, being also named "allopathic treatment". This method is used for a case whose signs are consistent with its essence, i.e., a cold syndrome is marked by cold signs, a heat syndrome by heat signs, a deficient syndrome by deficient signs, and an excess syndrome by deficient signs. Therefore, it is one of the commonly used therapies in clinic.

(2) Contrary treatment: In some complicated and serious diseases manifesting as some false appearances which are not consistent with the essence. Therefore, one should not simply treat cold for cold sign, or treat heat for heat sign, but should see through the false appearances to differentiate the real or false, thus treating the essence. So called "contrary treatment", being also named "consistent treatment", means to differentiate the disease nature of cold, heat, excess and deficiency by analyzing clinical symptoms and signs, and then treat the disease by going with the false manifestations of the disease. It is suitable for a case whose manifestations are opposite to the natures of disease. On treatment, treating hotness with the heat, treating coldness with the cold, treating obstruction with tonics, and treating openness with purgatives.

For example, in the stage of extreme internal heat of some exogenous diseases, because predominant yang rejects yin, there may appear cold sign of extreme cold limbs. This cold sign is false and the heat exuberance is true. So it still needs cold-cool medicinals for treatment. Therefore it is called treating coldness with the cold.

In some patients with yang depletion, because internal exuberance of yin-cold rejects yang externally, there may sometimes appear heat sign such as flushed check, and vexation. This heat sign is the false, and the yang deficiency with hyperactivity of cold is the essence. So the warm and heat medicinals should be taken for treatment. Therefore it is called treating hotness with the heat.

An abdominal distention and fullness caused by failure of the insufficient spleen to transport, because there is no stagnation of either water-dampness or indigested food, should be treated by strengthening the spleen and replenishing qi, or opening the obstruction by tonics. This is therefore named treating openness with purgatives.

For a diarrhea resulting from the affection of the transformation and transportation by the food stagnation, not only the antidiareics are contraindicative, on the contrary, the medicinals of digestant and evacuant need to be given to remove the stagnated products, and as such the effect can be got. This is known as treating obstruction with tonics.

In addition, there is another method which was classified as one of contrary treatments by ancient Chinese practitioners, which is to prevent vomiting due to repellence between yin and yang while taking the medicine in treating some great heat or cold syndrome. This is generally to add a small dosage of warm-natured herbs to a prescription which is greatly cold-natured or to take in a cold-cooled natured decoction as it is hot; or to add a small dosage of cool or cold natured herbs to a prescription which is greatly warm or hot natured, or taking in a warm or hot nature decoction when it is cooled. This is essentially some concrete methods in making formula or for administration of decoction. So they will not in detail discussed because it belongs to the scope of science of formulas.

8.2.2 Strengthening the Vital and Dispelling the Pathogen

The course of a disease, in a certain sense, is the process of the struggle between the two contradictory aspects of the vital and the pathogen. When the pathogen gains the upper hand, the disease will progress; when the vital gains the upper hand, the disease will subdue. Thus in treatment strengthening the vital and dispelling the pathogen should be carried out to change the ratio in strength of the two sides of the vital and pathogen, so that it is conducive for the disease to take a turn for recovery. Therefore, strengthening the vital and dispelling the pathogen are also an important principle in clinical treatment.

"Superiority of pathogenic qi leads to an excess and inferiority of essential qi leads to a deficiency". The superiority or inferiority of the vital or the pathogen decides the deficiency or excess of a syndrome. "Tonifying what is deficient and reducing what is excessive" are the concrete application of the principle of "strengthening the vital and dispelling the pathogen". Primary and secondary relationship between the vital and pathogen will change following the development of a disease. Therefore, there are the following aspects about the application of "strengthening the vital and dispelling the pathogen".

8.2.2.1 Strengthening the Vital to Dispel the Pathogen

This means assisting the vital qi, building up a good physique, raising the resistance of the body against pathogens and self-repairing power by applying various therapies of medicament, nutritional therapies and functional exercise so as to gain the goal of dispelling the pathogen and resuming the health. This is so called "strengthening the vital to dispel the pathogen" and "the pathogen will get out by itself as the vital is resumed" The measures for strengthening the vital are to reinforce the deficiency, they are mainly suitable for cases whose vital qi is deficient but the pathogen is not excessive, or in which there are exogenous pathogens but with the deficiency of the vital as the primary aspect of the contradiction. Clinically, according to the patient's concrete conditions different methods of replenishing qi, nourishing blood, supplementing yin, strengthening yang, etc., may be taken for their different presentations of deficiency syndrome. So that the substantial basis for functional activities of the viscera and meridians, namely, essence, qi, blood, body fluid are resumed.

8.2.2.2 Dispelling the Pathogen to Strengthen the Vital

This means to eliminate pathogens of disease by applying medicament, acupuncture, cupping or operation so as to get the goal of resuming the vital following the elimination of pathogens. This is what is called "dispelling the pathogen to strengthen the vital", and "the vital will resume as the pathogen is driven out". It is suitable when there is an excess of pathogen with no deficiency of the vital, or although the vital is deficient but the excess pathogen is still the primary aspect of the contradiction.

It is proved by practice dispelling the pathogen should be taken as the main in treatment of the contradiction of the vital and the pathogen. What is more, according to the clinical observation, most diseases caused by exogenous pathogens present with excess syndrome, and thus reducing the excess by eliminating the pathogen should be taken too. The methods should also vary with different pathogens in pharmacotherapy. So the methods to dispel the pathogen are many and varied, such as relieving the exterior, clearing heat, detoxification, purgation, dissolving phlegm, resolving dampness, excreting the water, breaking the stagnated blood, removing the stasis, dispelling the mass, eliminating insect, etc.. All of these belong to the category of dispelling pathogens, or the methods to eliminate the causative factors. They can be appropriately chosen according to the condition of an illness in clinic.

It should be pointed out that strengthening the vital and dispelling the pathogen are dependent upon and supplementary to each other. Strengthening the vital can enhance the resistance to eliminate pathogens; whereas dispelling pathogen can eliminate the interference to the vital and stop the injuries to the vital so as to help the recovery of the vital qi.

8.2.2.3 Dispelling the Pathogen before Strengthening the Vital

This is mainly suitable for the case with rampancy of a pathogen that needs urgently for dispelling the pathogen, or the case that the vital qi is deficient but it is not so serious and still can stand the reduction, especially for those whose deficiency of the vital directly caused by the pathogen. For example, in the process of heat disease by exogenous contraction, there occur abdominal fullness, distention and pain, and constipation due to accumulation of heat in the gastrointestinal tract; as well as red tongue with no moisture, brown, dry and black coating, dryness of the throat, even delirious speech and coma because of the injury of yin by the dryness transformed from accumulated pathogenic heat. This case should be emergently given purgation, or "attack before reinforcement". This is done for that the heat accumulation will become more and more serious due to constipation, and in turn, the body fluid will be more consumed. Therefore, urgent purgation to preserve yin is needed, and then the medicinals nourishing yin to produce fluid are used.

8.2.2.4 Strengthening the Vital before Dispelling the Pathogen

This is mainly suitable for a case with excess pathogens; however the vital gets too weak, in a grade of exhausting of yang or yin, to stand the attack. So strengthening the vital should be taken before dispelling the pathogen. After restoration of the vital to a certain level that can stand the attack, then the pathogen is considered. At present, for some cases of excess of pathogen with deficiency of the vital, such as syncope or sudden collapse of heart yang are usually treated based on the principle of "reinforcement before attack" in clinic.

8.2.2.5 Strengthening the Vital and Dispelling the Pathogen Simultaneously

This is mainly suitable for cases in which the conditions of both deficient vital qi and excessive pathogenic qi are similar in severity. However in the concrete application one should distinguish which aspect is prevailing, the deficiency of the vital or the excess of the pathogen. For a case of prevailing excess of the pathogen with deficiency of the vital, one should mainly dispel the pathogen with strengthening the vital as the subsidiary. If the disease lasts long, the vital will get greatly deficient, and the residual pathogen still exists, then one should mainly strengthen the vital with dispelling the pathogen as the subsidiary.. In conclusion, the principle of "strengthening the vital and dispelling the pathogen simultaneously" is most commonly used in clinic. And in making a prescription with medicinals one should distinguish the primary from the secondary and apply it flexibly according to the concrete condition.

8.2.3 Attaching Importance to the General Condition

The human body itself is an organic whole; every part composing the body is closely related with others. Any a disease or a local pathological change has close relation with the whole. In clinical treatment, one should neither only emphasize the local pathological change with ignorance of the whole body, nor only pay attention to the whole body with ignorance of the local pathological change. The best way is that, basing on the conception of holism, one should both attach importance to the local, and what is more, pay attention to the whole body, thus one can get an expected result by combining the two clinically.

The commonly used therapeutic principles in Chinese medical clinic are coordinating yin and yang, regulating the function of the viscera, and regulating qi and blood.

8.2.3.1 Coordinating Yin and Yang

The occurrence of a disease is essentially the outcome of the superiority or inferiority of yin or yang due to destruction of their relative balance. Therefore, coordinating yin and yang to remedy and restore their relative balance is one of the cardinal principles in clinical treatment. This principle can be divided into two aspects, i.e., "eliminating the surplus" and "supplementing the deficient".

(1) Eliminating the surplus: This means, in treating a case with an excess of yin or yang, the measure of "reducing what is excessive" is clinically taken. Clearing away yang heat with cold natured remedy is used for an excess-heat syndrome due to exuberance of yang heat, or "cooling what is hot"; and dispelling yin cold with heat natured remedy for a case of excess-old syndrome due to exuberance of internal yin cold, or "heating what is cold".

Since an excess of yin makes yang suffer and an excess of yang makes yin suffer, exuberance of yang heat can easily consume yin-fluid, and exuberance of yin-cold can easily damage yang-qi. So in regulating the superiority of either yin or yang, one should also pay attention to whether there is a condition of the corresponding inferiority of either yin or yang; if there is, one then needs to consider the deficient at the same time, appropriately using supporting yang or nourishing yin as the auxiliary.

(2) Supplementing the deficient: This means, in treating a case with an inferiority of yin or yang, the measure of "reinforcing what is deficient" is clinically taken. If yin fails to restrict yang due to its deficiency, which is often manifested by a deficient heat syndrome, it should be treated by nourishing yin to check yang; if yang fails to restrict yin due to its deficiency, which usually presents a deficient cold syndrome, it should be treated by supplementing yang to check yin. However, a case of yin or yang inferiority often leads finally to the deficit of the kidney yin or yang. Thus for a case of kidney yin deficit one should apply the method of "nourishing the origin of water to check the hyperactivity of yang"; and for a case of kidney yang deficit one should apply the method of "supporting the source of fire to expel the nebula of yin". For a case of both yin and yang deficiency, supplementing both yin and yang is needed.

Based on the theory of interdependence of yin and yang, the cases of inferiority of either yin or yang may involve each other. Therefore, in treating an inferiority of either yin or yang, one should also pay attention to "seeking yin from yang" or "seeking yang from yin." That is, when nourishing yin, herbs supplementing yang should be appropriately added to the formula; and when supplementing yang, herbs nourishing yin should be appropriately added to the formula.

In addition, yin and yang are the general principles for syndrome differentiation. Various pathological changes may all be summarized by an imbalance of yin and yang. Therefore such conditions as disorder of the exterior or the interior, turbulence of ascending or descending, as well as advancing or retreating of cold or heat, deficiency or excess of the pathogen or the vital, discordance of he nutritive and defensive phases, and disharmony of qi and blood are all the concrete manifestations of imbalance of yin and yang. Then in an abroad sense, such methods as relieving the exterior, pursing the interior, emesis and purgation, ascending the clear and descending the turbid, clearing away heat and eliminating cold, reinforcing the deficient and reducing the excess, harmonizing the nutritive and defensive phases, and regulating qi and blood all pertain to the category of regulating yin and yang.

8.2.3.2 Regulating the Viscera

The human body itself is an organic whole, there is cooperation and inter-promotion in physiology, and inter-influence in pathology between *Zang*-viscera and *Zang*-viscera, *Zang*-viscera and *Fu*-viscera, *Fu*-viscera and *Fu*-viscera. When one of the viscera has a disease, it will affect others. So on treatment of visceral disorders one should pay attention to regulating the relationships among the viscera instead of thinking one only. Therefore, there are principles of indirectly invigorating and purging, and treating sense organs based on the conditions of *Zang*-viscera.

(1) Indirectly invigorating and purging: This means that, when one viscus has a disease, it should be directly treated, besides, other viscera that closely related with the viscus needs also to be regulated. For example, a lung disease may be caused by the invasion of the lung by pathogens, but it also can be affected by diseases of the heart, liver, spleen, kidney and large intestine. For a case of panting and cough due to failure of the lung in diffusing and descending, which is caused by deficiency of heart yang with stagnation of heart vessels, the treatment should be mainly warming heart yang. For a case of haemoptysis due to adverse rise of qi and fire, which is caused by hyperactivity of liver fire, the treatment should be mainly reducing liver fire. For a case of cough with copious sputum due to failure of the lung in diffusing and descending, which is caused by accumulation of phlegm-dampness in the lung resulting from insufficiency of the spleen, the treatment should be mainly tonifying the spleen and drying dampness. For a case of dry cough and dryness of the mouth and throat due to

loss of liquid moistening of the lung, which is caused by deficiency of kidney yin, the treatment should be mainly nourishing the kidney and moistening the lung. For a case of panting with more exhalation than inhalation due to adverse rise of lung qi, which is caused by failure of the insufficient kidney to receive qi, the treatment should be mainly warming kidney to receive qi. For a case of panting due to failure of lung qi to descend, which is caused by accumulation of heat in the large intestine, the treatment should be mainly purging the *Fu*-viscus to clear heat from the large intestine. Another example, a spleen disease may be caused by, besides the illness of the spleen itself, the illnesses of the liver, heart, kidney and stomach. For a case of failure of the spleen in transformation and transportation, which is caused by failure of the liver to govern free flow of qi, the treatment should be mainly smoothing the liver. For a case of subjugation of spleen-earth by liver-wood due to spleen insufficiency, the treatment should be mainly supplementing earth (spleen) and restringing the wood (liver). For a case of failure of the insufficient spleen in transportation caused by declining of life gate fire with deficiency of heart yang, the treatment should be mainly supplementing fire (kidney yang) to strengthen the earth (spleen). For a case of failure of the spleen to transport due to ab normally descending of stomach qi, the treatment should be mainly descending stomach qi to coordinate the ascending and descending of qi dynamic of the spleen and stomach. The inter-influence among other viscera and harmonizing treatment are all like these.

(2) Treating sense organs based on the conditions of *Zang*-viscera: The five *Zang*-viscera have close relationships with the five sense organs through connections of meridians. The diseases of the five sense organs can also be treated based on the conditions of the five *Zang*-viscera according to the conception of holism in Chinese medicine. For example, because the liver opens its orifice in the eyes, an excess syndrome of eye illness may be treated with the remedy with actions of clearing the liver; and a deficiency syndrome of eye illness may be treated with the remedy with actions of tonifying the liver and nourishing blood. Another example, because heart opens its orifice in the tongue, soreness in the mouth and tongue may be treated with the remedy with actions of clearing heart fire and reducing small intestine heat.

In addition, the principle of choosing point in acupuncture may also according to the conception of holism in Chinese medicine. For example, an illness of the upper can be treated on points in the lower [Yongquan (KI 1) or Taichong (LR 3) is often taken to treat the dizziness with hyperactivity of liver yang type], an illness in the lower can be treated on the points in the upper [moxibustion on Baihui (GV 20) is usually used to treat rectal prolapse], points in the left can be taken to treat the illness of the right, and points in the right can be taken to treat the illness of the left (points in healthy side are often used as a subsidiary treatment of hemiplegia). Some other examples are choices of front-*Mu* or back-*Shu* points, *Yuan* (source) points, *Luo* (connecting) points; all these embody the principle of regulating the general condition.

8.2.3.3 Regulating Qi and Blood

Qi and blood are the material foundation for the functional activities of the viscera. Although qi and blood have their own functions, they help each other. When the relationship between qi and blood in mutual dependence and promotion gets disordered, various disorders of qi and blood will occur. Therefore regulating qi and blood is also an application of the principle of holistic treatment. Regulating qi and blood is mainly to apply the principle of "eliminating the surplus, supplementing the deficient", and thus restoring the harmonious relationship between qi and blood. For example:

Qi produces blood. A case of qi deficiency may lead to shortage of blood production, and finally resulting in deficiency of both qi and blood. The treatment should be mainly replenishing qi, with replenishing blood as the subsidiary, and no simply replenishing blood can be considered.

Qi circulates blood. A qi deficiency or qi stagnancy may cause sluggish flow of blood, and thus qi deficiency or qi stagnancy with blood stasis may develop, the treatment should be replenishing qi and circulating blood, or regulating qi and activating blood to dissolve stasis.

Disorder of qi dynamic may lead to disorders of blood flow. For example, if blood goes upward following adversely rising of qi, it will cause syncope or hematemesis, the treatment should be lowering qi to harmonize blood.

Qi controls blood. If qi gets deficient, its controlling action will be weak, thus there may occur various kinds of bleeding because blood escapes from the vessels, then the treatment should be replenishing qi to control blood.

Blood is the mother of qi. So blood deficiency may cause qi deficiency, blood exhaustion may lead to qi exhaustion. On treatment, replenishing qi to cure the collapse should be taken according to the therapeutic principle of replenishing qi first for blood exhaustion.

8.2.4 Treatment Suitable for the Season, Locality and Individual

This is to determine a suitable treatment for a disease according to differences in season, region, and the patient's constitution, sex, and age. The occurrence, development, and transformation of disease can be affected by many factors, such as season, climate, geographic environment, especially patient's individual constitution. So on treatment of disease, all these factors should be taken into consideration, analyzing the concrete conditions concretely, and thus making different treatments. Only in this way can the appropriate therapeutic plan be established.

8.2.4.1 Suiting Treatment to the Season

Climatic changes of the four seasons may exert a certain impact on physiological functions and pathological changes. A clinical principle established on the basis of the characteristics of different seasons is "suiting treatment to the season." Generally, in spring and summer, the temperature gradually changes from warm to hot, with yang qi rising and the striae of the skin and muscles loose and open. At this time, even a patient is suffering from contraction of wind-cold; he cannot be heavily given acrid and warm natured herbs with dispersing actions in order not to injure the qi and yin with too much dispersion. In autumn and winter the weather gradually changes from cool to cold, with yin prevailing and yang declining, so the striae of skin and muscles are compact and yang qi goes internally. In this time, if a case is not a syndrome of severe heat, cool and cold natured herbs should be carefully used in order not to damage yang.

Summer-heat pathogen has a remarkable seasonal pathogenicity and is often associated with dampness. So, in treatment, clearing away the summer-heat and removing the dampness should be emphasized. It is dry in autumn; acrid and cool natured herbs with actions of moistening dryness should be used for a case of exogenous warm-dryness. This is different in administration from wind-warmness in spring and exogenous contraction of wind-cold in winter. Acrid and cool natured herbs should be given for a case of wind-warmness, acrid and warm natured herbs should be given a case of wind-cold. All of these show that one should suit the remedy to the season.

8.2.4.2 Suiting Treatment to the Locality

A principle in deciding treatment based on geographic characteristics is known as "suiting treatment to the locality". In different regions and geographic environments, climatic conditions, and people's customs are different, so the people there are also different in physiological activities and pathological features. Thus therapeutic methods and principles should differ as well. For example, in northwest China the terrain is high and it is cold and dry with little rainfall, people there have the habit to take in more meat foods and dairy products, and have a stronger constitution; so they often suffer from invasion by exogenous cold and interior heat, the treatment should therefore be to eliminate the exogenous cold pathogen and clear the interior heat. In the coastal areas of southeast China, the terrain is low, and it is damp and hot with heavy rainfall, and people's constitution is relative weak, the striae of the skin and muscles loose and open, the diseases there are often carbunclely and ulcer, or exogenous contraction of seasonal pathogens. Because the yang qi easily escapes, interior cold is apt to produce. The treatment should be to astringe yang qi and warm the interior cold. In Chinese medical practice, sometimes different methods can effect a cure for the same disease, this is to suit the remedy to the locality. For example, for a syndrome caused by invasion of exogenous wind-cold, in cold areas of northwest China the acrid and warm natured herbs with actions of relieving the exterior should be used in heavier dosage, and Mahuang (*Herba Ephedrae*) and Guizhi (*Ramulus Cinnamomi*) are often taken; While in warm-heat areas of northwest China the acrid and warm natured herbs with actions of relieving the exterior should be used in lighter dosage, and Jingjie (*Herba Schizonepetae*) and Fangfeng (*Radix Ledebouriellae*) are often used. This is also the principle suiting the remedy to different geographic regions and climatic conditions. Briefly, one must suit the remedy to the locality in treatment of a disease.

8.2.4.3 Suiting Treatment to the Individual

A principle determining treatment based on the characteristics of the patient's age, sex, constitution, and customs is known as "suiting treatment to the individual."

(1) Age: In people of different ages the physiological states and abundance of qi and blood differ. So the differences should be considered in treatment. Aged people, whose vitality is in decline with deficient qi and blood, often suffer from syndromes of deficiency, or complicated by excess. In treatment, the reinforcing method should be used for deficient syndromes, but for a case with excessive pathogens that needs an attacking method, it should be taken with great caution, and the dosage of herbs should be lighter than that for young people. Children are full of vitality, but their qi and blood are not abundant enough and their viscera are delicate. Thus they are likely to suffer from cold, heat, deficient, or excess syndromes with changeable conditions of illness. Besides, infants cannot manage their lives by themselves, they are predisposed to starvation or over-fullness, cold or heat disorder, therefore, for children the drastically reducing remedies should be avoided, and the tonics should be carefully prescribed, and the dosage of herbs should be smaller. In conclusion, the general dosage of herbs should be used according to the difference of age; for too small a dosage will fail to treat disease, and too great a dosage will tend to injury the vital qi.

(2) Sex: Women differ from men physiologically. Women have their special conditions such as menstruation, leucorrhea, pregnancy and delivery, which all need to be considered when being given prescriptions. For example, drastic purgatives, stagnated blood breaking herbs, intestine lubricating herbs, and exciting herbs that might harm the fetus or are poisonous, should be forbidden or prescribed with great caution during pregnancy.

(3) Constitution: Because of the differences in innate endowment and health care after birth, individuals have different types of constitution such as cold or heat, and strong or weak. Generally, a person with a constitution of yang hyperactivity or yin deficiency should be carefully given warm and hot natured remedies. A person with a constitution of yang deficiency or yin exuberance should be treated with great caution by using cold and cool natured remedies. Therefore the remedies should be different among persons with different constitutions, even for the same disease.

In addition, some occupational and working conditions and emotional factors and living customs may also contribute to the occurrence of some disease. So these should be taken into consideration too.

In summary, suiting treatment to the individual means that, on treatment one should grasp the condition of whole body and individual characteristics instead of treating the disease alone. Suiting treatments to the season and to the locality emphasize the influence of natural environment. The principles of suiting treatments to the season, locality and individual fully embody the holism of Chinese medicine, and the principle and adaptability in clinical practice. Only by comprehensively observing the conditions, concretely analyzing the idiographic instance, being good at suiting treatment to the season, locality and individual to prescribe the formula, can one gain the better curative effect.

Review Questions

- What is the "treating the diseased"? How to make "treatment before a disease develops"?
- How to improve the resistance of the vital qi against the pathogen?
- What are the meanings of routine treatment and contrary treatment? Explain with examples how to apply them.
- What are the meanings of strenthening the vital and dispelling the pathogen? How to apply them?
- What is the principle of coordinating yin and yang?
- What are the meanings of suiting treatments to the season, to the local and to the individual? What cencept in Chinese medicine do they embody?